Butterworth Books is a different breed of publishing house. It's a home for Indies, for independent authors who take great pride in their work and produce top quality books for readers who deserve the best. Professional editing, professional cover design, professional proof reading, professional book production—you get the idea. As Individual as the Indie authors we're proud to work with, we're Butterworths and we're *different*.

Authors currently publishing with us:

E.V. Bancroft
Valden Bush
Addison M Conley
Jo Fletcher
Helena Harte
Lee Haven
Karen Klyne
AJ Mason
Ally McGuire
James Merrick
Robyn Nyx
JP Preston
Simon Smalley
Brey Willows

For more information visit www.butterworthbooks.co.uk

CHUCKING PUTTY AT THE QUEEN
© 2024 by Simon Smalley. All rights reserved.

This trade paperback original is published by
Butterworth Books, Nottingham, England

This is a work of non-fiction. While all the events in this book are true, some names have been changed to protect the privacy of the people involved.

This book, or parts thereof, may not be reproduced in any form without express permission by the author.

Cataloging information
ISBN: 978-1-915009-68-5
CREDITS
Editor: Nicci Robinson
Cover Design: Simon Smalley
Production Design: Global Wordsmiths

Best wishes,
Simon Smalley

CHUCKING PUTTY AT THE QUEEN

by Simon Smalley
2024

Acknowledgements

I offer my gratitude to every reader of *That Boy Of Yours Wants Looking At* who expressed their enjoyment in so many fabulous reviews from around the world. As a writer, to receive such wonderful validation is a phenomenally encouraging reward.

If, whilst reading this second volume of memoirs, you wonder about the depth of my recollection of events decades in the past, let me explain. I'm simultaneously blessed and cursed with hyperthymesia, an uncommon condition that enables people to recall life experiences with incredible (and some say, abnormal) detail. Over the years, old friends have displayed their incredulity at the things that I recount as if they'd happened the previous day, examples of ephemeral nothingness, details so inconsequential that they floated away from others like a dandelion seed on a gentle summer breeze. I only hope that this unusual ability will enhance your reading experience.

When my book was published, there was no crystal ball sufficiently powerful to show Caroline Barry's full-page interview with me in the *Nottingham Evening Post* or my future appearance as guest speaker to students on the Creative Writing in the Community course at Nottingham Trent University. My heartfelt appreciation goes to Bev Baker, Senior Curator and Archivist at the National Justice Museum for proposing me to Dr Sarah Jackson, Associate Professor in Modern and Contemporary Writing at NTU. I had to write that in full, you understand, as it was such a mind-blowing invitation.

Any amount of curiously arranged tea leaves in the bottom of my finest porcelain cup could never be interpreted as the many other engagements that I was invited to speak at, or even my book being stocked in Nottingham city and county libraries. No gathering of prophets, seers, and sages could have foretold how my teenage experiences and book would feature in the Punk: Rage & Revolution exhibition at the Backlit Gallery, for which I was interviewed by Panya Banjoko, poet, writer, and founder of *The Nottingham Black Archive*, and expertly filmed by Matthew Chesney, the gallery's founder and director. My inclusion would not have happened without Craig Humpston, who enthused about my book to Matthew.

Similarly, no amount of dark-eyed palm readers dripping with beads and swathed in autumn-toned crushed velvet could have prepared me for BBC radio's *The Late Show* invite to be interviewed by Becky Want. And as for Su Pollard and Tom Robinson reading and endorsing my debut memoir on its cover...

I offer my appreciation to Roger Hollier for inviting me to discuss my book and generally gab on about myself to a room full of men at Silver Pride, and also to Ross Bradshaw of Five Leaves Bookshop for including me in the "Reading Proud" event, and to Butterworth Books for including me in their roster of authors for the Queer the Shelves 2024 lit-fest.

Did those magical things really happen to me, that boy from St. Ann's who wanted looking at? How I wish that my parents were here to see the literary achievements of their youngest of six children.

With the cerise and yellow cover of my first volume blazing on bookshop and library shelves, there was no time for me to soothe my blistered fingertips in a shallow bowl of chilled lavender water. I immediately set about excavating more of my plentiful memories and began committing them to my hard drive. Some were traumatic to relive, and others more joyous. Once again, the latter allowed me to spiritually reconnect with those whom I've loved and lost.

Upon finishing *That Boy Of Yours Wants Looking At*, I received many emails from readers demanding to know what happened next. My original ending for this second compendium of my life was a similar cliff-hanger until my editor and publisher, Nicci Robinson, intervened. "Oh no, not this time! You can't leave the reader dangling again!" I took heed and therefore, within these pages the question of what happened next is answered—but please promise that you won't immediately flip to the final chapter.

I really hope that *Chucking Putty At The Queen* provides further entertaining insights into my earlier years. What a long, strange trip it's been.

Dedication

To my wonderful parents, Sid & Betty,
for their loving encouragement that
empowered me to follow my own path.

To W. Somerset Maugham,
whose canon inspires me to have faith in my own words.

To Joni Mitchell,
whose lyrical majesty provides me with continual wonder.

To Stella Gibbons,
a glorious wordsmith who is so much more than Cold Comfort Farm.

To Pete Shelley,
who glued me to the romance in punk and
gave me nostalgia for an age yet to come.

To Sylvester,
a fearless gay trailblazer and early AIDS awareness
campaigner, and who remains forever Mighty Real.

To Marc Bolan,
Sad to see them mourning you when you are
there within the flowers and the trees.

To Nicci Robinson, my editor and publisher,
for believing in me from the very start of my literary adventures.

To John Stanbridge, my raison d'etre since 1986,
"Hey feller, I think you're swell."

"When one has to suffer so much it is only fair that one should have the consolation of writing books about it."

W. Somerset Maugham

BOOK ONE

Before

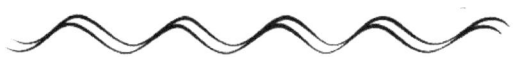

1

TEARS OF A CLOWN

Powerful hands on my shoulders forced me underwater. I couldn't prise the fingers away as I thrashed my head from side to side and flailed my legs, desperate for my feet to connect with a solid surface. My lungs were going to burst. Ignoring every screaming instinct not to, I surrendered and opened my mouth. But it was air, not water, that filled my lungs. I opened my eyes. Dad was above me, gripping my pyjama top as he shook me.

"Wake up, Son. You're having another nightmare." He wrapped his arms around me as I sobbed.

"It was the one about being drowned again, Dad."

He hugged me tighter. "It's all right, I'm here. It was just a silly dream. You're safe with me."

Every night since Mam's death two months earlier, my sleep was tormented by the same scenario until Dad woke me. "Will it ever stop, Dad?"

He stroked my hair. "Yes, and before you even know it."

I lay back down as he fussed and tucked the sheet around me. "Try to think of something nice. It's your birthday soon, and we'll do something extra special."

"What like?"

"How about a party?"

"But who would I invite?"

He pulled the silky eiderdown up beneath my chin. "That's for you to decide. Now try to get some sleep."

The next morning I thought about his suggestion of a birthday party as I half-heartedly helped him to prepare the Sunday dinner. Milky daylight struggled to enter our narrow kitchen, despite Tim having recently cleaned the small square windowpanes. Switching the overhead bulb on in the daytime only dragged the depressing shadows underneath the cupboards closer to me.

I was more under Dad's feet than being of help but earlier, when I

3

was sitting in Mam's chair with one of her cardigans over my lap, he'd squatted before me and gently persuaded me that he needed a hand.

So far, my contribution was an unenthusiastic washing of soil from the new potatoes which I'd then placed into a pan of bright, cold water. With my task completed, I looked out at the rectangle of earth in the back yard that Nick bombastically called "the garden." The satsuma smears on the marmalade cat from up the street seemed to glow as it twisted from beneath the sunless, evergreen depths of the privet bush. It paraded itself, rubbing against the bare sapling rising from the acorn that Mam and I had planted a couple of years earlier. How dare it? I rapped the bone handle of the carving knife on the gleaming glass in an attempt to shoo it, but it only quivered its tail and gave me the type of contemptuous look peculiar to felines.

Dad basted the leg of beef with its fragrant, mouth-watering juices then returned it to the oven because he was cooking it as Mam used to: "slow and low." At the side of the sink, a glazed earthenware pot contained a substantial dollop of creamy, homemade horseradish sauce. Dad had spent an eye-watering thirty minutes pulverizing the gnarled ivory root he'd bought from Arthur Smith, the greengrocer at the bottom of the street. Gran, somewhat sternly, judged Arthur as "a character" whom she wouldn't trust with her life savings, but I preferred to believe the opinion of my always exuberant Aunty Lu, who said that he was "a right bleddy bogger, and no mistake." This was true, and his jovial patter and entertaining dexterity whilst selling his wares was legendary in the network of streets that surrounded his shop. On this morning, when we'd bought the horseradish along with our other fruit and veg, he'd tried to make me laugh by using two carrots as legs that he walked up my torso before he pulled a brussels sprout from behind my right ear. My laughter separated the mist of my deafness, and my hearing was focused enough to hear him ask Dad how he was coping.

He patted Dad's upper arm. "If there's owt that me and Sybil can do, just say so."

Walking the hundred yards home with our vegetable bounty safely within the stretched spider web of Mam's old string bag, Dad squeezed my hand and told me that everyone was being so kind, unlike his two brothers.

"I've not seen hide nor hair of Bill and Harry since—for ages."

I tiptoed around the cracks of the pavement not wanting to induce more bad luck whilst he tiptoed around mentioning Mam's funeral.

Back in the kitchen, Dad lifted the pan of spuds and with a screech of metal on metal, he slid it onto the trivet on the top of the stove. I stuffed my fingers in my ears and grimaced.

He wiped his hands on the tea towel tucked into the top of his trousers and leaned down. "Sorry, Son."

The bristly tickle of his handlebar moustache created a shiver down my spine. He'd placed his mouth so close to my ear because the responsiveness of my hearing continued to ebb and flow like the waves at Mablethorpe beach. It was improving and was better than the blanket of woolly deafness that wrapped around me immediately after Mam's death. Laborious medical tests had concluded that excessive trauma created a psychological mental block to prevent me hearing more destructive news. Sometimes I doubted the validity of the diagnosis. Maybe the tormenting kids at school were right, and I really was barmy and needed locking up in Mapperley Madhouse.

"That's a big sigh, Son. Are you okay?"

He'd already got enough on his plate, and I shouldn't burden him by confessing my exhausting sadness that this would be my first birthday without Mam.

"Why don't you go into the front room and play your records?"

Having always been kept "for best," a reverential, churchlike serenity softened the front room, further enhanced by the splodgy paint-by-numbers portrait of a salmon pink-faced *Madonna with Baby*, although that clashed garishly with the woodgrain wallpaper of the chimney breast. Beneath it, a bunch of daffodils in the aquamarine glass vase that Mam had so loved stood on top of the unlit gas fire as if upon an altar, their sprightly green stalks supporting the sunshine trumpets radiant in the diffused daylight through the net curtains.

I dropped onto the bashed settee, surrendering to the rush of bittersweet memories of the spring morning only twelve months earlier. Mam was busy in the kitchen making a fry-up breakfast, Tim was out buying a new reel for his fishing rod, and Nick sat with his elbows on the table, engrossed in his football magazine. The gentle spring rain was the type which saturated everything but wasn't so miserable as a relentless winter deluge.

Dad's face lit with a conspiratorial grin, and his eyes twinkled. "Shall we go down to Arthur Smith and buy your mother some flowers?"

"Oh yes, please!"

Dad called through to the kitchen. "Betty, I'm just nipping out on an errand with Simon. Won't be a tick."

"Oh, Sid, I'm just about to start frying the bacon."

As if anticipating Mam's next comment, Dad lifted his umbrella from its home, wedged next to the ugly grey bulk of the gas meter just inside the front door. He winked and whispered, "One, two, three..."

"And it's raining, you'll get soaked." Mam's words sizzled with the sound of hot fat in the frying pan.

"I've got my brolly, and we'll be back in two shakes of a lamb's tail."

Dad chuckled as he pulled the front door closed and thrust open the dark green waterproof canopy. For seconds on the empty street, the taut fabric temporarily obliterated the dreary sky, and it was as if it were just us huddled beneath the secretive coppices at Colwick Woods. The paving stretched ahead like an unfurled roll of grey silk towards the greengrocer's shop. I skipped the first few yards but pulled up short at the house where a pair of fearsome Alsatians lived. Every time I passed, they always advertised their presence by snarling and barking behind the window covered in their frothy spittle. Sometimes, the antagonistic owner sat on a chair in the open doorway with the ugly beasts laying at his side. Dad said that because this man was "a real short arse," he relished the fear his dogs produced in passers-by. If the confrontational trio were there when I was with Mam, she'd cross the road so that I was safely sandwiched between her and the houses. I clasped Dad's hand harder and moved my body as close to him as I could. Thankfully on this wet morning, the horrible man's front door was closed, and the grubby curtains were drawn so I couldn't see the dogs, and they couldn't see me.

With his head protected by a flat cap of tattered tweed and the collar of his thick brown overcoat pulled up, Arthur Smith stood behind an aluminium curtain of drizzle dripping from the edge of the navy-blue tarpaulin awning that bore his name in faded white letters. With its aged surface tarnished with verdigris, a conical copper urn was home to an explosion of pussy willow, the charcoal lengths bursting with silver-white furry buds. In smaller vases, delicate harlequin sprays of freesias glowed from shining, crisp cellophane, their colours hazily creating exquisite,

Chucking Putty at the Queen

spilled paint puddles on the drenched slabs. I didn't know which to choose, but my eyes were drawn to the cheerful clusters of canary yellow daffodils.

I skipped from beneath the protection of Dad's brolly to the dry safety next to Arthur and looked up to his unshaven face. "Dad's brought me to buy some flowers for Mam, but I'm in a rush because she's doing breakfast."

"In that case, you'd better be quick about it and choose a nice bunch for her. I know she likes daffs, don't she?"

When I'd carefully counted out enough burnished bronzed coins onto Arthur's leathery palm in exchange for the yellow treasure that he'd deftly wrapped in a page of the *Evening Post*, Dad and I set off home. With one hand in his and the bright blooms in the other, the elation of my eagerness to present Mam with the surprise floral gift made me recklessly not bother to avoid stepping on the glistening black cracks bordering the soaked paving slabs. Everyone knew that stepping on the cracks brought you bad luck, but I was so happy, I didn't care.

I threw myself through the front door whilst Dad vigorously flapped the rain from his umbrella, and I raced to the kitchen bearing the flowers like an athlete with the flaming Olympic torch. Mam stood at the cooker, one hand on the frying pan handle and the other holding the wooden spatula as she manouevred rashers of bacon in the sizzling fat. She didn't look around.

"Here you are. Thank goodness you were so quick. The bacon's just about done. What have you two been up to?"

"Mam, look. We've bought you some flowers from Arthur Smith!"

"So that's where you belted off to when I was cooking your breakfast. I hope those horrid dogs weren't out." She glanced at the small bouquet. "Oh, daffs. My favourite! But mind you don't get splashed by this spitting fat. Go and sit at the table. Sid, can you give me a hand, please?" Mam beamed at Dad when he entered. "You are a darling. That's such a lovely thing to do."

After breakfast, Mam placed the blooms into the aquamarine vase, and after she filled it with water from the kitchen tap, she puckered her lips as I turned my face to hers for a kiss.

That aquamarine vase was once more filled with daffodils and shone as a tormenting reminder of our loss. I wiggled the tips of my forefingers

7

in my ears. Was I really getting better? Since I'd got up, Dad's words weren't muffled and indistinct as if I had rubber corks stuffed in my ears and cotton wool wrapping my brain. I placed his favourite LP by The Platters onto the battery-operated record player. It was an unstated family Sunday morning tradition that Dad played the collection of sentimental songs just loud enough for Mam to hear in the kitchen.

In those unworried days, I loved to watch her slice carrots into chunky orange rings as she sang a few lines or peel spuds as she hummed along. In moments like that, with the smell of slowly roasting pork mingling with the fruity aroma of Dad's pipe smoke, and the lingering tang of the Brasso that Tim had used earlier to polish the ornaments, my life could not have been more perfect.

I desperately needed to hear the songs as a touchstone to those secure yet now suddenly distant happy mornings. My previously dependable, unchallenging routine had been erased and replaced with a topsy-turvy existence. Comfortably wrapped in the nostalgic, melancholy crooning of "I'll Never Smile Again," I jumped out of my skin when Dad pushed open the door and popped his head around.

"I thought that you'd be playing your new T. Rex single. Why are you listening to The Platters?"

He sat down beside me on the bristly 1930s settee and put an arm around my shoulders. I leaned into him and buried my sobs into the thick green threads of the jumper Mam had knitted for him, as if I'd be able to detect her beneath the comfort of his everyday musky tones of Old Spice aftershave. "It reminds me of before."

Dad stroked my hair. "I understand. I really do."

"It's not fair, Dad."

His sigh seemed without end as he pulled his handkerchief from his pocket and dabbed my tears. "I wish that I could wipe away your hurt as easily."

The back door banged, and Tim called from the kitchen. "Are you in, Dad? I've got some chitterlings off the market for you."

"*From* the market, Tim. Not *off* the market." Dad pushed up from the settee and folded his handkerchief into a neat, white square. "But on a Sunday? The market's closed."

"Yeah, Harry on the mushy pea stall held onto them for me."

"Thank you. I'll give you the dosh in a minute." He slipped his hanky into his back pocket, then squeezed my shoulder. "We should start planning for your birthday party next week."

"It won't be the same."

Dad lowered his eyes. "I'll try my best."

"Sorry, Dad. I wasn't being ungrateful."

"I know that. But I think that your mother would have liked you to have a party."

That afternoon, I helped him tidy his big black leather work bag. He'd just replaced his pair of beautiful Rolleiflex cameras, and I held a light meter as he continued to enthuse about the celebration.

"I'll get Sid Sharpe to design a bespoke invitation card for you."

I giggled. "Wow, Dad. Two Sids working at the same place."

"Yes, Son, but he's Syd as in Sydney, Australia, whereas I'm good old-fashioned St. Ann's Sid."

This colleague worked in the graphics department. Dad brimmed with enthusiasm for the talented artist and had mentioned him several times in the past, adding that he was impressed with my imaginative capabilities when Dad took my drawings to frame.

"It's obvious that you have an artistic bent, Son. You'll get on well with Syd and his friend, Bill. They're both graphic designers and are amazingly creative. You should see their bungalow. It's huge, and crammed with ferns and palms, and the walls are covered with panels of chocolate-coloured cork, and just about every available surface is filled with modern artwork and weird sculptures." He took a breath, his eyes shining with recollection. "And there are two enormous sofas made from emerald corduroy. You could fit five men onto each one. They almost swallow you up when you sit on them."

I handed him the light meter and giggled at his enthusiasm for the fabulous-sounding bungalow.

"And their hi-fi system is top of the range. They have more LPs than Nequests. Your eyes would fall out, as Aunty Lu would say."

The thought of someone having more records than the music stall on the Central Market was impossible for me to comprehend, and I daydreamed that one day I'd also reach such dizzying heights in record collecting.

On the Saturday before my birthday, there was an outdoor event at Dad's firm, and he was chief photographer. It was an occasion separate to their traditional summer fete and grandly named an "international relations drive" due to a liaison with a South African counterpart. I wasn't bothered about the justifications for the jamboree because it was the day that I was to meet Syd and his friend, Bill.

I perched awkwardly on a folding metal chair outside the refreshments tent next to the prickly bales of golden straw that corralled the donkey ride, although the hairy beasts had not yet arrived. Any backside-numbing discomfort I experienced was overridden as I proudly watched Dad duck and dive to obtain unusual shots of the activities at the coconut shy. I immediately loved the red-faced owner who wouldn't have looked amiss in a Victorian melodrama. The tips of his extravagant white handlebar moustache extended almost further than the rim of the straw boater atop his head, and his substantial girth was resplendently encased in a purple and orange striped waistcoat. The satiny material was as loud as his rambunctious hollers of "Roll up, roll up" that punctuated the muted thuds of the wooden balls hitting the canvas backdrop.

"Oh, bad luck, young sir!"

"Huh, it's a swizz." The forlorn boy shuffled away.

I giggled, remembering how Mam used to say that the coconuts were pressed onto pins that protruded from the wooden cups that they rested in.

Although it was only March, unexpectedly hot sunshine reflected and glowed from the highly polished brass valves adorning a nearby steam engine decorated with gorgeously ornate paintwork swirls and curls. I clapped my delighted appreciation when the cheerful tune that tooted from its organ segued into "Who Were You With Last Night?" The Victorian music hall song often featured on *The Good Old Days*, one of my favourite television shows.

Echoing around the vast sports field, a baritone voice announced that all attendees must take note that the St. John's Ambulance first aid facility was located next to the beer tent. The grey Tannoy speaker that boomed the instruction was high above Randy's Genuine USA Burgers 'n' Hot Dogs stall, where the stars and stripes flag nailed to the front drooped in a mist heavy with the tempting smell of frying onions. My stomach did flip-flops of hunger. To use Tim's words when he'd taken me to Goose Fair, I could just wallop off a hot dog. Dad was busy setting up his tripod and a silvery light deflector (or reflector; I could never remember which it was). He'd be busy for ages. I smiled at the proprietor, a heavy-set man whose oil slick of shoulder-length black hair slid from beneath a grease-stained chef's hat. Business must have been slow judging by his morose expression. He rested his chin in his cupped hands, anchoring the elbows of his tattooed, leg-of-lamb arms to the counter between the plastic tomato-shaped ketchup dispenser and a smooth yellow orb blighted by congealed mustardy blobs.

So deeply absorbed was I in my junk food contemplation, I almost slid from the metal seat when the wooden chuck smashed against the shiny circular bell at the top of the Test Your Strength attraction. The accompanying bellow of triumph made me turn around just in time to see an immense man whose ginger beard was so luxuriously hirsute that it seemed that only his eyes and nose were visible. He roared and shook his meaty fists skywards, stretching the white vest cladding his barrel chest so tautly that I expected the cotton to rip.

"Are you sitting comfortably?"

I pulled myself upright and looked up at a tall, balding man wearing thin wire-framed spectacles. The hair missing on his head was made up for by the thick black beard that wrapped his face and parted in a white slash when he smiled.

"I'm Syd—the other Sid, you might say."

At his side stood a burly, clean-shaven chap with an uncanny resemblance to a young Harry Secombe on the cover of his *Sacred Songs* LP that Dad had. When I was younger and learning to read, Dad asked me to choose a record to play, and I chose that one because I thought that it was called *Scared Songs*. My disappointment was immense when the stylus landed on the vinyl and "Jesu, Joy of Man's Desiring" played. The LP was a collection of religious songs and nothing at all about monsters, ghouls, and phantoms.

Syd bent down to shake my hand, the sun reflecting ruby flashes from the jewel set into the gold ring around his pinkie finger.

"So, at last, we meet the famous Simon! Your dad's told us a lot about you."

His voice carried the deep rumble of a passing tank that was part of the army display team. His hot, dry hand dwarfed my own smaller one as I thrilled at the knowledge that I was famous. He released my hand and laid it against his palm, gently bending my supple thumb backwards, away from my forefinger.

"Your dad's right. This indicates that you're artistic, just like him. When you grow up, you'll either play the piano or the guitar—or both!"

"Really truly?"

"Oh, yes. Or you may become a distinguished composer or a celebrated writer." Ivory flashed amongst the woolly blackness wrapping his face. "Definitely something to do with the arts and creativity."

He let my hand go, and I stared up into his twinkly eyes, wondering if he was having me on. "Wow, can you really tell that just by bending my thumb back?"

"Without doubt. And also, I've seen the photos of you wearing your mum's scarves and jewellery."

He flashed a glance at Bill, who chuckled and murmured, "Don't forget the high heels."

Syd laughed. "Your dad's given me a very special commission for your birthday, but you'll have to wait a short while longer, if you don't mind."

A couple of days later, when the evening meal plates and cutlery were cleared away and Tim and Nick had gone out, Dad placed a small box onto the white tablecloth. "Your invitations, sir!"

The contents of the mundane cardboard rectangle that bore a scuffed, frayed-edged Kodak sticker were akin to the discovery of King Solomon's treasure. Words of invitation as yellow as the daffodils in the front room were captured within the strokes of a stylised black S that dominated the snowy photographic card, whilst between them, lilac lines contained the date of the party. Dad explained how he'd photographed the original artwork and, after some rudimentary technical magic, had reproduced it onto the textured card then trimmed the edges with his small, ripple-edged guillotine. Head-swelling sophistication washed over me as I delicately held the card as if it were a sheet of centuries-old, mouth-blown Venetian glass. "Wow, Dad, it's fab! I bet that nobody else round here has ever had anything like it."

Dad grinned. "You're probably right, Son. But don't forget to arrange your guest list."

The size restrictions presented by our small front room necessitated a modest attendance, especially as Dad was going to borrow a folding table from Daisy and Rex, the landlord and landlady of the Devonshire Arms around the corner.

Chucking Putty at the Queen

I sat with my fingers poised above the white keys of my mustard-coloured Petite typewriter. Although this birthday party was to be a joyous occasion, I gritted my teeth and hunched my shoulders like a frustrated newspaper hack searching for the perfect headline. The guest list should have begun "Mam and Dad," but the events of January made that impossible. But why should it be so? I lightly pressed the M, A, and again the M just enough to slowly raise the metal rods. The typeface gently kissed the white paper, leaving only the faintest grey ghost of ink. "I've not forgotten you, Mam. You're always top of the list."

My typewriter melted into a sandy pool through my swimming tears. The weight of my sadness was as if great hands pressed down on my wrists, making it an effort to raise my fingers to the keyboard again. Salty wetness dribbled onto my top lip, and I furiously wiped my eyes with the backs of my hands. It seemed that I was always crying these days, concealing the shame of my wet face behind a wall at school or hiding in the toilet at the end of our back yard. I should heed Nick's repeated advice that I needed to grow up and act my age. After all, I was soon to be nine years old. I resumed my list, angrily jabbing the keys. Each black letter assaulted the Arctic white paper. Of course, for the next line, Dad was next. But it still looked wrong. The putty-coloured eraser that he'd given me was perfect for rubbing the word out. The cylinder clicked when I rotated it down, and I depressed the spacebar for four spaces past the feint "Mam" and inserted "and Dad" on the same line. That looked proper. They were together again.

My satisfaction instantly enlivened me, and I swiped the return lever to begin the next line. Penny and her husband, Mike, whom we affectionately knew by his nickname of "Meash." But who next? I stared at a cobweb in the top corner of the ceiling. There would be empty places. Marge was away working in London, and Steve was around and about, occasionally staying over at ours when he wanted to keep a low profile, which was not an easy task in our neighbourhood. I never understood why he considered hiding in the family home to be a clever idea. His nefarious reputation followed him around like the stench from the fish market dustbins on a sweltering summer day, and the eager fingers of those he'd aggrieved willingly pointed the police towards our front door.

The typewriter carriage flew repeatedly as I added guests. There'd be Tim, Nick, and Aunty Lu, plus the next-door-neighbours. I finished at the bottom with three asterisks that preceded *Official Photography by Sidney George Smalley* because of course, Dad would be armed with one of his trusty Rolleiflex cameras, poised to capture the occasion forever.

2

THE BIGGEST ASPIDISTRA IN THE WORLD

On the south side of the River Trent, there was a quiet, tree-lined street in which stood a small bakery owned by my new brother-in-law's father, Mr Howard. After their wedding, Penny and Meash lived in the flat above the office. One Saturday when Dad drove Mam and me to visit them, Mr Howard was there.

He shook our hands enthusiastically and grinned. "I'd like to donate to the Harvest Festival at Simon's school. Penny's been telling me how you volunteer there."

Mam blushed. "Oh, it's nothing, really. I just help a few kids who struggle with their reading and writing, and Sid takes in items of interest."

This was true. Dad provided myriad oddities and when Gran died, he hauled her mammoth aspidistra to the classroom.

My teacher, Mrs Greer, stared. "Gosh, that must be worth a small fortune."

It was a strange thing to say. I didn't know if she was referring to the plant or the vessel it resided in when she traced her forefinger over the raised ornate pattern on the blue and brown Victorian majolica cachepot. It stayed in the classroom until we broke up for the six weeks summer holidays.

I watched her struggle to load the aspidistra into the back seat of her Mini that she'd parked down the side of the building. "Where are you going with my gran's plant, Miss?"

"Oh, Simon, you made me jump. What are you doing here?" Her usually alabaster cheeks burned red.

"I'm on an errand to the secretary from Mr Walker."

"Well, get along, then."

"But what are you doing with it, Miss?"

"I'm taking it home for the holidays so that I can water it each day. Plants, like all of us, need love and attention."

"But my gran said that you shouldn't overwater aspidistras. That's why

they're called the 'cast iron plant.'"
"But you never know, Simon. We may have a heatwave."
That didn't sound right. "But what about my gran's posh pot, Miss? Wouldn't it be easier to carry just the plant?"
She slammed the car door. "They belong together. It would be a shame to separate them."
Neither plant nor pot were ever seen again because Mrs Greer taught at a different school when the holidays were over...
However, the simultaneously best and worst donation occurred when the Harvest Festival came around. Mr Howard had baked a loaf specially for me to put on the table with the contributions of produce which would be distributed amongst the local pensioners. When Mam walked me back after I'd had my dinner, Father Kean, the jovial, bespectacled vicar from St. Catherine's church was standing by the school gates.
"I hope that you haven't forgotten your donation to the Harvest Festival, Mrs Smalley."
"Don't worry; my husband's having the afternoon off work and will drive over to the bakery in West Bridgford to collect it."
Father Kean rubbed his hands together. "We're all looking forward to it immensely. It's a very generous offer, and I'm sure it will feed many grateful mouths—perhaps five thousand."
I pranced up the steps into the cool, dark foyer and skipped through the shadowed corridor into the brightness of the playground. I didn't know why Father Kean was so excited about a loaf of bread.
Instead of lessons, we congregated in the hall to sing hymns. My favourite was "We Plough the Fields and Scatter," even though I knew it was nature that fed and watered the land, not a fairy tale god. At opposing ends of a long table, stone jars burst with bullrushes and teazles that I'd collected on our countryside drives. Turnips, cabbages, leeks, and carrots necklaced an enormous pumpkin, and pyramids of tinned goods fronted wicker baskets crowded with apples and pears.
Heads turned towards the door. Mam and Dad carried between them an enormous wheatsheaf made of golden bread. *Now* I understood Father Kean's comment about feeding the five thousand. The wide-eyed children that encircled my parents rang my alarm bells. This unprecedented and unrivalled offering would drive a wedge deeper between me and them.
The loaf was held next to the smallest boy in the hall to demonstrate

that the top was higher than his head. Then it was laid on a table of its own, and at its crusty base was laid a rectangle of stiff white card, upon which the headmistress's beautiful calligraphy read, *Generously donated by Mr & Mrs Smalley.*

A few minutes after they left, a boy named Jimmy sidled up to me. "Mr Walker wants to see you in the loo."

"In the *loo?*"

"Yeah, right now."

The lights were off when I stepped into pine-smelling coolness. Three boys grabbed me and shoved me into a cubicle, and after unsuccessfully trying to push my head into the toilet bowl, they slammed me against the wall and repeatedly punched me in the stomach.

"My mam says you lot think you're better than everyone else with your posh talking."

"Here's one for showing off with your stupid bread."

That was the most vicious blow, after which I struggled to refresh my winded lungs as they ran off. These tough boys were experienced at fighting and knew what they were doing. Their punches were aimed to leave no visible marks. I turned on the cold tap and doused my hot face. I was fed up with being told that I was "la-de-dah" just because I spoke correctly.

Too many dreadful things had happened in the months since that Harvest Festival. But now Mr Howard had come up trumps again by baking me a birthday cake, and he'd certainly pulled out all of the stops. My eyes feasted upon the cream florets that decorated the edges of a confectionary number nine, and its sides were studded with a pebbledash of chopped nuts. Silver letters congratulated *Happy Birthday* and on the top of the immaculately smooth Wedgewood blue icing, a small toy car was parked beside nine white plastic daisies from which rose candles the colour of forget-me-nots.

Although it was still chilly for the end of March, Dad hadn't lit the gas fire due to its proximity not only to the table, but also to where the backs of my legs would be when, as host, I'd be sandwiched between the table and the metal bars of the fire.

I really wasn't fussed about a birthday party, but Tim had told me that I shouldn't let Mam's memory down by being sulky and miserable, so I decided to wear my favourite jumper, the one she knitted for me from the sandy balls of wool that we'd chosen from the stall on the Central Market. I was growing, and although there were four or five inches of my wrists protruding from the arms of the rib-crushing garment, I refused to allow Dad to donate it to the St. Catherine's jumble sale when one of the church ladies came collecting several days earlier.

I unclipped the lid of the portable record player and as the birthday disc jockey, I began with my most treasured possession, "Hot Love" by T. Rex.

"Give it a rest and put summat else on," Tim said after the fourth consecutive play.

Following Dusty Springfield's "Son of a Preacher Man," the debut LP by The Rolling Stones hit the platter. But even their rip-roaring rendition of "Route 66" that I loved so much failed to enthuse me. It wasn't just the net curtains that the deepening afternoon gloom outside the window darkened. There was one song that I had to play, one that Mam used to sing along with: "Wooden Heart."

Aunty Lu clapped her hands. "Lovely, a nice bit of Elvis the Pelvis."

Tim leaned over a plate, sniffing suspiciously at the concertinaed pastry tubes. "What's these then, Dad?"

"Vol-au-vents with cream cheese and chopped mushrooms."

"Vollo what?"

Nick butted in. "I go to grammar school and obviously, I speak French. I can tell you that literal translation is *flying in the wind*."

"Huh." Tim sniffed the crinkled pastry again. "More like they'd give you wind."

However, Tim's disdain was my awe. "Are they really French, Dad?"

"Yes, Son."

"Wow. French food at my birthday party. If Ma—"

Aunty Lu clapped again. "Ooh, these sausage rolls look good enough to eat." She laughed and popped one into her mouth. "Bleddy hell, Sid, did you use concrete instead of flour? I think I've lost one of me gnashers!"

I stared at her, wondering if she'd deliberately stopped me referring to Mam, but before I could think deeper about this possibility, she went boss-eyed at me and sucked the sausage roll in and out of her mouth like a pastry piston. Just like Mam, my bonkers Aunty Lu always knew how to make me laugh. But she still wasn't Mam.

Bathed by the shimmery light from the aquarium, a golden box of

Chucking Putty at the Queen

Terry's All Gold chocolates shone with luxurious warmth as I surveyed the feast that Dad had prepared single-handedly. Squirts of Primula cheese dotted fleshy slices of tinned Ye Olde Oak Ham, which Dad knew was a favourite treat for me, and fresh celery sticks stuck above the rim of a white mug. Jammy whirls of jolyrol slices were arranged as if sliced sections of a felled exotic, alien tree, and puddles of sloppy jelly glowed in molten jewel colours in bowls beside glasses fizzing with Dad's home-brewed ginger beer. Wooden cocktail sticks impaled pineapple chunks and quarters of fresh tomato, and a starburst of crispy pink wafers rested beside a jumble of fig rolls that nobody really liked but still added to their plates so as not to offend Dad.

My wonderful father had created all of this especially for me, and I was surrounded by the people whom I loved—even Nick at that supreme, overheated peak of my emotions. But there was one important person missing.

I looked up and saw Aunty Lu watching me. She rapped on the corner of the table with her knuckles, snatching me from the edge of the black hole that I was about to fall into.

"Come on, sexy legs! Blow out your candles and make a wish."

I blew on the tiny yellow flames and looked through the ascending smoky strands to the door. I knew what should happen next, as it always did in the daydreams that I'd luxuriated in during the days leading up to this party: the door would open for Mam to enter with the glamorous confidence of a film star at an awards ceremony. With her glossy raven hair swept back, her familiar wide smile framed by red lips, and her eyes shining as if made from polished jet, she'd hold her arms wide to welcome me, her youngest child.

But the door remained shut. My legs became as wobbly as the jelly in their bowls. I lowered my head and tried to focus on the wonderful blue cake, where one candle remained alight, its molten wax dripping down the thin blue shaft as tears slid down my cheeks. "Wooden Heart" had ended, and the record continued to revolve, the stylus clicking rhythmically in the run-out groove, marking the seconds of my wretched, sobbing anguish. My legs crumpled, and I lurched against the table. Dad was instantly beside me and hugged me to him.

"It's all right, Son, I know what you wished for, and if only I could have made it come true, then you know I would."

3

THE SUN AIN'T GONNA SHINE ANY MORE

A FEW WEEKS LATER, AUNTY Ann travelled up from her home in rural Kent. Dad had already proclaimed this Saturday morning occasion "the royal visit." I remembered Mam telling him that after her sister married money, she thought she was better than everyone else.

"We'll just about have time for breakfast before she arrives." He headed into the kitchen and took the frying pan from the top of the Formica-fronted cupboard just as Tim announced his decision to clean the living room windows. "Can't you wait until after breakfast, Tim?"

"It's okay, Dad. It won't take long, and I'll be finished by the time the sausages are ready."

"Oh, really, Tim. I'll get the house smelling nice and foody, and you'll cover it up with the stink of chemicals."

"Give over, Dad. It won't pong that badly."

Armed with an old mutton cloth rag and a bottle of shocking pink Windowlene, he set to work on the four large panes. I loved the astringent smell that Dad complained of because it whisked me back to when Mam had undertaken this task, often drawing a face in the smeared liquid with her forefinger and once, even writing "bum" in big letters as I giggled my approval.

"Hurry up, Tim, the sausages are almost ready. Aunty Ann will be here before long, and you've not tackled the outsides yet."

"Hold up, Dad, I'm just about done in here." Tim stepped closer to the glass and huffed on the bottom corner of the top left pane. He rubbed with a vigorous circular motion before stepping back and smiling at his handiwork as if he were Rembrandt, certain that he'd completed a masterpiece. "Tell you what, Dad," Tim tossed the pink-stained cloth into the open cupboard next to what used to be Mam's chair, "I'll do the outside tomorrow before I clean the brasses." The late spring sunshine emphasised the dullness of the metal ornaments on the mantelpiece over the fireplace. Cleaning and polishing them was Tim's Sunday morning routine that he'd neglected since that dreadful day at the end of January. He nudged the cupboard door shut with his foot. "But they look lovely from here. Mind you, I don't know why I've bothered, 'cos Mam—"

I ceased trying to balance my knife through the prongs of my fork. As I stared at Tim's face, Gran's phrase—"You look like you've been caught doing something that you shouldn't be doing"—sprang into my mind. In these awkward weeks since Mam's death, there was an air of embarrassment whenever she was mentioned, which I tried to avoid doing as I was convinced to do so would upset Dad. My discomfort was engendered by the spiteful playground helpers at my school, Mrs Grey and Mrs Black, who'd tried their hardest to convince me that I had contributed to Mam's death because I didn't behave like "a proper boy."

Tim jutted out his chin. "Mam always said that if you clean the windows, you can guarantee it'll rain."

I turned away from the hurt that showed in his eyes. Light filtering through the half-cleaned panes fell upon Mam's empty chair. It was a pre-World War Two maternity recliner on which she'd nursed all of us. After I was the last of her six children to be born, it became her favourite seat in the cramped house. Each side bore a dark mahogany trough in which various items could be stored for easy reach. Since her death, the contents remained undisturbed like precious relics in an Egyptian tomb and, with a befitting reverence attached to the inexpensive items, none of us would dare to remove them. Next to a rolled copy of *Woman's Realm*, slender grey needles speared a small ball of sandy wool left over from when she'd knitted my jumper and matching bobble hat.

I stared into the empty fireplace. "It feels like it's always raining now. Even when the sun shines, there are black clouds."

Dad extinguished the flames beneath the frying pan. Three paces brought him next to me, and he cuddled me to his side. "There'll be sunny days again, I promise."

"Yes, Dad. I believe you. Honest."

"Come on, Son. The sausages are ready, and the eggs are like mini sunshines, so why don't we start there? Your mother used to say that you'll never feel happy on an empty stomach."

Dad, Tim, and Nick had finished breakfast and left their empty plates on the table with knives and forks tidily arranged like clock hands pointing at twenty-five past five. Dad always waited until I'd finished before he cleared the crockery away. Nick lounged in Mam's chair reading the football magazine he'd bought with his weekly pocket money that he ostentatiously referred to as his "personal allowance." Muted thuds and bumps from the top of the house indicated that Tim was preparing to go to town and spend some of his wages in the boutiques before embarking on a lunchtime boozing session.

The sunlight that came in through the open back door, weakened by clouds filling the sky, illuminated Dad from one side as he tucked a green and white striped tea towel into the top of his trousers to function as an apron. It was no longer snowy white, and the embroidered legend, *Property of Nottingham City Baths*, betrayed its origin.

Dad's delicious fry-up revived my spirits, and I prolonged my savoury enjoyment by delicately nibbling my remaining sausage. The flavoursome zingy herbs and spices continued to explode in my mouth, lining my palate with a fizzing sensation not unlike when I'd recklessly emptied a whole tube of Sherbet Fountain onto my tongue. High above me, the volume of the old Bakelite radio in the top room increased to such a level that those of us below had no doubt that Mick Jagger could get no satisfaction. It was one of my favourite songs by the Rolling Stones, and I accompanied the repetitive guitar motif by tapping my knife against the edge of my plate.

"I'm quite sure that we can live without your contribution, Son."

"Sorry, Dad."

"When you've finished tip-tapping like Ringo Starr, can you manage another banger?"

"Ooh, yes, please!"

Nick glanced over the top of his magazine. "Can I have one as well, Dad?"

"No, sorry. There's only one left, and Simon's having it."

Nick scowled and shook his magazine noisily. "It's not fair; you're always spoiling him."

"Not necessarily, Nick. And if I was, then you're old enough to understand the reason why." Dad smoothed the barely noticeable creases from the tea towel and stepped back into the tiny kitchen.

Nick snorted. "I'm going to call round for Stephen." He rose from the chair, jabbing his right elbow into the back of my neck as he passed me. "Little tin god."

"Dad!"

Nick jabbed me again. "Don't you go snitching on me," he hissed and headed towards the bottom of the stairs.

He paused and glared at me.

Dad appeared in the kitchen doorway, making the sausage dance in the frying pan like a ball on a tennis player's racket. "What is it, Son?"

"Ringo's the drummer in the Beatles, not the Rolling Stones." I could almost touch Nick's heavy sigh of relief. He turned and shoved through the curtain. Seconds later, the front door clicked shut.

Dad harrumphed. "Rolling Stones, Beatles—they're all the same to me: long-haired layabouts."

This deliberate use of his generation's idiom for any male without a short back and sides haircut made me giggle, and his twinkling eyes and the wide grin beneath his handlebar moustache confirmed that he was determined to make me laugh.

"Mind your backs. Important sausage delivery coming through."

He deposited the final fat banger on my plate, causing the spitting fat to alight in tiny pinpricks on the back of my hand. "Ouch!"

"Sorry, Son. It's a bit well done."

"It looks perfect to me, Dad."

"Be careful; it's hot."

Piercing the sausage skin with my fork released a moist pop, and pearly dribbles of hot fat fell onto my plate. From the kitchen, a ferocious bubbling was joined by an atomic cloud of steam when Dad dunked the heated frying pan into the washing up water. The volume of the music from the top of the house increased, and it was hard to resist resuming my cutlery percussion as I clamped the hot sausage between my teeth. Crikey, Dad was right. It *was* hot, but he would have a fit if I let it drop onto my plate. I held my breath as fire spread through my teeth into my gums.

Dad slipped past me. "You look like Winston Churchill chomping his cigar. Don't burn your mouth." He yanked open the heavy curtain and called upstairs. "Tim, turn it down a bit, please. The neighbours don't want to hear your music at full blast."

I dropped the sausage onto my plate with a greasy splat and sliced it to create three manageable chunks. Noisy footfall descended the uncarpeted top stairs, followed by four heavy steps across the back bedroom directly above my head, then the door grated on the floorboards.

"You what, Dad? I couldn't hear you. I had the radio on. Hold up, I'm coming down."

An army platoon wearing hobnailed boots couldn't have been louder. Tim's disembodied head poked through the curtain. The flowing dark auburn locks framing his rectangular face reminded me of the Punch & Judy man on Brighton seafront when Mam took Nick and me to visit Aunty Fran, another of her sisters. When the anarchic show ended and the children dispersed, Uncle Billy poked his head through the red and yellow striped curtains. To my surprise, it wasn't a wizened old man controlling the vaudeville puppets as I'd expected, but a long-haired teenager, vacuously chewing gum.

"What's up, Dad?"

"I think that everyone else within a five-mile radius could hear your radio."

Dad wasn't really cross, just mindful of the neighbours, and he returned to the kitchen. Tim scowled at me; his brow crumpled just the way Mam used to look when something annoyed her.

He nodded at my plate. "You filling your face again?"

I gulped the remaining inch of cooled sausage before he could steal it. "There was one going spare, so Dad gave it me. Aunty Ann's coming soon."

"I know. That's why I'm pissing off down town. I don't want her getting onto me about how long my hair is. She was bad enough at Mam's fune—" he looked at the empty chair beneath the window, "the last time she was here."

I hated the pussyfooting around Mam's cremation and wanted to scream, "Funeral!" at the top of my voice. Instead, I watched him tuck his white cheesecloth shirt into his jeans.

"Right, I'm off. Catch you later." He slammed the front door behind him.

Mam always said he didn't know his own strength.

Seconds later, Dad called from the kitchen. "Have you finished?"

The only evidence of my delicious breakfast was a few rose petal smears on the white plate where I'd used a crust of fried Sunblest to mop up the juice from the plum tomatoes. "Yes, ta, but I could eat it all again."

"Sorry, Son, you're out of luck."

With the washing up done, Dad stood on the back doorstep. "Hmm, it looks a bit black over Bill's mother's."

I loved the colloquialism for impending bad weather. I slipped my hand into his, and he squeezed my fingers with rapid, tense pulses.

"When's Aunty Ann coming round, Dad?"

"Any time now. And to be honest, I could do without it. I've got enough on as it is."

A noise behind us made me whirl around. Nick stood in the doorway of the living room.

"I thought that you'd gone to Stephen's."

"I did, but he wasn't in, not that it's any of your business. Hey, Dad, Aunty Ann's standing outside on the front."

Dad let go of my hand and smoothed my hair. "Come on, Son, let's get this over and done with, then we can get up to the woods."

"Dad, wait." I nodded down to the front of his trousers where the old tea towel hung.

He whipped it away, folded it, and laid it on the draining board. "Thanks, Son. It's a good job your aunt didn't see that, or she'd think that I'm totally incapable."

After making sure that his tie was tightened, he twisted the ends of his handlebar moustache and led the way to the open front door, where Aunty Ann stood with an umbrella hooked over one forearm and her white-gloved hands clasped as if she were a Jehovah's Witness.

"Hello, Ann. Why on earth are you standing out there?"

"I shan't stay long, Sid, so I won't come in. I just wanted to say my farewells and to see if you've given any more thought to..." her dark eyes flashed at me, *what we were talking about.*"

Above the lead-grey expanse of the factory roof, the sky swelled with clouds of charcoal. There was a deep rumble, then the paving slabs blotched as if a steamroller had squashed hundreds of juicy black grapes. I clapped my hands. "Mam was right! Tim cleaned the windows, and here comes the rain."

But Aunty Ann didn't share my jubilation. "Blast it. I only had my hair done yesterday." She pushed past me. "I *will* come in, Sid, thank you."

Dad closed the front door, repelling both the rain and the dismal daylight, then clicked on the side lamp, instantly transforming the room into a cosy grotto. The rough upholstery of the armchair beneath the window prickled my bare knees as I knelt on it and slipped my head and shoulders under the net curtain that smelled of the previous summer's fly spray. On the other side of the rain-rippled windowpane, two girls huddled in the factory doorway singing, "Rain, rain faster, ally ally aster."

The ferocious downpour abated as quickly as it had begun, and the street brightened as if the clouds were blown away by a Norse god. The girls fled from their shelter, now chanting, "Rain, rain go away, come back another day." *Make your mind up.*

Dad tugged open the front door, allowing the linen-fresh smell of wet pavements to instantly invigorate our stuffy front room, and we stepped out onto the paving slabs that shone as if they'd been replaced with neatly ordered rectangles of greaseproof paper.

"Ann, let me drive you to the train station."

"It's okay, Sid, really. I'll walk. I'll enjoy the exercise."

She watched Dad as he stared down the street. "Come on, Sid, you know how I feel about it. You look worn out, and it would help Simon too."

"What would help me, Aunty Ann?"

"I was talking *about* you, not *to* you."

Dad put his arm around my shoulders as she began to enthuse about her plan. And the more she enthused, the more horrified I became. She wanted Nick and me to go and stay with her in Kent.

"Don't worry, Sid. It's simple. You put them on the train here, and I'll meet them in London."

Nick sidled from the doorway and joined us on the pavement. "I've been to London, and actually I didn't reckon much to it myself."

Dad squeezed the bridge of his nose and muttered, "Here we go again."

"In fact, it's highly overrated, and I think you'll find that Buckingham Palace is nothing more than a glorified bungalow. It's quite a letdown, actually."

Aunty Ann stared at him as if she'd never met him before.

I didn't believe him. "Don't be daft."

"I saw it from the coach. *You* haven't because you've never been to London."

"I have, then! Remember when Mam took us down to Aunty Fran's at Brighton? We changed trains in London."

"That's just changing at a train station. It's not like spending an actual entire day there, like I did."

He always had to have the last word and, obviously seeing his retort as a success, turned his back on us and slipped indoors.

"Regardless of Nick's opinion," Dad turned to Aunty Ann, "it's a lot to organise, because—"

"Not really, Sid."

Dad sighed as if he knew he was beaten. "Well, leave it with me for a few days, and I'll let you know."

Refusing to hear any more, I sauntered to the corner shop next-door-but-one to divert my worries by examining the galaxy of confectionary.

"Simon. Aunty Ann's off now. Come and give her a kiss."

This wasn't the end of the matter. She continued to badger him by telephone at work, and his irritation doubled when she left a message for him with Daisy and Rex at the pub. Then, nothing more was mentioned until one evening when he came in from work. The last time I'd seen him looking so uneasy was on the terrible Sunday when he'd told us Mam had died.

"I've been thinking, and your Aunty Ann's right. It would be marvellous for you two to spend a couple of weeks with her in Kent."

This was worse than any nightmare, and one which no amount of Dad's shaking would free me from, because he was its creator. But I knew one thing: I wouldn't leave Dad. I wasn't sure where Kent was and vowed to consult his roadmap once Nick was safely out of the front room. If I asked him, he'd go all superior on me. But no matter in which part of the country it lay, there was no way I was going. I was staying here with Dad where I belonged.

4

GET IT ON

I TRIED TO BE GROWN up when Dad reiterated the itinerary that he'd devised for the journey that Nick and I were to make. He suggested that I imagine it as an Enid Blyton adventure, but I just didn't want to go. I'd be away from him, away from home, and I'd have to sleep in a strange bed. After Mam died, I'd begun sleepwalking and, terrified that I'd tumble down the steep stairs during one of these somnambulistic wanderings, Dad decided that I should sleep with him. I was comfortable with my reassuring new routine and couldn't bear the thought of being so far away from my nocturnal security.

"Dad, Simon's crying...*again*."

"Nick, do something useful in the other room. Stop being so spiteful. You're old enough to understand what's happened. Simon isn't. And you should know better."

Nick stomped from the room as Dad sat on the edge of the chair. He placed his hands on my shoulders and pulled me to him.

"I know, Son, I know. But you'll have a lovely time. Kent's a delightful part of the country, and there'll be lots of exciting things to do. There's a farm next door with cattle and another nearby with boys the same age as you and Nick. Aunty Ann's going to take you for days out to Canterbury and to the seaside at Margate. It really will be just like one of your Enid Blytons."

I remained unconvinced, despite this bucolic *Famous Five* enthusiasm. "Dad, I'm not being rude, but I'd rather not go. I'd prefer to be here with you." I pulled away when he chuckled. "What's funny?"

"Sorry, Son, I'm not laughing at you. But sometimes the way you speak is so old-fashioned." He tousled my hair. "You will enjoy it, honestly. It's beautiful in Kent."

"What about my T. Rex single? I can't live without it." Surely my melodramatic statement would put the brakes on this journey.

"Don't worry. I've already told Aunty Ann how important it is to you.

She says it's fine for you to take the little record player."

"Hasn't she got one of her own?"

"I guess not."

"But what about batteries, Dad? They'll run out before the two weeks are over."

"You won't need them. I've got something for you if you'll fetch my work bag, please."

I lugged it over to him, struggling as if it was full of house bricks. He removed the contents as if he were a magician with a top hat: assorted flashbulbs, a roll of Scotch masking tape, a leather-bound book bearing the Rolleiflex logo embossed in shiny silver on the front. I half expected him to pull a bouquet of plastic flowers and a white rabbit from its seemingly bottomless depths.

"Here we are. For a second, I thought I'd left it on my desk."

He laid a small, orangey-red plastic box onto the chair arm. Its top bore a small white switch and a protuberance that resembled a red American hard gum. From one side, a wire protruded and at its end, a small silver spindle shone. From the opposite side, a similar wire led to a three-point mains electricity plug.

"No need for extra batteries because this is a transformer. I had Reg in the lab make it specially for you instead of paying me for photographing his daughter's wedding."

"What does it do?"

"You plug this end into the record player, and then plug the other wire into the wall socket. It transforms the current and bypasses the battery facility." He pointed to the American hard gum. "And this then lights up red to show you that it's working."

This was all too thrillingly Doctor Who for me. "Wow, Dad. That's amazing. Thank you."

Dad looked at his watch. "Crikey, Son, it's nearly time for T. Rex on *Top of the Pops*."

"Get It On" was at number one, and I sat cross-legged on the carpet like a devotee in front of a shrine, transfixed by the black and white images of Marc Bolan on our bulky old, rented television. Dad turned to a sweating, red-faced Nick who'd just entered the back door with a football, which he carefully placed in the corner of the room as if it were the FA Cup. The aged joints of the dining chair next to me made an ominous splintering sound when he plonked himself down.

"Just in time. Nick. I want you to take Simon into town tomorrow and buy him this record to take to Kent."

"That's not fair, Dad. What about me? How come he gets everything he wants?"

"He doesn't get everything he wants. Your mother and I treated you all fairly and squarely. You've just had a three-speed racer."

Nick had already moaned to me that the beautiful Raleigh was second-hand from a man at Dad's work whose son had died aged twelve before he'd even had chance to ride it. I hoped he wouldn't be so callous as to vocalise his ingratitude to Dad.

"Yeah, but..."

"Nicholas, I could do with a bit of help. I don't ask for much, and it would be nice if you thought of someone else for once."

Nick stared at the carpet. "Okay, Dad, I'll take him in the morning."

Dad dug into his pocket, removed one of the new fifty pence pieces that had replaced the ten-shilling notes since the advent of monetary decimalisation a few months earlier, and placed it on the sideboard. The next evening when he came home from work, I was already waiting near the back gate, eager to show him my new T. Rex single. I'd read aloud every detail from its labels before he'd reached the back door.

5

HEAR MY TRAIN A-COMIN'

As Dad drove us to catch the train, he jovially reiterated how lovely Kent was. Too soon, he'd parked on Station Street. Our footsteps echoed as we crossed the cathedral of arrivals and departures, then clumped down the wooden steps to the platforms. I gripped Dad's hand harder than I ever had before, fighting to keep my tears locked up. His other hand grasped the strap of the portable record player, and Nick brought up the rear, bumping the old suitcase against his left leg, moaning about its weight. He'd insisted that as the more grown-up of us two, he would be in charge of it, so I wasn't going to give him a hand. Let him do it himself if he was that much of a clever clogs.

We joined the scattered crowds beneath the canopy where the early morning sun created angles of shadow. Pigeons paraded and pecked at fragments of crisps that a young boy tossed to the ground. I was miserably reminded of the black and white images of child refugees in Dad's book of war photography. As if he knew my thoughts, he squeezed my hand.

"You'll love Kent, Son, I'm sure. And don't forget that, on Thursday, you'll be able to see T. Rex in colour for the first time."

Once more, the carrot on the stick dangled in front of me. Carriage doors slammed shut, indicating imminent departure. People hugged and kissed, shook hands, and promised to write. Coughing loudly as if to draw attention to his Falstaffian magnificence, the elaborately moustached guard slid a gold watch from the pocket of his waistcoat. The links of its chain shone across his black serge girth as he looked up at the platform clock that glowed like a harvest moon amongst the stark metal branches in the wooden canopy.

"Departing for London St. Pancras. London St. Pancras."

A tall, thin man stumbled from the open doorway of the buffet lounge and onto the platform, a sandwich clamped between his teeth and his unbuttoned grey mackintosh flapping behind him like seagull wings. In one hand, he carried a briefcase, and in the other, a white plastic cup, which spilled its contents over his fingers as he athletically leapt into the train.

The whole scenario was one of urgency, departure, and sadness. Mam's words vibrated from the past: "London is all hustle and bustle. Give me home any time." A couple of days earlier, Aunty Mary had called round to our house and related a selection from her library of maudlin anecdotes, this time concerning a boy who was lost in London and taken away by strange men, never to see his parents again. New panic seized me. What if Aunty Ann wasn't there to meet us? What if Nick fell under a train and was killed? I would be stranded in London just like the unfortunate boy in Aunty Mary's woeful tale, and I'd be taken away by strange men. I'd never see Dad again. I looked around to check that he was still there. He was staring to where Nick lounged against the buffet window frame, picking his nose.

"Nick. Get your finger out. I mean that in two ways because I'm trusting you to look after Simon. And please don't cause Aunty Ann any trouble."

Dad stepped forward with his arms wide, but Nick formally held his hand out.

"I'm not a little kid anymore, Dad. I'm fourteen. I don't need cuddles, unlike *some people*."

"Nicholas, I know that it's difficult. It's been difficult for all of us, and your aunt's only trying to help. Please remember what I said: look after Simon."

Dad grabbed the suitcase and with the record player in his other hand, he boarded the train. Relief overwhelmed me. He'd been kidding about just us two brothers travelling to London. My mind raced ahead as he strode along the corridor. He'd hire a car in Kent, and we'd go exploring and have those Enid Blyton adventures that he'd convinced me awaited in the lush countryside. "Are you coming with us, Dad?"

"No, Son. I'm just making sure these are stored correctly."

When he leaned down and kissed me, I wrapped my arms tightly around him and unsuccessfully tried to link my fingers behind his back. Memories of being left at the children's hospital when I was younger burst and released my tears. "I don't want to go, Dad."

The train shuddered, and the coupling chains clanked as the buffers connected, making us stumble.

"Don't worry, I promise I'll phone you from the Devvo tonight at eight."

Chucking Putty at the Queen

Dad's limited finances didn't stretch to the luxury of us having a phone at home, so Daisy and Rex suggested him using theirs in their living room at the pub. It would be more comfortable and private than Dad standing in the phone box down the end of the street endlessly feeding coins into the pay slot.

Dad mussed my hair. "Cheer up, Tatty Head. I'll phone you tonight."

The train vibrated and when he stepped down onto the platform, he became as unreachable as Neil Armstrong descending from the Apollo space module onto the moon. A shrill whistle signalled it was time for the grubby diesel locomotive to depart. The guard slammed our carriage door shut, incarcerating me as his prisoner. I was trapped. When the train heaved and lurched again, we fell into our seats. I pressed my face against the glass just in time to see Dad blow a kiss, then our carriage was enveloped by the short, dark tunnel that ran beneath the station.

Dad was gone.

The railway sidings soon gave way to patchwork strips of back gardens in rapid shutter glimpses of private lives and before long, open countryside, edged by a pink ribbon of rose bay willow herb, replaced domesticity. Each time the train slowed to pull into a station, I kept my eyes on the yellow record player on the rack above us. There was no way anyone other than me would disembark with it. I'd refused when Nick ordered me to put my records on top of it, and I continued to defiantly clasp them to my chest. Even though I knew every detail of their labels, I periodically scrutinized them, speaking the words under my breath as if they were an incantation to protect Dad from the evil that had caused Mam's death.

My boredom rose with the increasing temperature of the stuffy carriage, and the harsh seating itched the sweaty backs of my bare legs, just as the covering on the chair in the front room at home did. How I wished that I were sitting there reading, knowing that Dad was in the kitchen instead of being captive within this stifling jail on wheels. Dad had suggested that this railway journey would be an adventure, but it was more like the ghost train at Goose Fair. Nick was engrossed in his football magazine, and I couldn't even have a sweet. Dad gave us a bag of humbugs which Nick commandeered, and only occasionally let me have one. The last of these bulged beneath his cheek like a grotesque abscess. Maybe I should have one of the potted beef sandwiches that

Dad wrapped in greaseproof paper. Nick had devoured his within ten minutes of us leaving Nottingham station. He closed his magazine and like Hungry Horace in the *Dandy* comic, he eyed my unopened, neatly wrapped snack resting on my lap.

"You going to open your sarnies yet?"

"No, I'm saving them."

"Till when? Come on, open them. I'm starving."

"Get lost. You've had yours already."

"Don't be so mean."

"Mean? You've eaten nearly all the humbugs." I patted the crispy grey greaseproof paper. "I'm saving mine 'til we see Aunty Ann. I'm going to give her one of them."

He snatched the package from my lap and ripped it open. "Don't be stupid. She's too posh for potted beef sandwiches. I'll have it."

As I went hungry, the train ate up the miles as it raced closer to the capital until we slowed and stopped beneath the enormous glass canopy. We were in London. I'd been here before but that was with Mam holding my hand. Without her, it appeared even more busy and made Nottingham station look like a model railway kit. Bossy Nick took charge of our luggage, and we joined the shuffling snake of passengers sliding towards the open carriage door. When I gripped the back of Nick's jumper, he rested the record player on a recently vacated seat and slapped my hand away. I clutched my singles tighter to my chest. Something up ahead brought us to a standstill, giving me the chance to peer through the window. Where was Aunty Ann?

My fears of being lost and abducted by strange men vanished when the crowd parted, and I spotted her. She scanned the train windows, and I rapped on the dirty glass with my knuckles, but she didn't hear me and almost bumped into a metal Wall's ice cream sign when she stepped back to allow a porter to pass with a wagon loaded with suitcases.

I giggled, remembering Dad's earlier warning: "Aunty Ann has become very toffee-nosed. She works hard at wiping out where she comes from and will pretend not to know certain words."

"Like what, Dad?" I'd asked as he leaned over the suitcase, packing my spare pair of plimsolls because I was to wear my new ones for travelling. Before Dad closed the lid, I'd made sure that the wooden Dr Scholl sandals Penny had given me were safely at the top of the case for easy access.

Dad stood up and pressed the palms of his hands into his lower back.

Chucking Putty at the Queen

He stretched backwards and gave a blissful groan as he rocked his head from side to side. "Please don't ask her for a sucker. She'll probably faint or go all hoity-toity and call it an iced lolly."

My feet had barely connected with the platform when Aunty Ann rushed forwards and pecked our cheeks.

"Gosh, boys, it seems you've grown in the past few weeks," she said, enthusing in a jolly hockey sticks tone. "You must be hot and thirsty. Is there anything you'd like from the buffet?"

Oh, this was too wonderful an opportunity. "May I have a sucker?"

She didn't faint but grimaced as if I'd asked for a sandwich filled with cold tripe and onions. "A what?"

"You know, a sucker." I moved my fingers to my face as if holding a wooden stick and made slurping noises whilst performing exaggerated licking motions.

"Oh, you mean an *iced lolly.*"

In a rare moment of brotherly unification, Nick and I exchanged the quickest of satisfied glances.

"Come along, boys. We've got twenty minutes before the connection, so you can have—" she shuddered as if someone had dropped one of her iced lollies down the back of her neck, "a sucker."

Ten minutes later, I tugged her sleeve. "Aunty Ann, don't forget *Top of the Pops* on Thursday. I'm going to see Marc Bolan in full colour for the very first time."

"Yes, yes, your dad told me about that."

"Promise you won't forget."

"I promise." She pushed through the bodies. "Now come along. Gilbert's waiting for us at my house. You'll have such fun when we get there."

I was already rather scared of my taciturn uncle-by-marriage. On one of their visits to Nottingham from their home in Nairobi, the temperature seemed to plummet when Gilbert entered. I'd tried to be polite and offered him a Garibaldi biscuit on a plate. "The black bits are raisins, not squashed flies."

He dismissed me with a regal wave, not even deigning to look my way. "It is my firm belief that children should be seen and not heard."

Instinct told me that fun was the last thing we were going to have when we got there.

6

EVERY DAY IS LIKE SUNDAY

THE TRAIN FOR THE second leg of our journey was not so packed and considerably slower than the one we'd just endured. At our destination, I successfully pleaded with Aunty Ann to let me change into the Dr Scholls that I adored so much, then we crammed into her car and left the small local railway station. After several minutes, we parted company with the dusty-edged, grey ribbon of a minor road when Aunty Ann hauled the steering wheel to the left.

"Not long now, boys."

I held my breath as we sped along a bumpy lane between hawthorn hedges interlaced with pinky-white blooms that shimmered in the heat. I'd discovered refuge within the pages of my Enid Blyton books from the ghastly reality of Mam's death, and Dad was right, the pastoral beauty of my new surroundings wouldn't have been out of place amongst the page-turning prose. The families in the stories were wealthy and existed within a comfortable village lifestyle that was completely divergent to my working-class environment. I frequently wished that we lived in such a blissful manner, and although those wishes for my emotional and spiritual salvation were granted, albeit temporarily, I was already missing Dad; what would he be doing? We were gradually beginning to navigate our new family routine since Mam died, and this separation had rocked the boat of my fragile mental stability.

A hare bounded from the dark green shadows of the hedgerow, and I screamed when Aunty Ann jammed on the brakes.

"Silly creature."

I didn't know if she meant me or the hare but from thereon, she moderated her speed, and we slowly bumped along between high, grassy verges. I'd never seen so many poppies before; they burned like a scarlet wildfire beneath creamy clouds of cow parsley. I clung to the wrinkled leather strap on the inside of the door with one hand and pressed my precious T. Rex singles flat against my lap with the other. I couldn't afford for them to be damaged during this rutted ride. The hot breeze swayed thousands of oxeye daisies and through the open windows, blew over my face with the fragrance from untamed twisty tangles of wild honeysuckle. As we slowly journeyed, the sinuous tendrils seemed to writhe like grass snakes amongst the spires of dark nettles that rose from an abundance of buttercups.

Then there it was. My home for the next fortnight was an enchanting, chalky cottage settled amidst a bowl of dense, secretive woodland. It was the antithesis of the regimented rows of soot-grimed terraced houses crammed into the narrow streets of home. Framing the front door and windows, crosshatches of trellis supported sturdy stalks bearing roses that glowed like hot coals against bottle-green, spear-blade leaves. Sunlit diamonds glinted on the dimpled windowpanes, and a gentle breeze made the frilled lace curtains undulate and froth from the open casements bordered by threads of light yellow jasmine.

Dazed by such perfection, I slowly slipped from the car and floated towards the cottage. "I wish that Mam could see this."

"Well, she can't. She's dead. So stop moping and get the suitcase."

Nick's cruelty smashed my reverie. How dare he speak to me like that? "Get it yourself."

He stomped to the car as I wandered over to the green suede lawn contained by sun-bleached ornamental grasses, lost in my enchantment at the delphiniums that shot in blue skyrocket trails from islands of plump burgundy dahlias. To my delight, a twisty path descended past the cottage towards the indigo shadows of dense woodland from where a mist of apple-scented wood smoke drifted towards me. I quickly slipped the Dr Scholls from my feet and hooked the straps over each forefinger before stepping onto the path. The sun-warmed pebbles scrunched and shifted, massaging my bare soles like thousands of tiny pressing fingertips. A slender gap between the peeling bark of several silver birch allowed me to glimpse the rooftops of a nearby farm where, despite the heat, a thin pearly cord spiralled from one of its cluster of four terracotta chimneys. The serene scene only served to increase my sense of disconnection from home. The malaise of melancholic loneliness sabotaged my peace, and as the infection of homesickness consumed me, I wandered back to where Aunty Ann and Nick stood by the car.

Nick tapped his foot against the portable record player. "I've taken the suitcase in. Are you going to carry this or not? It was your stupid idea to bring it."

"Yes, of course I am." To my astonishment, when I bent over to grasp the carrying strap, the usually slothful Nick jogged on the spot, then raised his arms above his head.

"Aunty Ann, I need to stretch my legs. Is it okay if I go exploring?"

"Yes, but don't go far, and if you go onto the lane, only go to the end. Do *not* go onto the road, because tractors come around the bend before you know it. Gilbert's already had a couple of close calls in his car."

Our brotherly relationship was not the best, yet I didn't want him to leave. Already I could see his body splattered on the front of a tractor, and that would be another member of the family killed. First Gran, then Mam, and now Nick. I had to look after him. "I'll go too."

"No!"

Aunty Ann looked up. "Whatever's the matter, Nicholas?"

Nick scowled. "Nothing. I just fancy being on my own for a bit. I am fourteen, after all. I'm not a baby like—"

"I know, like some people." God, sometimes I hated him so much. "Go on. Go on your own. See if I care. Serve you right if you get squashed by a tractor."

Nick sauntered away, his hands in his pockets and whistling as if he hadn't a care in the world. I jumped when Aunty Ann rested her hand on my shoulder.

"You come indoors with me. Don't worry about Nick. He's a teenager and needs his own space. You'll find that out in a few years."

In the long, low-ceilinged room, I lowered our portable record player to the shag pile carpet and stared at a pair of loudspeakers that stood each side of a gleaming turntable and amplifier. "You've got a record player!"

"Yes."

"But I thought that you didn't have one, and that's why I had to bring ours." I skipped the few paces and lifted an LP sleeve that lay on the shiny Perspex lid. "Ugh! Oh, Aunty Ann, you've got Roger Whittaker." I'd hated the South African singer's joyless single "New World in the Morning," which always seemed to be on the radio around the time when Gran died.

Aunty Ann gently took the record sleeve from me and placed it back on the lid. "It's not mine; it's Gilbert's. And before you get any ideas, he won't allow vulgar pop music to be played on his system. That's why I said that you should bring your own."

Ignoring this slur on my musical taste, I knelt before the amazing stereo with the reverence of a worshipper at the feet of a priest. As I examined the knobs and switches, I knew that my "vulgar pop music" would sound fabulous on this space-age hi-fi. Dare to ask the laconic Gilbert if he'd let me have a go?

Aunty Ann tapped my shoulder. "Now, you're all right just looking. But don't fiddle with anything. I'll know if you do because I'll only be in the kitchen preparing a macédoine."

The word sounded like it was some kind of poultice for an injury, and although I was reticent to display my ignorance, I just had to ask. "A *what*, Aunty Ann?"

"A macédoine of cherries, melon, blueberries, tangerine, pineapple, strawberries, and raspberries."

She sounded as if she were Fanny Craddock addressing a television audience. I giggled because Mam would never have used such an elaborate word. "Oh, you mean a fruit salad. Will there be Carnation milk with it as well?"

Aunty Ann shuddered. "We don't have condensed milk here. We have fresh cream from Zig Zag."

She could have been talking Martian for all I knew. "From Zig Zag? Is that a shop, like Fine Fare?"

A kindly smile lit her face and for the briefest moment, Mam was in the room. "No, it's the farm across the fields. We buy fresh cream from them."

With a jangle of the metal bracelets that she'd brought back from her earlier life in Nairobi, she swept past me towards the kitchen, glancing at herself in the long rectangular mirror. The low bulb from a yellow-shaded table lamp cast a wan glow over the floral print chair covers and doubled the black shroud of shadows. This was such a posh and alien environment, and we just didn't fit in.

With my hands stuffed into the pockets of my shorts to prevent me from succumbing to the temptation of touching things, I approached the television near the window. Its cyclops eye reflected me as a ghost in an unfamiliar grey room. On the polished veneer top stood a silver art nouveau frame. The picture within was obscured by the afternoon light that shone on the glass. I'd only seen a real colour telly in the window of the Rediffusion shop in town when Dad and I went to pay the rental on our black and white set every Saturday morning, and that always had the BBC test card showing the girl and her creepy looking doll posing at the side of a chalkboard. With the stealth of a burglar, I crept towards it, but as I closed in on my target, the sunlight obscuring the contents in the ornate frame vanished. There was Mam when she was younger, smiling from beneath the brim of a large straw hat.

A dizzying fuzzy glow surrounded the picture, and I stumbled backwards, falling into the floral quicksand of a luxuriously stuffed chair. I allowed myself to drown in a gorgeous daydream that Mam had placed the photograph there herself because she and Dad really lived here, and I'd been born in this idyllic rural hideaway. But if that was the truth, then the cottage definitely wouldn't be infused with the edgy atmosphere trapped beneath the low ceiling as if the dark Tudor beams were fingers pressing down on me.

Angry voices from the kitchen warned me that something was wrong. I hauled myself from the upholstered softness, slunk towards the louvered doors and crouched so that I could peep between the angled wooden slats. Only a few inches away, my aunt and her husband faced each other.

Aunty Ann banged a green plastic beaker onto the work surface. "It's not your problem? They're my dead sister's children, for Christ's sake!" She banged the beaker again. "What was I supposed to do? I had to do *something*."

I couldn't discern Gilbert's mumbled response.

"I've told you already: just view them as a temporary inconvenience. It's all right for you; you don't have to see them. You can be in the garden all day or off with your chums swilling scotch at the golf club. I'm the one who has to entertain them for the next two bloody weeks."

The cruel starkness of this exchange, particularly referring to Mam as her dead sister made me regret eavesdropping. Gran had been right: people who listen at doors never hear anything good about themselves. Beneath that guilty weight, I slunk back to the living room as a door slammed. I dropped onto an uncomfortable bentwood chair in front of the bay window and stared at the carpet. Why had Aunty Ann been so determined that we stay with them if we were so unwanted?

"We've worked hard for all of this."

I almost fell from the chair. I'd assumed that Gilbert had left the house, but it must have been Aunty Ann storming off. I slid from the highly polished seat and stood to attention. With long, tanned fingers, he firmly packed treacle-coloured strands of tobacco into the bowl of his metal pipe, a pipe so unlike Dad's, which was carved from a cherry wood branch and buffed to a warm glow from years of use. It fitted comfortably in his hand, and I loved the way his handlebar moustache twitched when he puffed on the mouthpiece to draw the air through, creating a minuscule bonfire in the bowl. His tobacco was deliciously fragrant and softly masculine and reminded me of the autumn bonfires of damp smouldering leaves that the park keeper cautiously tended. In brash contrast, Gilbert's pipe resembled a part of an industrial machine that had fallen off, and its starkness reinforced the intimidation he projected. Furthermore, the noxious, burning old bike tyre stench of his tobacco made me gag. I disliked his bloodhound eyes and horsey teeth, and the paisley cravat that covered his long, saggy neck, and his unpronounceable surname that reinforced his lineage of French nobility.

In a last, desperate attempt to get out of coming to Kent, I'd confessed these concerns to Dad. He'd hugged me and reassured that Gilbert was well known for being last in, first out.

"What do you mean, Dad?"

He chuckled. "Before you were born—before Nick was born, actually—whenever a few of us drove out to the Vale of Belvoir for a beer, he would be the last to enter the pub. There was always something to delay him: he'd forgotten his matches, or he'd dropped his keys. Any tactic to ensure that someone else got the beers in. Similarly, when the beers were low, instead of offering to stand his corner, he'd be first out of the door, saying ridiculous things like he felt faint and needed fresh air, or one of the cars looked as if it had a flat tyre, or that a village child was messing around by the boot. He had a reputation for having short arms and long pockets, so don't be intimidated by his bladdy long-winded froggy name."

Despite storing the knowledge of Gilbert's unsociable parsimony, I instinctively withdrew from the tall, thin man. "Pardon?"

He looked down his equine-length nose at me. "I said that we've worked hard for all of this."

Several horse brasses and a copper bed-warming pan hung beside the wide mouth of the fireplace and above it, with the bottom of its gilt

Chucking Putty at the Queen

frame slightly scorched from the heat of log fires, an oil painting became my focal point as he droned on. In an unwelcoming landscape, a derelict windmill stood on barren, wintery marshland, replicating my bleak emotions in oil paints before my eyes. I was equally as distanced and was only just aware of Gilbert's voice. It was like how it was when Mam died, the sense of being underwater and everything dull and disconnected.

The sharp poke on my forearm with the end of his pipe reconnected me to my present surroundings.

"I say, old boy, snap out of it. Are you paying attention?"

"Yes."

"Were you admiring my artwork?"

"Did *you* paint that?"

"Yes, do you like it?"

"No, it gives me the willies."

His glare could have stripped the paint from the canvas. "This leads me onto the subject of property. It would be appreciated if you didn't touch things that do not belong to you." With his haw-haw tones, he could have been formally addressing fellow diplomats at a meeting of the League of Nations. "Next on the agenda: my grounds."

His grandiose appellation made me think of the posters advertising Kew Gardens that I'd seen upon our arrival at St. Pancras station. Again, I stared at the miserable painting. I hadn't noticed a lone man bent almost double from the weight of gathered reeds strapped to his back, labouring with his burden against the wind that pushed the rushes at an acute angle. It was a painting full of hopelessness and despair, and I could have been that forlorn-looking figure, struggling forwards in my life. Gilbert was still waffling, but I wasn't paying attention until he raised his voice.

"Are you hard of hearing or just plain rude?"

I looked up at the heavy-lidded eyes. "My ears, when... After..."

"After what? Come along, spit it out."

And so, I spat out the horrid words, intended to hurt someone else as much as they hurt me. "After my Mam died." There, they were out, but I didn't feel any better. I tried again. "When Mam died, my hearing went funny, and I had to see a special doctor about it."

"But you can hear now?"

"Sort of, on and off. Sometimes it goes all like...like being underwater."

He shook his head. "If you can hear me now, then I hope you'll pay attention." He waved his pipe in an arc. "To recapitulate: the majority of my garden is out of bounds, but you *are* permitted to walk along the path to the lane. However, you must *not* go onto the road, because there are tractors and other farm vehicles, and the farmer isn't used to," his dark, rheumy eyes first dropped to Mam's tricoloured silk scarf that I'd tied around my right wrist and then down to Penny's old Dr Scholl wooden sandals that adorned my sockless feet, "strange boys wandering around."

"I'm *not* a strange boy, and anyway, Aunty Ann told us about the tractors already."

"And now *I'm* informing you of them. Also, take note that the lawn that you see to the front of the house is of too steep an incline to play football on."

I stepped backwards. "Good. I hate football."

"I beg your pardon."

"I hate football."

He clenched the steel pipe with his gruesome, gravestone teeth and left the room, trailing an evil-smelling cloud of purple-grey smoke. I sighed, remembering how Dad had chivvied me that this holiday in the pastoral delights of the Kent countryside would be like an Enid Blyton adventure. But he was wrong. It was the start of a horror story, and I didn't want to turn any more pages.

7

OUT IN THE COUNTRY

IN WHAT APPEARED TO be a neglected, unforgotten corner far away from the cottage, the unclipped branches of a young lime tree touched the ground, creating an irresistible green cave. I dropped to all fours and shuffled inside. Away from the unforgiving summer sun, the cool, slightly moist earth and dried remnants of the previous year's leaves that crackled beneath my bare knees was a delicious reminder of glorious afternoons spent in Colwick Woods with Mam and Dad.

The knowledge that Nick and I were in the way was too much to confront. How I wished that I could take a time machine back to when everything was all right. But I'd wished that so many times since Mam died that I knew it was futile. I pressed my eyelids closed as the gentle drift of breeze through the leaves became the sound of waves.

I stood on a beach. On the horizon was the derelict windmill from the painting that hung on Aunty Ann's wall. I was alone and looking for Mam. The sand stretched forever, and a distant sapphire shimmer hinted of a remote ocean. A familiar voice carried on the breeze. Sweat rolled into my eyes, stinging them as I squinted into the heat haze.

"Simon, where *are* you?"

"I'm here, Mam! I'm over here!" I spun around and around, trying to see her, but the sand and cloudless sky dominated my sight. The light was so bright that I had to shut my eyes. A dog barked repeatedly with growing insistency, and I opened my eyes to green shadows. The Jack Russell terrier from the nearby farm yapped excitedly as I lay on my back beneath the ground-scraping lime tree branches.

Gilbert's furious features broached the leafy curtain. "Come out of there at once. What the hell are you playing at? Your aunt's deranged with worry."

Nick looked over his shoulder. "I told you the farmer's dog would find him."

Trying to keep my fingers away from the snapping teeth of the liver and white terrier, I picked up my singles from where I'd carefully laid them next to a cluster of red toadstools, then shuffled until I pushed through the low-hanging branches onto where the loam gave way to the immaculately mown lawn.

Aunty Ann rushed forwards, her face drained of colour. "Simon! We've been looking for you for ages. You didn't answer my shouts. I thought you'd run away or been down the lane and had a mishap with a tractor. Gilbert says you're disobedient. He even drove up and down the road. What on earth were you doing under the tree?"

I tried to blink away my tears. "I'm tired. I'm just so tired of everything. I only went under the tree for a little sleep."

"Just look at your shirt. It's covered in bits. Come here. I suppose I'll have to wash it now, not as if I don't have enough to do. You *are* tiresome."

As I stepped forwards holding my precious T. Rex singles, she stared. "What's that inside your shirt?"

"Nothing." I looked down at my new plimsolls. The tips resembled meringues that had been dunked in tea from where I'd dragged them across the decomposing organic debris covering the moist topsoil when I'd crawled beneath the tree. They'd need whitening.

"Come on, it's all right. You can show me."

I withdraw the small, silver-framed photograph of Mam that I'd taken from the top of Aunty Ann's colour television.

Gilbert exploded. "Theft now. Obviously, a family trait."

Aunty Ann glared at him. "Not now!" She daintily squatted, put a finger beneath my chin, and lifted my face to hers. "You're not in trouble. I just need to know why you took it."

If only I could return under the tree where it was quiet and just be left alone until it was time to return home to Dad. That's all I wanted.

"Come on, Simon, you can tell me."

Tears drenched my cheeks. "I'm so unhappy, and I just wanted..." The leaves shushed me. She wouldn't understand.

"What did you just want?"

"I just wanted to go to sleep with Mam like I used to."

Nick sniggered, then gave my shoulder a shove. "See? Didn't I tell you he's crazy?"

A couple of days later, Aunty Ann's cat-like eyes peered over the rim of her cup of Earl Grey tea. We only had PG Tips at home, and the exotically scented beverage invigorated my curiosity. When we got back, I'd ask Dad if we could have some, but I guessed that the corner shop wouldn't sell it. I'd go in and ask them for it anyway, just for the reward of seeing the surprised look on their faces. But what if we never went back home? What if this visit to Kent was already a new life for me, one without Dad? Doubt tightened around my throat like a hangman's noose because Nick had frequently warned me that Dad was going to put me into an institution for unwanted children. Each night as I lay in bed, I imagined standing in the pouring rain outside an orphanage as Dad drove away forever. Was my being here the result of an elaborate ruse concocted between Dad and my aunt to get rid of me? Or was it just Nick being his usual spiteful self? I remembered Mam's words of advice after yet another of his lies was revealed: "Don't believe a word Nick says. He'd tell you that black is white if he knew it would upset you."

"Are you listening to me, Simon? We'll go and see our friends the Thompsons today. They're lovely people and have two sons your ages."

I shrugged off my ridiculous fears and got ready to go to Aunty Ann's car. Dad wouldn't do that to me. He just wouldn't.

Nick bagsied the front seat of the car because he was the eldest, and I sat in the back holding my talismanic T. Rex singles. The clock inset into the polished wooden dashboard marked the twenty minutes we journeyed along narrow lanes until Aunty Ann pulled up beside a wide, white-painted five bar gate. Stretching beyond it to a vanishing point were two rows of beech trees, their bark the dusky lilac-grey of a wood pigeon's feathers.

"Here we are, boys. Open the gate, please, Nicholas."

Nick scowled as he alighted from the car and I grinned, revelling in his hatred of being addressed by his full name.

"And don't forget to close it."

Every bone in my body became jellified as we juddered along parallel ruts in the dry, dark earth that led into the distance like the train tracks that had delivered us here to Kent, so far away from Dad. With a teeth-gripping grinding of gears, Aunty Ann manoeuvred her immaculate car, a shining incongruity amidst the agricultural anarchy of rural muck, and only just avoided colliding with a mud-spattered, olive-green Land Rover parked beside halves of barrels bursting with blood red geraniums.

At the end, a vast, square farmyard sloped, bordered on two sides by low stables, their rust-hued pantiles edged with spongy velvet lines of green moss. Swallows and swifts swooped. The feathered zephyrs darted through smoke that rose from a smouldering heap of golden straw, which I guessed was something to do with the piebald horse grazing in the adjoining paddock.

I'd instantly liked Aunty Ann's dreamy cottage, but I fell head-over-heels in love with this three-storied Georgian farmhouse. The mellowed red brickwork suggested a comforting reliable permanence. My imaginings of Mam and Dad owning Aunty Ann's picturesque cottage went out of the window. This was far more like it, and just the ticket. I could see Dad in his tweed hacking jacket and flat cap, pulling up in his Alvis Firefly and opening the door for Mam, delightfully summery in a floral cotton dress as she held onto a white, wide-brimmed hat, having just come from the county farming show where she'd won a prize for her homemade rhubarb chutney. My latest daydream exploded with a volley of resonant barks from a trio of black Labradors bounding from the farmhouse doorway.

Dad's suggestion that this holiday could be an Enid Blyton adventure was finally justified when a plump lady emerged from the shadows, wiping her hands on a blue and white striped apron. Just as in those stories that I loved, this was my favourite authoress's archetypal farmer's wife with dark hair worn in a bun and a smiling face that resembled a browned scone set with blackcurrants for eyes.

She yelled at the dogs to be quiet, then called over her shoulder, "Alistair! Roger! Our guests are here."

Aunty Ann wound the driver's side window down. "Hello, Dolly."

Nick guffawed and I exploded into giggles. That film had been on the telly and even in black and white, I was knocked out by Barbra Streisand's sumptuous frocks and extravagant hats. I wondered if this homely-looking farmer's wife had a wardrobe in which such apparel hung. The thought of her milking cows in an ostentatious hat was too much. I clamped a hand over my mouth.

Aunty Ann twisted around.

"Now then, you two. Remember your manners."

Her glare could have cut sheets of metal. Once again, the familial similarities came to the fore and for the briefest moment, it was Mam's dark eyes warning me.

Chucking Putty at the Queen

The farmer's wife folded her arms across her ample bosom. "Good morning, Ann, dear. You're as punctual as ever."

"You know me, Dolly, I've no time for shilly-shallying. As arranged, these are my nephews, Nicholas and Simon. I'll be back later to collect them."

Anyone would think that she was having her shoes re-soled. The farmer's wife smiled as we alighted. We'd only just closed the car doors when, after another grating of gears, Aunty Ann sped from the farmyard, leaving behind the feint smell of burned rubber.

"Always in a hurry, your aunt. My husband says that one day she'll meet herself coming back. Now, boys, I'm very pleased to meet you. We don't stand on ceremony here. Make yourselves at home, and please, you must call me Dolly. My husband is Arthur, but he's away fixing some broken stock fencing around the big field yonder."

She waved vaguely towards the distance. I'd never heard anyone say yonder before and promised myself that I'd begin using it when we got home.

"Roger, Alistair, our guests are here!" she called even more loudly.

Two boys sauntered from the shadow of the doorway. Uncertain of what to do, I clutched my records hard against my chest. The older brother, Roger, was thickset and dark, with sideburns already crawling down his cheeks and a smear of dark hair on his top lip. I was a bit scared of him as he looked very bad-tempered and reminded me of a tough lad called Billy who lived round the corner from us at home and whom Mam said was "a born troublemaker." If I ever saw him when I was in the corner shop with her, I tried my hardest not to look at his surly face. I didn't want bashing up at school any more than I already was. On the other hand, Alistair was fair and stout, with small blue eyes shining in his remarkably pink face. With his cropped strawberry blond curls, he reminded me of a bull in one of the antique oil paintings in the Castle Museum at home.

With introductions over, my face remained warm with embarrassment. I'd never been in the company of farm lads before. A pair of wood pigeons cooing at the apex of a barn made me realise that my hearing had returned to one hundred per cent efficiency. I wished that it hadn't when to my horror, Roger nudged Nick and whispered, "Do you want a fag?"

Nick grinned. "Not half. I'm gasping."

51

"Come on then."

When they sauntered away, I wriggled my toes against the smooth wooden ridge on the Dr Scholl sandals. Nick shouldn't have a cigarette. He shouldn't. Cigarettes were bad. One evening, I'd watched with fear from the front window at home when two boys from my school lurked in the darkened doorway of the factory, passing a cigarette back and forth. Mam caught me watching and told me that I must never ever smoke. *Mam*. It was always Mam in my thoughts.

"They're not going to be much use here."

Alistair's voice jerked me from our front room window and back to the Kent farmyard. "Pardon?"

He nodded at my feet. "I didn't know you can get them for boys. Do y'know, I've seen hippies wearing clogs? They come here to buy milk. Dad charges them a few bob to put their tents up in the bottom field." He chuckled. "They say, 'Thanks, man' to him, and one girl called him groovy."

"Oh, they're not for boys. They were my sister's. She let me have them when she got new ones. Those are the latest model; they have blue straps. I tried colouring these the same with a felt pen, but it didn't quite work out how I'd hoped and washed off the first time it rained."

"Oh." He shrugged, smiling. "Fair enough. But you won't get far in them on a farm. You can use my spare wellies." He strode to the farmhouse and returned with a pair of mud-crusted wellington boots. "Why have you got those records?"

"Because they're my favourites. It's T. Rex. 'Hot Love' is the old single, and my dad bought me their new one 'Get It On' specially to bring down here, and I can't wait till tomorrow 'cos I'm going to see Marc Bolan singing it in full colour on Aunty Ann's telly." I stopped to draw breath and witness his admiration, but he shook his head.

"Never heard of him, but I'm not interested in music. I like tractor engines. Do you know my dad lets me help him strip our Massey Ferguson down?"

I had no answer to this statement. He held out his pink paw.

"Pass 'em here, and I'll hold them whilst you put my wellies on."

"No." I jerked backwards and one of my singles slipped and connected with the hard cobbles. My scream soared above the terracotta pantiles.

Mrs Thompson rushed from the doorway. "Whatever's the matter?"

Alistair squatted. "It's okay. Simon dropped his record, that's all."

"Thank goodness. I thought there'd been an accident. Just you two take care." She returned indoors as Alistair stood upright and blew on the Fly Records label. 'Hot Love.' Is that your new one then?"

"No. I just told you, didn't I? My new one's called 'Get It On.'" I snatched my treasured disc from him and slipped it from the white paper sleeve. A jagged-edged chip blemished the rim of shiny black vinyl. Tears bubbled around my eyelids.

Alistair was contrite. "Sorry, that was my fault. Is it broken?" He peered at the record. "It doesn't look too bad, just the edge. We don't have a record player, otherwise you could check it's okay. We've only got a radio. It's not a transistor." He gave an awkward chuckle. "My granny calls it the wireless."

I appreciated that he was trying to make it all right. "Yeah, my gran used to call hers that as well."

"Used to? Hasn't she got it anymore?"

"She died in September. And my mam died in January."

He jerked a thumb towards the farmhouse. "They told me. I'm sorry." He placed his hand on my shoulder. "I say, that's rotten bad luck. I've still got my parents and both sets of grannies and grandpas."

"I've got no grandparents. It's just Dad now."

"And your Aunty Ann."

"Yeah, and Aunty Ann. And some other aunts as well."

"Are they all as bad as her, rushing around?"

"No, but Aunty Lu's ever so funny. She puts her hand up my shorts and says, 'Bitta cock, bitta cock.'"

"That sounds a bit odd. Is she funny in the head?"

"No, she's not bonkers. She's just funny. I love her to bits." With my records once more securely against my chest, I steadied myself by holding onto his shoulder as he helped me put on his wellies. Alistair carried my Scholls as I clumped behind him into the coolness of the farmhouse.

Kilner jar islands dotted a white linen cloth that covered a huge table, and a shaft of light through the large window smeared the whiteness with jam and marmalade colours as if the preserves were spread on a giant's slice of bread. Within the vast fireplace, charred chunks of logs protruded from the grey ashes that softened the bottom of the sharp brickwork corners.

Nick and Roger returned, and when Nick exhaled as he dropped onto the chair next to me, I hoped that Mrs Thompson would not be able to detect the lingering cigarette smell as easily as I could.

Instead, she smiled and nodded at the two T. Rex singles that rested on my lap. "I'm sorry that we don't have a gramophone. You watch you don't drop jam or crumbs on those recordings." She held a plump hand towards me. "Shall I put them safe for you, up there on the mantle?"

"Don't bother, you're wasting your time. He won't let go of them." Nick tapped the side of his head. "He's not right. Everybody back at home says he's got a screw loose. He takes them all over the place with him. It's T. Rex this, T. Rex that. It would be a shame if something unfortunate happened to them. He'd cry like a girl."

His threat made me transfer my singles from lying flat on my lap to being clamped in the vice of my bare thighs.

Mrs Thompson patted my shoulder. "You do what makes you happy, dear."

Despite Nick's nasty interjection, this overall relaxed atmosphere was far preferable to the "Look, don't touch" antique shop environment of Aunty Ann's house, where I wouldn't have been surprised upon our return to see signs warning that all breakages must be paid for. I loved being in this mellow old farmhouse, sitting amongst the untidy, unbothered family whose old tabby cat lay curled asleep in the dimple of the worn, baggy seat of a high-backed, oxblood leather armchair. It was the amiable opposite of when I'd sat cross-legged on my aunt's thick Axminster carpet. "Sit on the chair, not the floor. You're not in St. Ann's now, you know," Gilbert had chided.

The cat awoke, unfurled itself, and arched its back, shuddering with ecstasy, its tail a quivering question mark. Dare I suggest to Aunty Ann that we stay here in this red brick cauldron of hot summer sun, wrapped in farmyard smells and the aroma of baking bread? It would be just like a *Famous Five* adventure…but we had to return to the uptight atmosphere within her immaculate showroom home where it was obvious that we were an intrusion.

8

THE HISSING OF SUMMER LAWNS

AS WE'D WAITED ON the platform of Nottingham station for the arrival of the London train, Dad reassured me that he'd alerted Aunty Ann of my need to watch *Top of the Pops* because T. Rex were number one in the charts with "Get It On."

"Don't worry, Son. She won't forget, so don't pester her. I told her that it will be the first time you've seen them in colour."

But I did pester her. For the first half of our inaugural week in Kent, I'd fizzed with anticipation and, ignoring Dad's instruction, reminded Aunty Ann several times each day until finally she snapped under my nagging. She slapped the long knife that she was using to slice a cucumber onto the work counter with a resounding crack.

"All right, all right, *all right!*"

Within a minute, she'd jotted it on her kitchen notepad that hung from a hook next to the huge white fridge freezer, which evidenced her prosperity. We had no such luxury, and like everyone around our way, in hot weather we resorted to submerging our bottles of milk in a bucket of cold water in the shade.

After an achingly impatient wait, Thursday evening finally arrived. The sun's persimmon rays smouldered between the tree trunks and leaves, creating shadows that neared the cottage with the inevitability of an incoming tide. Above the water butt at the corner of the kitchen door, a restless squadron of tiny midges darted in the still air, and through the half-open side window, the grandfather clock chimed seven times. I hugged myself. The twenty-five-minute countdown to *Top of the Pops* had begun.

Gilbert had turned on his lawn sprinkler, sending hissing silver rods of irrigation around the perfectly mown summer lawn. The artificial rainfall instantly roused a dormant memory of when Mam took Nick and me to Brighton to see Aunty Fran. As we picked our way across the pebble-encrusted beach like storks through lily pads, Mam announced, "I've got something really special to show you."

Up on the promenade, the heat from the concrete transferred through the rubber bottoms of my plimsolls to be quickly absorbed by the soles of my feet. For the last few paces, Mam covered my eyes with a hand that smelled of the Nivea cream she'd lightly spread on my face to prevent me getting sunburned.

"And...open!"

We stood before an enormous white marquee, whereupon an ornate sign proclaimed, *Dancing Waters*. Mam paid the entrance fee to a lady in a smart yellow uniform trimmed with gold piping, and once inside the coolness of the tent, I was captivated by the watery display that synchronised to Grieg's "In the Hall of the Mountain King," a favourite of mine that accompanied our energetic Movement to Music classes at school. I held Mam's hand, transfixed as the water bubbled, gushed, spouted, rocketed, and churned until they unified in a breath-taking silver wall before abruptly losing their liquid life.

"Oh, Mam, they really did dance. I loved them!"

She'd squeezed my hand. "I knew you would."

Two summers later, the garden sprinkler in Kent was no *Dancing Waters*, but nevertheless, I whirled and twirled beneath the hissing jets, wishing that Mam could see me. The stupefying rays of the descending sun enhanced the beds of red salvia, and for a few seconds, my floral intoxication gave me the sense of being the only person on the planet—until Aunty Ann startled me from my reverie, tramping over the lawn from the side of the cottage, a violet turban covering her hair.

"Oh, there you are, Simon. You've not got soaked, have you? It's almost time for your programme."

"No, I'm quite dry, thank you."

With increasing excitement at the thought of seeing Marc Bolan on a colour television for the first time, I followed her indoors so closely that I could have been her shadow. The television awaited me in the cool twilight of the living room. I sat cross legged before it.

Aunty Ann shook her head. "Don't sit on the floor, *please*. I know that Gilbert's told you off about this already."

I jumped up. "Sorry, I'll sit on the settee."

"I've told you before: it's not a settee, it's a sofa. *Settee* is very council. Sometimes I wonder if you say things to deliberately annoy me."

She reached over and twisted one of the knobs on the front of the

Chucking Putty at the Queen

veneered box and returned to the kitchen as the amazing television bloomed into colourful life. Before long, I was gawping at my musical hero's face framed by liquidly corkscrew curls.

Nick entered from the garden and glanced at the television. "Aunty Ann, come quickly."

She rushed in from the kitchen, clutching a tartan tea towel. "What on earth's the matter?"

Nick gestured to Marc Bolan. "Can you believe that's supposed to be a man? It looks more like a woman to me."

"Oh, really, Nicholas. Is that all? I thought that something was wrong." Aunty Ann bent towards the screen. "Is he crying?"

"No." I clapped with delight. "It's glitter under his eyes."

"Whatever next?" Aunty Ann shook her tea towel and returned to the kitchen.

All too soon the performance was over, and I was as exhausted as a salmon returning to its birthplace after an epic journey across oceans. I couldn't wait for Dad's eight o'clock phone call when I could tell him all about it.

In the opulent cottage, the grandfather clock continued its comforting slow marking of time. I stood in the hall beside the white-painted ornate swirls of the iron table, its amber glass top dimpled as if created by hundreds of thumbprints. Aglow with evening light, a spider web stretched in prismatic colours across the shadowed curtain of ivy that clambered around the narrow rectangular window. From a hook in its white wooden frame and bound tightly by knotted string, a trio of fishermen's floats hung in orbs of blue, green, and mustard coloured glass. On our first day of exploring our temporary home, Aunty Ann had caught me with my face up close to them, trying to see if there was anything inside. She'd placed her hands on my head and gently moved me away, explaining that they were used by Turkish fishermen. Waiting for Dad's call, I was just as transfixed by the colours and jumped out of my skin when the phone rang.

For the past evenings, Aunty Ann answered. Then, after talking with Dad, she'd let Nick and then me speak to him, always urging me not to talk for too long as phone calls cost money, and it was good of Daisy and Rex to let Dad use the phone. But this evening, still effervescing from seeing Marc Bolan in full colour, I needed to get in there first. The phone was on its third ring as our aunt appeared from the kitchen. I hopped from foot to foot. "Aunty Ann, may I answer, please?" I'd never taken a call on a real phone, only on the pretend switchboard that Mam and Dad bought me for my fifth birthday, and more than ever, the need to hear Dad's voice and to tell him about my colour televisual treat was already driving me nuts.

Nick appeared and butted in. "I'm the oldest, so if anyone's going to answer the phone first, then it should be me."

The sixth ring. Gosh, I wish someone would pick up the receiver.

Aunty Ann smiled. "Just this once, Simon, and remember it's not a toy."

At the end of the eighth ring, I cleared my throat just as Dad did and tried to deepen my voice by pulling my chin into my neck. "Good evening."

"Oh, hello, Son. What a surprise. I was expecting your aunt. How are you today?"

By the time I'd finished, I was giddy and breathless. "You wouldn't believe it, Dad. It was magical. It's easily the best part of being here."

Aunty Ann snatched the telephone receiver from me. "Well, there's gratitude for you. After all I've done. Go and sit on the sofa."

With a regal wave of her hand, I was dismissed.

"It's settee, not sofa!" Elation from speaking to Dad and watching T. Rex in colour had emboldened me, and I ducked as the damp tip of her tea towel whipped past my head. My aunt's quick temper was another indication of how much in the way we were, and despite the gorgeousness of the countryside, it made me yearn all the more to return to the narrow, paved streets of home.

9

WHEN THE TRAIN COMES BACK

THE NEW SCHOOL TERM for the autumn of 1971 was upon us, and my emotionally challenging holiday in the Kent countryside already belonged to a distant age. We rejoined the harsh routine of life in St. Ann's, where the demolition of the neighbourhood crashed and thudded closer to our street. It was an inescapable fact that I'd soon be uprooted from where I was born and our home would join the anonymous mountains of rubble that rose around us.

I didn't have a house key, so after lessons, I sat with the retired couple next door to wait until Nick arrived from his grammar school a couple of miles away. Although I didn't particularly care for my brother, if he wasn't back by a certain time, the belief that he'd been killed overwhelmed me. On five afternoons each week, I sat next door with my eyes on their clock as if I were a frustrated factory worker waiting for his tea break.

This remained the case until one afternoon when I stepped from the small terrace at the top of our street and saw Dad standing at our front door. I hurtled towards him with my parka flapping against the backs of my legs. "What's up, Dad?" Puffed from my efforts, I rested my hands on my knees, panting. I wished I hadn't asked the question because I was already frightened of the answer. Since the beginning of the year, the gripping hand of the grim reaper was never far from my overworked, bereaved mind, and my imagination ran riot. Nick had been run down, or worse, it was Tim. He'd been killed in an accident at work. A chisel had slipped and cut his jugular vein open, and he'd bled to death.

Dad hugged me. "No, Son, there's nothing wrong. I had the afternoon off work because of something here that I had to deal with. Come on in and take your coat off. I've made you a special tea."

Alarm bells clanged. I didn't believe him. Something was terribly wrong. Dad didn't just have the afternoon off work during school term to deal with things and to make me one of his special teas. Perhaps it was Penny or Marge that disaster had stricken, or Steve was locked up in prison again. Dad being home early was all wrong, and with trembling arms and legs, I shucked off my parka.

Dad stepped into the living room, ceremoniously holding the curtain to one side to allow me to enter. The unusual aroma of oranges perfumed the air. The table was set with a plate of sandwiches and a small porcelain tray bearing neatly arranged vol-au-vents. The afternoon light from the back window fell on Mam's best cut glass bowl filled with orange jelly with several small shapes inside. Dad was behaving oddly, and against the murmur of horse racing commentary from the corner of the room, he directed my attention to the table, pointing out this and that as if he were a curator at a museum.

"You didn't really enjoy your birthday tea, did you, Son? I know Tim and Nick walloped off the vol-au-vents pretty sharpish and you only had one, so these are all just for you. Nine of them, to match your age. I'm sure that you'll be able to manage them."

He remained at my side, indicating the bowl of jelly, explaining that he'd been busy. He'd popped down to Arthur Smith's shop and bought a tangerine. When he'd peeled it, he'd carefully threaded cotton through the juicy segments and suspended them from a slim length of dowelling balanced across the rim of the bowl. Once the jelly was almost set, with tiny jerks, he was able to carefully extract the cotton, leaving the tangerine segments in the jelly which created the floating illusion of goldfish in an orange pond.

"Oh, it's supercalifragilisticexpialidocious!"

Dad cleared his throat. "I'm glad that you like it...but the real reason I had the afternoon off was *this*." He stepped aside.

In the corner of the room, instead of our cumbersome black and white television, there was a slim, modern set. The multicoloured silks adorning the jockeys flew across the screen like wallflower petals blown on a breeze as they raced their galloping horses along an incredibly green racetrack.

Dad grinned. "When you came back from Aunty Ann's, all you did was talk about seeing Marc Bolan in colour. You didn't stop talking about it for ages. It cheered you up so much that I thought it was time we got with it, and so I ordered this."

"Do Tim and Nick know?"

"They don't. You had to be the first, and I couldn't wait to see your face. I kept it a secret and organised it all by telephone from work. Tonight, we can watch *Top of the Pops* in colour here at home."

"Oh, Dad!" I threw my arms around his waist but kept my eyes welded to the colour set. The race was over. Snorting, steaming horses crowded the screen, mad-eyed and sheened with sweat.

"You know, you were always your mother's baby, and over the past months, you've had a hell of a lot of growing up to do. It was hard for me to let you go to Kent. I didn't know if it was a good or bad idea. I was still trying to find my way. At times, I was at my wit's end. I know your Aunty Ann was only trying to help, and it is a beautiful part of the country. I thought that a change of environment might do you good."

I was shocked at this unexpected forthrightness, with my father talking to me like I was a grown-up. It was wrong. I wanted to remain a boy and for him to be my protective dad. I pressed my face harder against his belly. "It did, Dad, honestly." I daren't tell him of the angry exchange I'd overheard and how my whole body had ached with the need to be at home with him. Nor did I confess how, after he'd phoned each evening, my desolation doubled with the ping of the handset being returned to its cradle.

He pulled away from me. "Now, Son, before you get square eyes, how about tackling the tea that I made for you? What did you call it?"

"Supercalifragilisticexpialidocious."

"You tuck in, and I'll make a cuppa."

But before I set about devouring my feast, I sat in Mam's chair. I would be the adventurer who would finally excavate the untouched memory treasure. I reached into the wooden trough and pulled out the ball of desert-coloured wool and two turquoise plastic knitting needles. There were several dozen stitches bunched up. I caught my breath, remembering that after completing the jumper and bobble hat, Mam planned to knit me a pair of mittens. That would never happen now. Everything that was familiar in my life was being destroyed. An uncertain future without Mam lay ahead, and I didn't want that thought in my head.

I returned the knitting to its wooden trough and sat before my banquet. I plunged my spoon into the sea of orange jelly in my first attempt to retrieve a fruit fish. For a few moments, I didn't care about anything. I was back home with Dad, although at bedtime, my mind would overflow with thoughts of Mam, and my cotton pillowslip would be moist with tears. But right now, the whole street could fall down around us, leaving only our house standing, just so long as we could remain together watching the silent faces on the fabulous colour television.

    Triumphantly, I extracted my tangerine trophy and smiled because right then, life was perfect. "Oh, Dad, you always make everything all right."

10

TAKE ME BACK HOME

The balmy summer of 1971 mellowed into bronzed autumn. The demolition of St. Ann's encroached closer to our house and with each twenty-four-hour cycle of the mantelpiece clock, Dad increasingly worried that the council had not yet offered us new accommodation.

Those who'd already relocated to the new houses loyally returned to the Devonshire Arms around the corner. They arrived as if adventurers from distant lands but instead of bearing chests laden with jewels and exotic spices, they brought with them reports of instant heating at the flick of a switch, of upstairs bathrooms fitted with ceramic baths, handbasins, and toilets, and the ultimate outrageous extravagance: a separate downstairs loo located off the hall. The thought of a hallway alone made me giddy with longing, because here in our Victorian two-up, two-down, the front door opened straight onto the pavement.

However, a psychological change had already affected these voyagers, and their social familiarity appeared to have dissolved with the increase in physical distance. Within the ever-lingering stench of smouldering bonfires, they stood on our doorstep bearing fond adieus, stamping to free their shoes of the ochre brick dust that was as pervasive and unstoppable as the cockroaches that infested the now-empty houses. Smiling and nodding, they awkwardly shuffled as if desperate to return to the freedom of the luxurious new neighbourhood and the plush wall-to-wall carpets of which they boasted. My admiration of such sumptuous floor coverings had prompted Dad's scornful remark as he closed the door on the latest visitors. "It's all on the never-never, Son, and that's a fool's game." He and Mam never had anything "on tick." Our belongings were mainly second-hand, and my parents asserted that what we didn't have, we didn't need. These visits to see the few of us left clinging to the life raft in a sea of destruction became fewer until they stopped completely.

The mandatory evacuation of our immediate area hadn't yet begun, but corner shop gossip assured us that it wasn't far off. Although I didn't want to leave the house I was born in, thus being irrevocably removed from my last physical connection with Mam, as I pushed the creaking door of our outside toilet shut one afternoon, I remembered the tales the visitors had imparted. I couldn't wait to experience the new lavatorial luxury.

On this particular afternoon, my football-obsessed brother Nick lounged against the rickety fence between us and next door, its drooping length as supportive to his weight as a sagging washing line would be to a baby elephant. I hoped that the rotting timber would snap, and he'd land on his bum. Better still, if he broke his neck, I'd finally be freed from the mental and physical torment that he inflicted upon me in varying degrees of severity each day.

He seemed on edge and glanced furtively down the yard to the back window. "I want a word with you."

His shove propelled me into the secrecy of the narrow recess between the brick outhouse and the engulfing dark green shadows of the overgrown privet bush.

He looked over his shoulder, then pressed a forefinger to his lips. "Dad told me not to tell you this, but there's something you need to know."

After Mam died at the beginning of the year, I was shackled to my fears of Dad's unexpected death, and my months of worry and depression coalesced into a disgusting knot in my throat. "What's up? You're scaring me." I tugged at the sleeve of Nick's dark blue grammar school jumper, and he jerked his arm away as if my fingers coursed with electricity.

"Get off! Don't you go blabbing to Dad about what I'm going to tell you, okay?"

"Yeah, okay."

"Good. Because if you do, it will cause all sorts of trouble."

"I won't say anything." A tug of war between wanting to know and remaining ignorant pulled across my thoughts. "Is he really poorly, like Mam was?"

"No. There's nothing up with him medically." Nick poked me in the chest. "It's you that's the problem."

"*Me?*"

"Yeah, you. Dad told me that he needs some time to himself."

"You what? What do you mean?"

"You've been getting under his feet and clinging to him ever since

Mam died."

I gulped, but the billiard ball in my throat refused to budge. "He told you that?"

Nick leaned closer. "Yeah, and just you remember what I've told you before."

How could I forget? After that cataclysmic day when Mam died, Nick had frequently taunted me that I was just a step away from Dad putting me into an institution for unwanted children. At nights when I lay in bed, a familiar picture developed. I stood outside the enormous oak door of a foreboding Gothic hall, a battered suitcase at my feet. I sobbed, watching Dad drive away beneath the tempestuous black clouds that unleashed a torrential downpour. My thin cotton shirt was ineffectual against such a hatefully cold deluge. Had I been wearing my duffel coat then I would have pulled up the hood in a tortoise-like attempt to escape whatever horrors awaited me inside the orphanage.

"I don't understand." I bit my bottom lip, hoping to halt the tears of panic that were accumulating.

"Listen. He doesn't like you being around all the time. He wants some Saturday afternoons to himself, and he told me to take you down Meadow Lane to the County matches with me as a favour to him."

I frowned because Dad knew that I hated football just as much as he did. "When did he tell you that then?"

"The other day. It'll give him a rest, so think of Dad for once instead of always thinking about yourself." He poked my chest again. "And don't you let on to him that I told you. I'll pretend that it's your idea."

Now I was really confused and struggled to comprehend the situation. Nick said it was Dad's idea, but I was to pretend that I didn't know that? I gave up worrying about the complexities of this fraudulence and was determined not to badger Dad, because I didn't want to upset him and be put into a children's home.

From thereon, each alternating Saturday over the winter of 1971, I endured the misery of being a part of the mob going to the Notts County match. Upon returning home and wrapping my arms around Dad with relief to see him, I feigned football fan excitement to mask the wounding confusion of what Nick had told me about him not wanting me around.

***

It was Saturday 19th February 1972, two months since we'd moved to the new house. The first anniversary of Mam's death a couple of weeks earlier had passed unmentioned, although Tim told me Dad requested that Little Nancy, who played the out of tune upright piano at the Sycamore, give a rendition of "Harbour Lights," which was his and Mam's song. Then he'd bought a double brandy, raised it aloft, and knocked the bronze liquid back in one go. This uncharacteristic behaviour scared me. Dad was a moderate drinker and never touched spirits, and I worried that his bereavement was driving him to drink just like it did to people in soap operas.

I still believed that it was my fault that Mam died, and once more I sought solitary solace in my records. I'd lugged the Dansette upstairs and was listening to my only T. Rex album, *Electric Warrior*, as I sat cross-legged on the bed with a sheet of writing paper resting on a *Rupert* annual. Lilac ink flowed from my fountain pen as I wrote my weekly letter to Mam, telling her what I'd been doing and how much I missed her. I signed off in the usual way, even though it was daytime: *Night-night, Mam,* followed by four evenly spaced kisses. I wasn't too bothered that the ink blurred from where my tears had landed. My secret letters were never posted because there was nowhere to post them to. Mam was dead and gone forever, but I just liked writing letters to her.

Heavy footsteps on the stairs alerted me, and I slipped the paper between the pages of the book and slid it under the pillow just before Nick burst into the bedroom with the furtiveness of an escaped convict, his eyes darting around as if searching for a hiding place.

"What you up to?"

"Nothing."

"Then why aren't you ready yet?"

"What for?" I rearranged Mam's jazzy headscarf around my neck, hoping that my unpreparedness would preclude me from the afternoon's events. Despite Nick's insistence that my presence on Saturdays was a hindrance to Dad, it was about time I found a way out of going to the football matches that I so heartily despised. Maybe I could spend the afternoon in the library since it was open until five. I wouldn't be at home under Dad's feet, but I wouldn't be at the football either.

"Don't play stupid with me. You know it's match day. Who are we playing?"

I hated it when sports-mad people said, "we're playing" or "we won" as if they were active participants instead of just being part of a paying audience. Although I would have loved to have been in T. Rex, I hadn't jubilantly proclaimed, "We're number one" when their latest single "Telegram Sam" hit the top of the charts a couple of weeks earlier.

"Come on, who are we playing?"

"York City."

"Hooray, the fairy got it right at last. Take Mam's scarf off, put this on, and show some enthusiasm for the beautiful game at least once in your pathetic life." Nick tossed a length of black and white knitted wool at me.

"Why should I?" I deliberately didn't catch it, and it fell to the floor as he punched an invisible target a few inches above his head.

"Because you're going to see the Mighty Magpies thrash the Robins."

This excited ornithological explanation far from stimulated me as much as it obviously did Nick, whose eyes bulged above his glowing cheeks.

"Put the scarf on."

"What for?"

"So that you fit in with everybody else going to the match."

"But I don't want to fit in with everybody else, and I don't want to go to the match. I hate football." I took a deep breath. "Do you know what the best thing in the world would be? What I really want to do most?"

"What?"

"I want to stay here with Dad and play my records."

Nick leaned over to the bed and growled. "Now, listen, you little prick. How many times do you need telling? Dad told me he doesn't want you under his feet all the time. You're going to the match. No more of this poncy T. Rex shit, wearing glitter and sequins. You're an embarrassment, and you need to grow up."

His punch to my shoulder made my tears well up so easily, as they had ever since Mam died.

"And don't start crying like a girl again."

"But me and Dad go shopping on Saturday mornings, and when there's no home match on, he helps me make my stuff."

"Yeah, that's another thing. He doesn't like you doing all that puffy crap. He wants you to be more like the lads round here."

"But I'm not like the lads round here."

"I know you're not, and so does Dad. He says it's about time you were. Don't you see that he's ashamed of you? He says that going to watch County is your chance to start behaving like a real boy. But like I told you before, don't let on you know what he said, all right? He swore me to secrecy."

"Why would he do that?"

"To stop you crying all over the place." He snickered. "You even started blubbing over 'Two Little Boys' when it was on the radio the other day. He's fed up with it."

"I can't help it." And I couldn't. The slightest thing set me off. By the time of the final verse of the mawkish, oversentimental number one single from a couple of years earlier, I'd collapsed onto the armchair, sobbing into the cushion Mam used to put behind her head when she was "having a minute."

He turned to leave and tugged my Electric Warrior poster pinned to the back of the door, but it didn't move. "And you are *not* wearing those fucking women's boots to the match. Put something normal on."

Several minutes later, he pointedly looked at his watch as I shrugged into my parka in the hallway.

Dad grabbed the metal tab and zipped it up for me. "Now, Son, are you really sure that you want to go?"

"Yes, Dad. Honest."

"Hmm. I'm not so sure. I still think that you're just saying it. You've been to a heck of a lot of football matches. Wouldn't you rather stay here with me and make a new cardboard guitar? I've got those four knobs from that old developer at work that we could use as volume controls just like on Marc Bolan's."

He knew me so well.

On the top of the record player was the LP *I Want to Stay Here* by the easy-listening duo, Miki and Griff. Dad had played it that morning, and the title had never been more apt than at this moment. But I knew I mustn't rescind my untruth as confusion swirled; why was Dad offering me the choice to stay at home if he wanted me to go the football and get from under his feet? "Of course, I want to go. We're playing York this afto."

Dad kissed my forehead and turned to Nick. "I've told you before, and I'll tell you again. Don't expose Simon to any trouble."

Nick snorted. "It's County, not Forest. *We* don't have boot boys."

Chucking Putty at the Queen

But I knew otherwise.

As soon as we were out of sight of the house, Nick pulled a gold packet of Benson & Hedges from his anorak pocket, withdrew a cigarette, and jammed it between his lips. Further fumbling produced a box of matches. Once the cigarette was lit, he dragged hard and after a couple of seconds, expelled the smoke through his nostrils. His casual arrogance so close to home shocked me, and he stared when I stopped in my tracks.

"What's up with you?"

"You're smoking!"

"So what?"

"But...you're *smoking*."

"What's your problem? Don't you go getting all little tin god on me. And keep your trap shut. Dad doesn't know."

"I bet you he does. He knows everything."

"So? Who cares? It doesn't matter. I can do what I want to. I'll soon be old enough to leave home."

I wish you would.

"Tell you what. We're playing Mansfield Town next week. I'll ask Dad if you can come on the coach trip with me." He dragged deeply again, then blew smoke upwards like the steam billowing from the funnels on the trains that Mam took me to watch in the now-demolished Victoria railway station. "Your first away match. It'll be great. You'll love it."

I wouldn't.

On this cold day, I despised being a foot soldier in this pavement-wide army of soccer fans marching along London Road, bordered on one side by cars and buses and on the other by the motionless mirror sheen of the canal. The weather had begun to clear, revealing a metallic sky smeared with patches of pink, yellow, and orange as if a rag dipped in watercolour paints had been dragged across the thinning clouds. It was what Mam used to call "a cold sky." The unmoving water reflected this exquisite diaphanous palette, transforming the black canal into a stretched ribbon of wintery colours. I was swept across the canal bridge on the wave of ardent football fans and looked down to where a solitary fisherman sat on a camping stool, hunched over his rod like an enormous garden gnome. If only I could find such escape from this crowd. The bewitching odour of fried onions from the hot dog wagon outside the football ground wafted greasily through the chilly air, provoking a deep grumble in my stomach.

Nick always had dosh—more than the pocket money that Dad gave him—and a couple of times, he'd flashed a pair of pound notes at me, twitching them between his fingers like a magician with playing cards. It was only later in the year that I learned Nick's supplementary income originated from the drawer in Tim's bedroom where he deposited his wage packet every Friday.

"I'd kill for a hot dog."

Nick smirked. "You'll be lucky. Just get in the queue for the match. I want to get a good spot."

As soon as we'd passed through the clicking turnstiles and were on the packed terraces, Nick negotiated our way through the crammed bodies right down to the front. I pressed up against the metal restraint as he began to chat animatedly about football fixtures with Bill, a burly mechanic who always stood in the same place and who vociferously shared his opinions on the progress of the match.

I survived the boredom of the first forty-five minutes by daydreaming about how I could have been snug in the house with Dad, making a new cardboard Gibson Les Paul guitar together. There was a tin of bronze spray paint in the shed left over from Tim's attempt to invigorate the frame of the antique oval mirror that survived the move from the old house. We could spray the cardboard body of the pretend guitar and with the knobs from the developer Dad had, it'd look authentic, just like Marc Bolan's.

"Oi, ref! Use yer bleedin' eyes! Do you want to borrow my specs for the second half?"

My delicious reverie was shattered by Bill's bellow as he pulled a chrome hip flask from the darkness of his heavy serge overcoat. The ingrained oily grime of his big fingers attested to his profession as a mechanic as he removed the stopper. Without taking his eyes from the action on the pitch, he tipped the vessel and swigged, then after smacking his lips so loudly that I could hear it above the clamour of the crowd, he thrust the flask to Nick.

"Here yer are, youth. Have a nip of this."

As Nick raised the rim to his lips, I tugged his anorak sleeve. "No, don't, you mustn't!" It was bad enough him smoking but to drink booze so brazenly horrified me. Nick shoved my hand away, pursed his lips as if he was about to play a trumpet, and swigged from the flask until Bill tugged it downwards.

"Steady on, youth. Whiskey costs money." He offered the flask to me. "Are you gonna have a nip an' all, young un? It'll put hairs on yer chest."

I snorted and looked at him as if he was offering me battery acid. "Certainly not."

"Suit yerself." Bill returned the flask to his pocket as Nick gripped my forearm.

"You'd better not go blabbing about this to Dad, okay?"

Seven-inch singles danced before my eyes. "How much is it worth?"

"A smack in the teeth, that's how much it's worth. Don't go getting clever with me. You'll regret it."

"And if I tell Tim you've been threatening me, he'll duff you up."

Nick harrumphed, then cupped his hands to his mouth. "Come on! Pass the ball, pass the ball!"

I took that to mean the subject was closed.

Although this was the last place I wanted to be, the miserable righteousness of my sufferance surged through me so forcefully that I imagined everyone else could see the golden halo forming above my head. I hated being here, but at least I was out from under Dad's feet so he could enjoy time to himself. Obeying Nick's orders, I was thinking about someone else instead of myself.

The shrill blast of the referee's whistle announced half-time, meaning that after the break, I must endure another tedious waste of my time. I was so cold that my eyeballs hurt. When my peripheral vision began to flash like silver sequins beneath a strobe light, I fell into another daydream of what I'd could have been doing if I'd stayed home. Dad always baked bread on Saturday afternoons, and I'd eagerly await the moment when he'd slice off a thick crusty end, smear it with butter, and present it to me on a plate. Oh, to be there now, warm and content, listening to *Electric Warrior* and making a fabulous new cape from an old net curtain, revitalising it with an eye-popping rainbow of glitter. But those visions were nothing more than wishful thinking, and as the teams trailed off the pitch, the refreshments staff shoved their galvanised metal trolleys from the shadows and began their rounds.

As well as announcements and half-time reports from other fixtures, records were broadcast through the public address system. I always hoped to hear T. Rex, but my desire was never fulfilled—until now, when

"Telegram Sam" crackled from the loudspeakers. In the limited space, I began to wriggle and pout, tossing my imaginary corkscrew hair. My potent imagination transformed the cold Meadow Lane football ground into the Hollywood Bowl where, beneath the blazing Californian sun, I was Simon Bolan performing my new single to a capacity audience.

Nick clouted me on the head, smashing my dream and rudely returning me to my miserable reality. "Pack it in."

"Give me a suitcase, and I will." I was rewarded with a second clout.

"Stop pratting about. What do you want from the refreshments bloke?"

"I'll have one of those dinky little packets of Ritz crackers with the cheese triangle and two silverskin onions inside. Oh, and a can of Fanta, thank you very much."

"Do you think I'm made of money?"

"It's not your money. Dad gave you it for both of us." Every time we came to the football, the same scene played out. I'd make my request and would only receive a disgusting hot drink.

The refreshments sellers were probably in their fifties but as they advanced, doggedly pushing their silvery-grey carts, to the nine-year-old me, they appeared as decrepit as the doddering troops on the end credits of *Dad's Army*. The chunky, black rubber tyres trundled over the frosted beige path. I hated the formality of the immaculately mown pitch and the regimented order it represented. It was so boring. I wanted reckless, glam excitement. In the cold afternoon air, I half-closed my eyelids until the unblemished iced white spikes around its edges sparkled like an incredible length of silver tinsel.

"Uh-oh, here he comes again; Old Misery Guts, with the Elbow Caff on wheels," a gruff voice called from behind me, provoking a turbulence of chuckling in the chilly air.

The Elbow Café was a popular greasy spoon that was sandwiched between Mansfield Road and Huntingdon Street. I'd dined there on a couple of non-footballing Saturdays when Tim insisted that we go for a cup of tea and a sausage cob, even though it hadn't been long since breakfast. I giggled, recalling his words when he shoved the door open on my first visit: "The tea's like gravy here. It's lovely. Nice and strong, not like that wazzy stuff Dad squeezes out of the pot."

Finally, the shining cylinder was a few feet away. The sputtering mercury drops of boiling water reminded me of the coins thrown from

the stands as the opposing team approached the green rectangular battlefield. When I'd first witnessed this spectacle, I clapped my hands.
"Oh, how lovely, they're throwing money to them as a thank you."
"Of course they're not. Don't you know anything?"
"What do you mean?"
"They file the edges of the coins until they're sharp."
"Why would they do that?"
"Hoping it'll do some damage."
"To what?"
"Faces, legs, arms."
"But they could blind someone."
"If they struck lucky, yeah."
The refreshments man was upon us. His absurdly oval head was crowned by a black and white striped bobble hat with what should have been Mighty Magpies stitched in thick red woollen letters. The embroiderer must have been dyslexic as it spelled Mihgty Magpies, and this misspelling always provoked catcalls from the crowd. "Ayup, mih-gitty magpies!"
Laughs rippled around me as the wag in the crowd continued. "D'ya want me to take it home to my missus, and she'll do it proper?"
The miserable vendor glared. "Piss off and shut yer cakehole, unless you want all boiling water chucking over yer."
He gave the trolley a hard shove to propel it forward. One solid tyre met with an obstruction, making the hot water tank wobble dangerously. I was scared it would topple over onto him and indulged in a moment of dramatic fantasy, visualizing the stark black headline on the front page of the Nottingham Evening Post: *HALF-TIME HORROR,* and beneath it, in smaller type: *Pensioner scalded to death in tea urn disaster.*
A multitude of hands stretched towards him with the urgency of religious devotees desperate to touch the hem of the Pope's cassock, but Nick was there first.
"Two Bovrils, mate."
I stared at him. "*Mate?* You'd best not let Dad hear you call people 'mate.' You're not on a building site, you know."
"Shut your trap and take this. Quick, it's burning my fingers."
Nick handed me the drink bought with the money Dad gave him.
"And ten Benson's, *mate.*" Nick smirked at me as Old Misery Guts

frowned, sliding a golden packet from beneath a tea towel. "Don't go shouting yer gob off about me fags."

Nick sniggered. "Like everyone doesn't know." He nodded to a man a few feet away.

Enlightenment blinded me as powerfully as the floodlights above us. Nick was purchasing cheaper drinks to keep the change and augment his cigarette-buying fund. Sensation revisited my fingers when I clasped the flimsy milky-white plastic beaker overladen with steaming deep brown liquid. I hated the foul drink, which smelled and tasted as if it were a bag of beef and onion crisps dissolved in hot water. The inadequate thickness of the beaker forced me to make a claw of my hand, awkwardly gripping the reinforced rim with my fingertips as I attempted to maintain as little flesh and plastic connection as possible.

I was trapped in a hubbub of debates on football fixtures, and the prospect of the following week's away game against Mansfield Town. Maybe I'd be able to slyly dribble the drink onto the ground without Nick seeing. But bodies surged from behind. A scalding wave sloshed over my fingertips. My hand splayed open, and the beaker plummeted to the iced gravel. I watched, delighted, as Bovril spread like oil leaking into the sea from the hull of a damaged tanker.

Old Misery Guts was quick to reprimand me, his veiny jowls glowing pink from the cold. "You can't have another un, and you're not getting your money back. It's your own fault you dropped it."

A high-pitched woman's voice made me wince.

"Mind your back, ducky. Can I just squeeze through before he boggers off?"

Thrusting between Nick and me, a black and white mittened hand awkwardly offered coins, palm upwards.

"Giz a tea, duck, and one of them little Kit Kats for me daughter, though why she thinks she deserves treats, I don't know."

Another surge from behind shoved the crowd into me, and the woman's money fell to the ground, landing in the remnants of the horrid beef drink.

"Now look what you've gone and made me do. I've dropped the last of your Christmas box what you got from your gran."

I twisted around to watch as the woman berated a girl of about my age.

"It weren't my fault, Mam."

"Yes, it was, you clumsy sod. You're always in the bleddy way, getting under my feet."

As if someone in the crowd had knifed me, the woman's words reminded me why I was suffering yet another ghastly football match. My heartbeat fluttered as I thought about what Dad might be doing. Baking bread, preparing our tea, or tinkering under his car, or doing some clothes washing by hand in the sink as we didn't have a machine. Whatever he was engaged in, he wouldn't be idle. If only I'd stayed at home, we would have made a cardboard guitar together, and I'd be happily gyrating with it in the back yard, pretending to be number one on *Top of The Pops*.

Despite her neck being swathed with coils of a chunky-knit scarf in the obligatory black and white stripes, the girl's bloodless face indicated her low body temperature. She shivered, then squeezed in next to me and smiled. "Ayup."

"Good afternoon."

When she peeled off the red and white Kit Kat wrapper and let it flutter to the ground, I nudged her and pointed to the message displayed on one of the large advertising hoardings. "You know you really oughtn't do that. We're supposed to 'Keep Britain Tidy.'"

The girl shrugged. "It don't matter. Everybody else does it."

I puffed out my chest. "That doesn't make it all right. If everybody else did it, as you suggest that they do, then we'd soon be drowning in an ocean of rubbish."

Her dirty thumbnail sliced through the silver foil with the ease of a scimitar, revealing the dark chocolate bar within. "You're dead funny; you sound like a teacher." A deft movement snapped the biscuit-filled fingers in half. "Do you want a bite of me Kit Kat?"

After my mini lecture, I couldn't possibly accept a snack from a litter lout. "No, thank you, I'm quite all right."

"Suit yerself." She noisily crunched the bar with her mouth open, obviously relishing the taste. "It's cold, int it."

"Yes, there is somewhat of a chill to the air but only to be expected, given the time of year."

She stopped chewing. "You don't half talk posh. Are you going to Mansfield next week?"

"Unfortunately, yes. Although to be perfectly honest, it's not really my scene."

"Oo-er! What is your scene then?"

I drew myself up and sucked in the frigid air, filling with self-importance at the chance to lecture this lip-smacking girl about my musical hero, but Nick's heavy slap to the back of my head stopped me before I'd begun.

"Don't be such a queer. You'll enjoy it."

The girl giggled again before cramming the remaining finger of Kit Kat into her mouth and turning back to her mother.

The onslaught of cold permeating from the concrete terraces was too severe for the thick soles of my fell boots to repel. I repeatedly stubbed the rubber tips against the low wall separating the fans from the pitch to see if I could feel my toes. It was the kind of deep chill that Mam would say froze her right through to her marrow. The second half was soon underway, and a new energy invigorated the men around me into a barrage of insults directed at the pitch.

"Pansies!"

"Nancy boys!"

"Queers."

"Puffs."

I was all of those names they yelled. A rip in the grey sky allowed a sliver of weak sunshine to momentarily bathe the ground in front of me, but instead of it being uplifting, a deep melancholy enveloped me, and within the thousands of fellow human beings gathered here, I'd never felt so alone.

How I dearly wished that I wasn't here, one speck of colour in a sea of black and white, engulfed by the developing atmosphere of violence once the raucous chants began. They were the antithesis of the fantastical descriptions that my corkscrew-haired pop hero sang as he shimmied in his Anello & Davide women's shoes. Instead, these intimidating chants were yelled by skinheads stamping in the wooden stands with their cherry red Doc Marten bovver boots. Their words confrontationally lampooned "The Tennessee Wig Walk":

> I'm a bow-legged chicken, I'm a knock-kneed hen.
> I ain't had a fight since I don't know when.
> I don't care where and I don't care when.
> 'Cos I am a County boot boy!

Chucking Putty at the Queen

And another, more succinct one that was delivered with the determined strength of a male voice choir and an accompanying barrage of artillery-strength clapping:

You're gonna get your fuckin' heads kicked in.

The shrill note of the referee's whistle ended the match, making it a two-all draw, and under the canopy of midwinter darkness, I marched homewards with the army into which I had unwillingly been conscripted. The canal shone with a sinister blackness, indicating bottomless depths and bringing to the front of my mind Aunty Mary's horror stories of tragically adventurous boys who had drowned there. A forceful wind had picked up and pushed ripples across the water, reflecting the sodium streetlights as distorted, undulating orange lines. They seemed to pull me towards the sinister Boots factory and warehouses that loomed on the horizon, and wouldn't have looked out of place in Fritz Lang's *Metropolis*. Even on the sunniest day, those eerie structures gave me the creeps and for as long as I could remember, the austere geometric simplicity of the narrow rectangular windows made me worry how people inside would escape should there be a fire.

Seven days later, it was the end of my first visit to an away match, a one-all draw against Mansfield Town. I couldn't wait to get on the coach and go home. Being the first on board, I headed for the back seats and sat next to the emergency exit. Nick dropped down at my side and began to play with an empty Coke bottle.

The door next to me flew open, and I stared into manic eyes.

"Fucking County bastards!"

Silver flashed. Nick lunged and whacked the knifeman's hand with the Coke bottle. The skinhead stumbled backwards and with enormous effort, Nick pulled the door shut. The thug hammered on the window with both fists for several seconds until the coach pulled away from the car park and headed back to Nottingham.

Nick's face was drained of colour. "Don't tell Dad, or he'll never let you come to a football match again."

But he didn't ask if I was all right and an hour later, my legs were still made of rubber when we walked up our front path. Dad was in the window, watching for us.

Nick hissed a reminder. "I told you, don't say anything, okay? Or he won't let you come to another match."

Dad beat us to the front door and stood on the step beneath the canopy.

"Hello, lads. Simon, you look perished. How does poached eggs and baked beans on toast grab you?"

"Not half. What a tip-top tea."

Dad unwrapped the scarf from around my neck and looped it over the coat hooks at the bottom of the stairs. "You won't be needing that for another week. Did you have a nice time at Mansfield?"

"A skinhead pulled the coach door open and tried to stab me with a knife."

"*What?*"

"We were sitting on the back seat, and he pulled the emergency door open and tried to stab me. It was a *massive* knife, Dad, though it was more like a Zulu spear." The way Dad stared at Nick told me that I was on the way to scoring the match-winning goal. I gave an extra hard kick. "And I'm sure there were all bloodstains on it."

"I thought that I told you not to let Simon get into any danger."

"It wasn't *that* bad; he's just making it up. It wasn't a Zulu spear at all." He glared at me. "It was more like a penknife."

"Whichever kind of knife it was, you still put Simon in danger. Right from the start I had my reservations about allowing him to go to football matches with you, but you insisted that he'd asked to go. I see clearly that I was stupid to believe you. Your mother always said that you're a liar." Dad placed an arm across my shoulders. "That's it, Son. No more football matches for you. From now on, you stay at home with me on Saturdays."

I really had scored the winning goal, and I went upstairs and put *Electric Warrior* on the Dansette, lay a fresh sheet of paper upon the *Rupert* annual and began a new letter.

"Dear Mam, you won't believe what happened today…"

11

ALONE AGAIN (NATURALLY)

In late September 1972, I was undoubtedly one of "all the young dudes" as I reclined in the front passenger seat of Dad's black Rover 95. I adored the fab single by Mott the Hoople that blasted from the car radio, and that it namechecked T. Rex made it all the more special for me.

There'd been no radio when Dad bought the car, but he managed to get one from a bloke at work who owed him a favour for photographing his second child's christening. It was for a different make of vehicle, but in his typical Heath Robinson manner, Dad created a bracket from a sheet of aluminium, assorted bolts and hooks, and a length of conduit. From my viewpoint on the pavement, I'd clapped and pirouetted when he'd screwed it beneath the dashboard, and after a period of grunting and groan-filled fiddling, he succeeded in connecting it to the cigarette lighter electrics. Of course, I was allowed first go. I pressed the power button and twiddled the tuning knob, skipping stations until I heard the honeyed American tones of DJ Emperor Rosko.

"We've got a radio in the car," I said, intentionally loud so that it would reach a gaggle of staring boys nearby. They lived a few streets away, and I hoped that, like the young dudes of the song, they'd carry the news of our wonderful vehicular addition back to their area.

Resting against my thigh was Mam's white buckskin handbag. Sumptuously lined with folds of peachy-orange silk, I'd claimed it as my own soon after she died. There were two reasons that made possessing this item imperative. The first was the cachet of owning such a sophisticated accoutrement so redolent of Hollywood leading ladies. The second, more precious motivation was that each time I split the gleaming clasp and parted the two halves, the delicate fragrance of her face powder escaped. I'd greedily inhale, luxuriating in a dreamy return to a time before her death, when my world was less emotionally precarious. Her subtle bouquet of lily of the valley temporarily soothed my grieving mind and once more, she was tucking me in between crisp sheets that had been boil-washed that morning, then blown dry on the backyard line. It was an irresistible indulgence which I had to ration, fearing an incremental diminishing of its potency. Not wanting to distress Dad, I hadn't told him of my covert aromatic gratification, and he was happy to let me use the handbag in my make-believe popstar life.

Inside its silken depths, my fingertips brushed the pen that Penny and Meash presented to me as a thank you for being pageboy at their wedding. I had meticulously unpicked the sticky tape, then ironed away the creases of the pink and orange striped paper with the palm of my hand. I'd never seen such chic wrapping before. Penny explained that she'd bought it in Brixham, the picturesque Devon coastal town where they'd honeymooned. But she wasn't too pleased when she found out that I'd told people they'd spent their first week of married life in Brixton, the deprived, socially challenged south London suburb.

Inside the leather-effect box, a stylised golden dart radiated from a bed of elderberry felt. "Oh, it's fabulous! It's so groovy." I rotated the shaft and depressed the tiny button at the top several times, loving the assertive click it made when the ballpoint nib projected from the opposite end. "Thank you. Oh, thank you. It's...it's just like a ray of sunshine that's broken off and been turned into a pen."

"You're always writing things, so we thought that you should have a pen of your very own, and you could begin your first book."

I grabbed the wrapping paper and turned it to its white side. "I'll start now."

After a couple of seconds, Penny glanced over my shoulder. "'*The Psychedelic Day*.'"

I was proud that I could spell the long word with ease, although my schoolteacher told me that I used it far too often in my speech.

Penny nudged me and laughed. "Which day was that, then?"

I carefully laid down my golden pen and fussed with Mam's yellow, red, and green paisley scarf that she'd arranged around my neck earlier that morning. "Oh, *really*." I shook the chunky amber, lime, and coral Bakelite bracelets that Aunty Lu gave me for my dressing-up. "Every day's psychedelic to me."

With their second wedding anniversary approaching, that gilded reward for my ceremonial participation was there in the handbag, easily accessible for when I signed autographs for the hordes of adoring fans that only my eyes saw.

    Mam's face powder compact also lived within the sumptuous satin folds. I pulled it out and flipped it open. My captured reflection within the shining circle reassured me that my cheekbones shone with just the right degree of silver glitter. Too much would be vulgar. I wanted to look as if I was sprinkled with fairy dust, not covered in Bacofoil. The only downside of my glamour was that the smooth skin of my jaw was rasped by the white and yellow crêpe paper boa that I'd created the previous evening. Also, my toes were numb because I'd crammed too much scrunched newspaper into the end of my shoes. Nevertheless, it really was the most fabulous footwear, and I'd hardly believed my luck when Marge offered them to me. She would soon be emigrating to Australia and couldn't take everything with her. When she'd asked me if I wanted them, I'd jumped at the chance as if she'd told me that she could bring our mam back from the dead. They really were the blue suede shoes of rock and roll legend, and each toe was augmented by an appliqued scarlet flower with a mimosa yellow centre. Setting them off were two-inch beige heels that tapered to a one-inch sole. I knew this because I'd measured them with Dad's metal ruler, anticipating the day someone would enquire about them, so that I'd be able to announce the specifications with casual confidence.

    A hectic schedule controlled my fantasy world from the moment I awoke that morning. When Dad had cleared the breakfast things away from the table, he'd assumed the guise of celebrated *New Musical Express* reporter Charles Shaar Murray. Using his hefty Philips reel-to-reel tape recorder, he conducted a relaxed interview with me about the forthcoming tour to promote my new chartbound LP with my group, *Electric Sequin*.

    I sat confidently in one of the four ornate dining chairs, my shoulders draped in an appropriately sequin-dotted cape made from an old nylon curtain. My head was crowned with the top hat Dad helped me create from stiff black card, embellishing it with lick-and-stick golden stars, silver diamonds, and orange crescent moons. Contemplatively pouting between delicate sips from a glass of fizzing champagne—pineappleade—I haughtily answered the questions that I'd prepared and written on a note pad for Dad to read from. Once the list was exhausted, he captured this landmark moment with one of his Rolleiflex cameras in his alternate occupation of rock star photographer. I couldn't wait for Monday when he'd take the film to work, develop it, and bring back the prints.

His chameleon-like involvement in my skewed reality also transformed him into my part-time chauffeur. We drove to lunch at Claridge's where I joined Zandra Rhodes, Molly Parkin, and Andy Warhol. This was followed by a shopping expedition within the art deco glory of Biba on Kensington High Street. However, surrounded by the inner-city grimness of the real world, Dad was actually driving through the streets of St. Ann's to see his friends Ken and Evelyn, who still lived on The Promenade, the long row of once-elegant but now worse-for-wear Victorian dwellings that had been spared in the mass demolition of our old area. Each Saturday they'd meet in the Vine pub at one o'clock, and I'd sit outside in the back of the car with a bottle of champagne and a food hamper from Fortnum & Mason. At my side was a pile of glossy photographs of me in concert which I signed for my fan club staff to post to the legions of my devoted followers. But should anyone peep in, they would have seen a ten-year-old boy, his head covered with a bizarre wig made from multi-coloured strips of crêpe paper, holding a crusty cheese and onion cob in one hand and clasping a bottle of Apollo fizzy lime and lemon in the other as he read the latest copy of *NME*.

When Dad delivered my lunch, he always asked, "Are you sure you're all right out here, Son? Wouldn't you prefer to be at home with your records?"

And I'd always say, "I'm okay, honestly, Dad."

Even though he sat with the door to the pub ajar so that he could see me, he sounded unsure. "I really don't like you sitting outside the pub in the car, but I understand why you want to."

I gazed over the wrecked streets to the back of Lymn's funeral parlour. Amongst the rubble lay a navy blue shoe, its strap twisted and snapped. One slingback was no good to me but what it rested upon piqued my curiosity. I slipped from the car, smiling and waving at the music press photographers, whose flashbulbs dazzled my eyes when I crossed the street. I pulled the object free. Once I'd blown away the coating of brick dust, I saw that it was a wallet made from plastic crocodile skin. What a find! It was the perfect item to stuff with my homemade currency that I'd named Bolan dollars.

Originally, I'd made only one banknote: a slip of paper upon which I'd drawn Marc Bolan's head enclosed in an ornate oval line made of five-point stars. I wasn't much cop at portraying eyes, and after several frustrating attempts which depicted my pop hero staring with the glazed look of a dead sprat, I decided to adorn his face with sunglasses. The denomination *One Million Bolan Dollars* decorated the top in stretched letters. I preferred to use American tender to complement the images of pink Cadillac glamour and transatlantic decadence rather than the staid, stiff upper lip connotations of our British culture. Dad took my original drawing to work and photographed it. Conjuring up his darkroom alchemy, he then transferred the image onto something that resembled light green rice paper and reproduced it dozens of times until I was rich with a fortune of meaningless money.

But until now, I'd had nothing to contain the cash and had stuffed it into my pockets as if I were the celebrity "spend, spend, spend" football pools winner, Viv Nicholson. Once we were back home, I commandeered the sink where Dad was about to wash soil from the carrots that he'd bought from the bloke who sold vegetables from his allotment around the pubs. I rinsed the artificial reptile skin in hot soapy water, then dried it carefully using Tim's hairdryer switched to its coolest setting to avoid melting the scaly-patterned surface. When my fingertips could no longer detect any damp inside, I stuffed it with Bolan dollars until it bulged satisfyingly with my imaginary wealth.

Flush with fantasy financing, I promoted Dad to the position of my full-time chauffeur and continued to accompany him on his Saturday visits to the Vine. I had the brainwave of transporting his reel-to-reel in the back of the car. I'd tape my LP of T. Rex's *Electric Warrior*, and with the car windows wound down, everyone would be aware of my presence. But Dad nixed this idea with his usual logic.

"You'd need an electricity supply for that, Son."

Momentarily thwarted, I proposed that we take the portable battery-operated record player on the back seat next to me but again, he pointed out the impracticality.

"I'm sorry, Son, but the arm will just bounce and skid around all over the place."

After another moment of thought, I had the answer to my publicity predicament. "You know, Dad, I'll just sit there, and people can look at me. If I had music blaring, it would look like a cheap gimmick."

Dad chuckled. "You're probably right, Son."

On one of those Saturdays, I'd insisted that Dad detour through the sad remnants of our old neighbourhood. My imagination thrust into overdrive, we prowled the desolate streets in our sleek black car moving at a kerb-crawler pace, the engine purring as if a hundred stowaway cats were beneath the bonnet.

"Pull over, driver!"

Responding quickly, Dad drew the car up to the kerb. Nature had worked quickly to reclaim the streets. Dandelion starbursts, straggly, yellow-topped ragwort, and pink spears of rose bay willow herb sprouted from the cobbles. The weight of lorries, bulldozers, and cranes bearing wrecking balls had pulverized the once sturdy slabs into the fractured fragments of an iced cake dropped to the ground.

I wound down the rear passenger window and beckoned to a figure shuffling towards us. It was Kipper Feet Elsie, a lugubrious lady thus nicknamed by Mam and Aunty Lu because of the flattened, brown leather carpet slippers that she always wore, whatever the weather. Mam told me that during one heavy snowfall she'd seen her wearing a pair of oversized wellington boots as she entered the corner shop.

"No slippers today, Elsie?"

"Oh, yes, Mrs Smalley, I wunt be without me slippers. They're under these bleeders."

After the demolition of her house, she and her husband were staying with a friend on The Promenade. A couple of days earlier, Tim and I had watched a medieval adventure film on the telly. I'd loved the flowery speech and decided to address Dad in a similar manner. "Driver, pray toot thy hooter!"

A double beep caught Kipper Feet Elsie's attention and, obeying my regally summoning hand, she shambled more quickly towards us. Recognition quivered her hangdog features.

"Oh, ayup, Mester Smalley."

I'd once tried using the local colloquialism mester instead of mister, thinking that I was being clever, but Mam had clipped me round the ear and told me not to let Dad hear me speaking like that.

Now Dad wound his window down fully. "Afternoon, Elsie. How's Bill?"

"He int too bad, duck, and he int too good. Can't shift that bleddy cough of his, but I mustn't grumble. There's worse things what happen at sea."

"Give him my regards, won't you?"

"I will do, duck. Are you settling into your new home then?"

"Yes, thank you. Although it was a great upheaval."

"And how's your youngest now? He went a bit bleddy barmy after you lost your wife, didn't he?"

The short length of cigarette that was permanently glued to her bottom lip almost fell when I leaned out from the back window. "Coo-ee! I'm here." My crêpe paper hair rustled like dried autumn leaves when I vigorously shook my head again and smiled. "I know you can't believe your eyes, but it *is* me. Touch my hand if you want to make sure. Here, have some Bolan dollars and have a fabulous life. My new album's out soon."

With arthritic fingers like knotted rope, she grabbed the sheaf of pretend bank notes when I thrust them towards her. After gawping at them, she shook her head and gave Dad a pitying look. "You want to get him looked at, Mester Smalley."

Regardless of this judgement, and to my delight, she stuffed the notes into her tatty brown handbag, shut the clasp with a sharp click, and traipsed off without farewell. I demanded that my chauffeur drive on, and when Dad slid the car away from the overgrown kerb, I lounged in the back, submerged in wonderment at living the stupendous superstar lifestyle of my own creation.

***

For tea, a few weeks later, Dad cooked tripe and onions for Tim and himself, and fishfingers, chips, and peas for Nick and me.

Tim pointed at me with his knife. "That bloke Don down the flats who worked on the bins told me you cheeked him the other day."

"No, I didn't."

"He said you tried giving him some of that pretend money of yours."

"Oh, yeah, I did that. But I didn't cheek him."

"Well, you don't just go up to someone who you don't know and who's been made redundant and say, 'Our Tim says you've been sacked, so here's some Bolan dollars. Have a fabulous life.'"

I speared a chip with my fork. "I thought it would make him happy."

Tim shook his head and smeared a golden blob of mustard onto his tripe. It looked so disgusting, I wanted to vomit.

"You're bleddy barmy, you are. Fancy going up to someone and saying *that*."

I stared at my reflection in the large picture window which was still steamed up after Dad's cooking. I couldn't make out my features, only the sparkling glitter beneath my eyes.

Dad looked up from his plate. "Cut him some slack, Tim. His heart was in the right place."

Hidden by the table, Nick pressed his shoe heel onto my sock-clad toes. Despite the pain, I knew better than to wince or to snitch on him.

"A shame his brain isn't in the right place. He's always doing stupid things like that and showing me up."

"How was I showing you up with my generosity? Anyway, you weren't even there."

"I mean showing me up by walking around dressed like that, with sequins and glitter on your face and wearing those women's boots and all that."

"This is T. Rex glamour."

"You look like a puff. Everyone says you're Albert Brown's boyfriend."

"That's enough, Nick." Dad's face was impassive as he sliced a triangle of tripe on his plate. "We'll have no more talk of Albert Brown."

Albert Brown was a diminutive, middle-aged man who wore his hair in a pageboy style and dressed in tartan miniskirts, silky blouses, white pop socks, and patent leather girls' shoes. He was regarded as an oddity and tormented as a figure of ridicule. It was common for members of the public to yell at him on the street: "Oi, Albert. Give us a whoopsie!" and in response he'd flick one of his legs backwards, lift the back of his tartan mini skirt, and flash a pair of frilly lace knickers as he trilled, "Whoopsie!" When I told Tim that I thought that he was fab, he'd frowned. "Don't you ever go near Albert Brown. He's a queer." And now my own appearance aligned me with this local legend. I excitedly squeezed my arms into my sides. What an accolade.

Tim screwed the lid onto the Colman's mustard jar. "You know what you need to do, don't you?"

"What?"

"You need to get out more with other lads—*proper* lads. There's that youth club down the King's Hall Methodist Church on a Tuesday night. You wanna go and make some real friends instead of living in a bleddy daydream." He lifted his knife from the side of his plate and jabbed the top of my left arm with the rounded tip of the blade. "Are you harkin'?"

"Go and get lost. I'm not going to church." The fish finger I was chewing muffled my words. "You know I don't believe in all that crap about God and Jesus."

Dad cleared his throat. "Simon, remember your manners. Don't talk with food in your mouth, and please don't tell someone to 'go and get lost.' I didn't teach you to speak like that, and neither did your mother. And I don't want to hear you say 'crap' ever again. You're not American."

My cheeks burned partly from the reprimand but mostly from the mention of Mam. "Sorry, Dad."

Tim wasn't giving up. "You won that Bible at school, didn't you?"

"Yeah, but not because I wanted it. It's just 'cos I can remember things." And I *could* remember things, including all the insignificant details of my life that were of no importance to anyone but me. The only missing minutiae scattered in my wrecked emotions belonged to the several weeks directly after Mam died. They remained locked deep in my mind, no matter how hard I tried to recall them.

Tim gulped noisily, and I watched with revulsion as he prodded his fork into another slice of wobbly, bleached white offal.

"Go on, Dad, tell him. He needs to go and make friends with proper kids and stop pratting about with all this dressing up stuff."

Dad was busy with his food. "Leave it, Tim. He's quite all right as he is."

I smirked at Tim. "Yes, thank you, I'm quite all right as I am. I like dressing up."

"Well, down there, they've got darts and ping pong."

"How do *you* know? Do you slip in there for an hour before you go for a pint in the Chase?"

"Don't be so bleddy cheeky to your elders and betters. There's kids there that come from all over St. Ann's. Dad, tell him he's got to go."

As usual, Nick had to butt in. "And there's table football."

I rolled my eyes and coyly patted my hair. "Can you see *me* playing table football?"

Dad sighed and carefully rested his cutlery on the rim of his plate. "There's too much talking and not enough eating going on."

We fell silent.

Tim finished first and lifted the wide plate to his mouth to slurp the milky liquid. "Cheers, Dad, that was lovely." He stifled a burp and nudged me again. "There's a record player down there an' all, so you could take your T. Rex singles and make some friends."

Tim's insistence on my integration with unknown children was worrying as well as tiresome. I was okay on my own. All this chit-chat about me making friends caused an unsettling memory to stamp through my mind: that of a visit to the recently created adventure playground. I only went under duress from Nick, who had assured me that it was the place where I'd find the friends that I had absolutely no interest in finding. I was immediately frightened by the raucous gangs of screaming kids and horrified that several were swinging on an old car tyre attached to a rope above a twenty-foot drop.

This wasn't my idea of an adventure, and why anyone would choose to play amongst such an abominable landscape was beyond me. I loved gambolling and frolicking amongst the greenery when Dad took me up to Colwick Woods each weekend, and he'd laughed at my explanation for my arms-wide spinning and twirling. "I'm chasing the wind." It wasn't an effort for me to mentally ramble back to family picnics in lush green fields where, beside a shallow, gurgling stream that rippled and rolled with mercury sparkles, Mam would spread our glamorous leopard skin print blanket, then arrange on it our banquet of assorted sandwiches filled with potted meat, cheese and tomato, or fish paste. Sometimes we'd have haslet too. The stone stopper of a brown two-pint bottle of Dad's homemade bitter would be unscrewed for the adults, and his own ginger beer was available for us young ones. And slap bang in the middle of all this, Mam would ceremoniously place a small bowl in which thin slices of cucumber were submerged in malt vinegar, having miraculously survived the long journey along twisting lanes without any spillage.

But I was scared within this ghastly intimidating bombsite where kids jostled and fought to dangle from a metal pulley, shrieking as they whooshed along the zip wire stretched between a pair of old telegraph poles that rose from the battered ground. Dark with creosote, the upright columns reminded me of the grainy, desolate panoramas from the First World War in the photobook Dad brought home from work. At the old house, he kept it on the top shelf of the bookcase. "You're too young to

Chucking Putty at the Queen

look at it, Son." But by standing on the arm of the chair and stretching like mad, I was just able to reach it. The first photograph made me wish I hadn't. A double page spread displayed endless graveyard trenches amidst monochromatic, mournful acres of branchless trees that remained as if every charred stump defiantly marked the location of a soldier whose life was lost during the bombardment of artillery shelling. This playground was equally hostile and unwelcoming, and as soon as we'd arrived, I wanted to go AWOL and run home, fuelled by the cowardice of a deserter from the muddy dugouts six decades earlier.

Nick cleared off sharpish, and through the turbulent shrieking kids who danced around an old pram in which a fire burned, I saw him shake hands with a youth in a black leather bomber jacket. No doubt they were sloping off for a cigarette.

Now I was alone again and jabbed my forefingers in my ears when two girls stood either side of me and screamed before running off. When I unplugged my ears, I only just managed to dodge a barrel rolling down the steep hill. I did *not* want to be here. I scanned the terrain for Nick, but he was nowhere to be seen. I jumped out of my skin when a lad leaped from the pinnacle of an untidy black mountain of old car tyres and stood before me, his thumbs jammed into the pockets of his blue and purple split-knee corduroy trousers. Loads of the kids wore them, and how I wished Dad could afford to buy some for me, but I knew it was out of the question and would never ask him.

The boy snorted at the back of his nose and launched a glob of phlegm at my feet. "I'm the king of the castle, and you're the dirty rascal."

"How dare you? I'm no dirty rascal."

"You're not the king of the castle neither, so there. You got any fags?" He raised his fists.

I didn't want bashing up and saw a way out. "Actually, I have." For a second, I believed that my reply enrolled me into the ranks of cigarette-smoking young ruffians but just as swiftly, that fleeting inclusivity ended.

"Ooh, my lady. Hark at you. *Actually*." He sniggered, placed his right hand upon his hip, and flapped his left hand at shoulder height. "*Actually*, I'm a little teapot. Pour me out. *Actually*, here's my handle, here's my spout." He yelled over the cacophony of the adventure playground. "Oi, Gordon! This puff's got fags."

In the near distance, a skinny boy with a blond basin haircut popped up from an oil drum. On its side, a graffitied allegiance to Nottingham Forest Football Club was daubed in long-dried drips of blood red paint. He clambered out and trotted across the rough ground, repeatedly slapping his hip with one hand and holding the other at chest height as if grasping the reins of an imaginary horse. He galloped past three boys jumping up and down on a sheet of corrugated iron and when he got closer, I noticed his fringed novelty waistcoat, the scrap of chequered material tied around his neck, and the grubby pink sticking plaster wrapped along the bridge of his circular wire spectacles. The resemblance to the child cowboy on the confectionary adverts was remarkable.

"Whoa, boy, whoa." He pulled up his make-believe steed and held out his grubby hand, palm side up. "I'm Gordon, and I'm the Milky Bar Kid, and this is a stick-up. Hand 'em over, or we'll duff you up."

I shook my head and tried to adopt the condescending tone of Father Kean, the vicar at St. Catherine's Church down the road. Mam and Dad had been friendly with him, and he'd often called round for a cup of tea and a natter, even though they weren't religious. "No, no, *no*. The Milky Bar Kid is a goodie, not a baddie, and he's certainly not called Gordon." I raised my eyes to the sky in despair, thinking of the cowboy films on the telly that Tim loved. "He's called Butch, or Rocky, or Chuck." I shook my head again. "And he doesn't hold up people, nor does he duff them up. He *helps* them."

"This one don't. Giz your fags or else."

I slid my hands into the side pocket of my parka, and both boys eyed me as if I were about to withdraw untold treasures. When I held out a packet of sweet cigarettes, the Milky Bar Kid shoved me hard on the shoulder.

"They're not proper fags, redskin."

His comrade snatched them from my hand. "But they'll do."

The rubber heels of my fell boots buffered against rubble when I edged backwards, my eyes scouring the depressing site in the hope that Nick would come and rescue me, but he was still missing.

The Milky Bar Kid shoved me again. "You'd best be here tomorrow with some proper fags, or we'll find you and kill you." He mimicked a pistol with his fingers and pointed them at my face. "Pyow, pyow, you're dead."

The pressure in my bladder was unbearable, but the gentlemen's public toilets was over the other side of the road. I certainly wasn't going to relieve myself here in front of these two, despite several splashed trails against the old doors from the demolished houses that were used for fencing the area indicating others had no such inhibitions.

The Milky Bar Kid's piggy eyes narrowed behind his spectacles. "Well, go on then."

"Go on then what?"

"Lie down on the ground."

"*Lie down on the ground?* Why should I?"

"Because I just shot you, and you're dead. So you gotta lie down dead."

"I'm not lying on the ground."

"Why not?"

"I'll get all muck on my bellbottoms."

A yell shot through the hubbub. "Oi, Gordon, Tony, come and see this."

The moment the boys turned around, I seized my chance and bolted downhill until I reached a gap in the makeshift fence, darted through, and hurtled straight across the road without looking. A car horn blasted, but I moved with the unstoppable velocity of the kids on the zip wire behind me. I bypassed the opening to the gents' toilets in the spike-topped green metal railings and didn't stop until I banged the front door shut behind me, thankful that I'd heeded Dad's words that morning: "If Nick's taking you to the adventure playground today, Son, it would be wiser if you wore your fell boots rather than your high heels."

Tim poked me again with the end of his knife, stabbing my attention back to the present.

"Are you harkin'? You could take your records."

Because of that incident at the adventure playground, I rejected his suggestion of taking my precious discs to the youth club. Maybe those two lads would be there and remember me, and because I hadn't returned with cigarettes, they'd probably steal my singles in revenge. But hang on, it was a church, and that meant it would be a safer environment. Also, it might not be such a bad idea for me to go there as it would provide a ready-made audience of new people to show off my homemade glam apparel to. My mind was made up, and this gig would be the warm-up for my nationwide tour. It wouldn't be long before my triple album rock opera was released, so this exposure was crucial. "Is it okay if I go down next Tuesday, Dad?"

He paused his spearing of opaque crescents of sliced onion and smiled. "I don't see why not, Son. You know my good chum Jim from work is involved in that church. You'll be quite safe with him there."

I drummed the ends of my cutlery on the table in celebration, already visualising the gawping faces when I swished around in my spangling finery. "But I'll need to make something to wear."

"Any idea what?"

"Don't know, but whatever it is, I'll need new sequins."

"Okay, Son. We'll have a look on the market on Saturday."

Tim shook his head and took his empty plate into the kitchen. "You're not bleddy right, the pair of you. You're not."

Saturday soon came and as usual, I accompanied Dad to the Victoria Market. This brightly lit facility was too sterile and characterless for me, and like countless inhabitants of our city, I mourned the bustling, atmospheric Central Market it replaced when it finally closed at the end of June. The loss of those charismatic Saturday morning shopping expeditions with Mam cut me deeply. I loved our joyful visits to my friend the ice cream lady, and then we'd push through the heavy swing doors into the coolness of the fish market. The fishmongers wore knee-length white coats and black wellies, and they sloshed the ground with water spouting from thick hoses as if they were wrestling monstrous relations of the slippery eels that lay shiny in death on the dazzling white marble slabs.

Unlike the old market, where skylights allowed natural illumination, strips of glaring neon harshly lit the aisles. Dad and I stood at the fruit and veg stall that he favoured because of a longstanding friendship that he and Mam had with the owners. It seemed that they had known everyone, whether in the city or out in the countryside villages we visited at weekends.

A wall of assorted fruit was displayed on individual twisted tissue paper saucers of clashing carnival colours. Grapefruit rested upon feathery flamingo pink; acid green apples nestled in petals of daffodil yellow; and oranges lay against clouds of sky blue. I adored the psychedelic wall of produce, but my impatience blossomed with the intensity of the gaily coloured gladioli displayed on the florist's opposite. I needed to get to the fabric stalls.

But Dad wasn't quite done. "Oh, and we'll have the radishes too, please, Jack."

Chucking Putty at the Queen

The stallholder's fingers were thick and rough like the carrots that the radishes rested upon. He blew the pinky vegetables in an attempt to dislodge the dusting of earth.

"These are the last ones, Mr Smalley. They're not from the wholesalers, you know? I lifted them last night from up me allotment. That's why there's still all soil on 'em."

An unusual figure rounded the corner of the stall and stood next to us. She was the real-life equivalent of the plump householder Mammy Two Shoes in the *Tom & Jerry* cartoons I so enjoyed watching. But unlike that character whose face was never shown, this woman, who wore an ex-army greatcoat, scowled and muttered from beneath a brown trilby hat. In the crook of one arm hung a substantial straw basket and to my astonishment, her feet were encased in a pair of steel toe-capped boots.

Jack was as cheery as ever. "Good morning, Eunice."

"Hush yuh mout'."

He winked at us. "Is that all, Mr Smalley?"

"Yes, Jack, thank you."

"I'll just reckon it up for you then."

As Dad tugged his wallet from the back pocket of his trousers, Eunice, took our bunch of radishes, and placed them in front of her. Dad casually lifted them and returned them beside our brown paper bags. Eunice grabbed them and slapped them in front of her. As cool as the glossy green cucumbers a few inches from my face, Dad once more retrieved the radishes and returned them beside our shopping. Eunice snatched them and slammed them in front of her.

She tilted her trilby hat right to the back of her head and glared at Dad. "Me dare yuh."

As if engaged in a game of chess, Dad picked the radishes up and once again put them with our stuff.

Again, Eunice grabbed them and slammed them onto the display. "Dem mah radish!"

Dad reached over, picked up the small bunch, and slipped them into the outside pocket of his jacket. "No, dem bladdy not. Dem *mah* bladdy radish!" He smiled at the stallholder. "How much do I owe you, Jack?"

But before Jack could answer, Eunice yelled, "Bastard bald head honky!" and after sticking two fingers up at Dad, she turned and stamped off until she was several feet away, then swivelled, and stood scowling at us.

Jack tapped the side of his head. "She's bleddy barmy. I can't be doing with her. She's always on with summat. The fruit's not ripe enough. The fruit's too ripe. She can buy it cheaper somewhere else. And she's always saying that I've shortchanged her."

Eunice's unrelenting scowl scared me, and I remembered Auntie Lu telling Mam about someone she'd had a run-in with. "Betty, if looks could kill, I'd have been dead on the spot." But Dad remained unfazed by the obvious dislike radiating from the strange shopper. He grinned, thrust his hand into his jacket pocket, and withdrew the radishes.

With a wicked glint in his eyes, he dangled them high in the air. "Would you like a radish, Son?"

Back home, with a sachet of sapphire sequins and a length of light blue tulle from our visit to the haberdashery stall, I had the rest of the weekend to create a new outfit to guarantee a memorable entrance in front of my new fans. Completing my task would be a doddle because I already knew just what to make: a cape of jaw-dropping glamour.

My *Electric Warrior* LP spun on the record player, providing musical inspiration as I transformed the delicate fabric with Mam's pinking shears. I snipped and cut until the straight edges became pleasingly ragged batwing shapes, and with it spread across the carpet, I carefully embellished it with sequinned letters spelling T. REX.

With only two days to get through, I organised my plan for Tuesday evening. I'd walk the long way to the church, a route which would take me around three sides of a long rectangle. I'd halt at strategic points and extend my arms to shoulder level, thus opening my astonishing cape to reveal the twinkling tribute to my musical obsession. In my mind's eye, I saw the awestruck pedestrians, bus passengers, and car drivers staring in disbelief. But why I was restricting my opportunities to show off my cape? I toyed with the idea of walking all the way with my arms constantly aloft. It would be well worth the effort just to hear the screech of car brakes and the thud of jaws dropping. However, after a muscle-fatiguing rehearsal that lasted less than a minute, I concluded that only Superman could keep his arms up for that length of time. Also, the building had several steps at its entrance, making it too challenging to climb them in my high heels and enter the church with my arms splayed wide as if I were the second coming.

Chucking Putty at the Queen

 By the time I was ready to go, the first intimation of salmon pink blushed the hyacinth sky as if the wispy clouds were made from rose petals. I carefully tucked my purple bell bottoms into the tops of the treasured high-heeled boots that Penny gave me, making sure that they ballooned Cossack-style over the leather tops, then I wrapped one of Mam's scarves around each wrist. Above the teardrops of glitter on my cheeks, the delicate dust of a crushed raspberry pastel crayon bloomed on my eyelids. To make sure that my wig-hat was just so, I'd re-threaded the dozens of multicoloured crêpe paper strands, fussing and fiddling until they resembled an exploded firework rocket. And, tied in a floppy bow, a wide blue ribbon secured my new sequinned creation around my neck. Time was marching on, and by quickly utilizing a pair of tiny silver safety pins, I fastened the batwing tips to the scarves that wrapped my wrists. I strode from the house, certain that the congregation at the church youth club would never have seen anyone so fabulous as me.
 Adhering to my itinerary, I took the unnecessarily long route to the church. At my pre-determined posing spots, I raised my arms and slowly rotated to display my glittering creation, expecting to hear cars crashing into one another as their drivers were distracted by my spectacular outfit. But there were no vehicular mishaps. At last, I reached the bullseye where I'd aimed my flamboyant arrow. The church wasn't of traditional Gothic design but in Art Deco style, with a trio of shops nestled beneath. On the tarmac-truncated remnant of a steep side street, a strawberry-blond boy rode an orange Raleigh Chopper pushbike in tight circles over the uneven cobbles. As I neared the steps I was surprised to hear Judge Dread's saucy ska single, "Big Six" sounding from a church of all places. Even though the BBC had banned the record, its suggestive lyrics were familiar to me as it frequently blasted from the open windows of a house near ours, but only when the parents of the older girl who lived there were out.
 This was it. Time for my superstar entrance. As if to fanfare my arrival, the thrilling double drum tribal thud of Gary Glitter's "Rock & Roll Part Two" replaced Judge Dread. During the past week, I'd transformed this church into Wembley Stadium, where earlier in the year, T. Rex had played two sold-out concerts in one day. The rapturous front-page report on the *NME* announced that Marc Bolan was the "unquestioned lord of them all," and with this in mind, I sashayed through the open doors with befitting

haughtiness as if I were approaching my own twenty thousand adoring fans.

The cacophonous energy died as if a plug had been pulled. The crowd parted like the fabled Red Sea, revealing a couple playing table tennis. They stared at me, bats mid-air as the white plastic ball rolled from the green surface and bounced on the scuffed wooden floor with an increasingly urgent staccato rhythm.

"Whatcha want?"

I stepped backwards and my high heel connected with something soft.

"Oi, do you mind? That's my foot you're treading on."

A shove thrust me towards a teenage girl wearing an enormous, crocheted cap in stripes of red, yellow, and green.

"Hey, Delroy," she screeched across the hall. "Come and look at the state of this."

A brutish youth lumbered over, his torso girdled by an over-tight, white T-shirt blemished with dark sweat stains beneath the arms. With his immense Afro, he reminded me of the lead character in the cartoon series, *Help! It's the Hair Bear Bunch*. He pulled the matchstick he was chewing from his mouth, looked me up and down with slow determination, then kissed his teeth.

"Who the fuck do you think you are, man? Adrian Street?"

This reference to the flashy wrestler whose camp mannerisms was a wonderful testimony to my couture and overrode any caution I may have had. I offered him my hand. "Pleased to meet you. I'm Simon Bolan."

The back of my head hit the floorboards. Stars shone with furious brilliance over his broad shoulders, where the evening sun illuminated a wall hanging that bore a biblical quotation exquisitely embroidered in gold and purple letters: "Although I walk through the valley of the shadow of death, I will fear no evil." I believed the Bible to be a ridiculous fairytale, its contents unbelievably embellished over the centuries. Yet, right here in the real world of 1972, the evil that I should not fear stood astride me with coal-black hatred in his eyes.

The club members gathered in a circle, laughing, whooping, and clapping. From the unseen record player, Dandy Livingstone's jaunty reggae hit single advised, "Suzanne, Beware of the Devil." He could have been just as easily warning me. When I hauled myself into a sitting

Chucking Putty at the Queen

position, a tall, toothy girl wearing a green tank top decorated with a large yellow smiley face pushed her way to the front and grabbed the arm of the big youth.

"Go on, Delroy. Slice him up."

"No way, man. I'm in enough agro with the fuzz as it is."

I didn't see the flick knife until he snapped it closed.

"You better fuck off, man, if you know what's good for you."

A cropped-haired youth in a Ben Sherman shirt pulled me to my feet and manhandled me towards the doorway, where a grubby poster reassured that Jesus Saves. Beneath it was the scrawled addendum, "But George Best scores on the penalty."

A push dispatched me down the steps and as my palms scraped across the gritty slabs, a wire rubbish basket flew past my head and rolled towards the main road. My high heels may as well have been roller skates for all the support they provided. The steps were now crowded with jeering, jostling youths who unleashed a barrage of gob.

"Go on, you freak. Fuck off and don't come back. We don't let queers in here."

I fled, trying to skip the stones that skidded past my ankles. Strips of crêpe paper stuck to my sweaty face as I stumbled uphill, pawing at the pebbledash walls for support until I reached home. In the shadowed porch, I shook so much that I couldn't depress the handle.

The door opened. "You're back early, Son...and your eyeshadow's running."

I touched my hot face with my grazed fingertips. When I looked down, they were red and wet. Dad tugged me into the brightness of the living room.

"What the bladdy hell happened? Who did this to you?"

He lifted my face as I sobbed the events.

"Tim and his bright ideas. You're not to go again."

"Don't worry, Dad, I won't." I brushed away the glitter that had transferred from my cheeks to his shirt. "Not even if Marc Bolan was there."

Dad separated the sticky crêpe fronds and kissed my forehead. "I'll tell you what, Son, why don't you take your wig-hat off and wash your face in cold water? I'll make us a radish sandwich. There's a few left over from Saturday."

97

We grinned at each other. "Dem mah radish!"

I didn't need an adventure playground or a stupid youth club. I was perfectly happy at home with Dad and my records, sequins, and glitter. The rest of the world could all go and get lost.

12

LATE AFTERNOON LAMARTINE STREET

IF THE WIND COULD own a voice as it gusted across the bleak bombsite terrain, then this early May tempest carried the boisterous shouts and yells that once resounded through these streets. The previously animated neighbourhood crammed with houses, corner shops, pubs, and factories had been obliterated into an impotent landscape of rubble. The wretched atmosphere of futility evoked the black and white photographs of Hiroshima and Nagasaki in Dad's *Book of Knowledge*. Their achromatic brutality stood in high contrast with the delicate wildflowers that we'd collected during our countryside excursions. Upon our return home, Dad helped me to carefully position the dainty blooms within sheets of tissue, then record the date and location onto a slip of paper. The floral treasure was pressed between the pages of the heavy volume and returned to the shelf. Time dragged endlessly until Dad announced that they were ready to be viewed, usually in the midst of winter when the moistureless colours still glowed like jewels amongst the lines of black text.

However, unlike the annihilated cities in that book, the destruction of St. Ann's was not created by the megawatt explosion of atomic bombs but by the council's order to eradicate a vibrant part of Nottingham that they'd deemed a slum.

Still kidding myself that I was taking a shortcut home from school, I passed the top of our old street, fighting the urge to look down to where our house had been. Instead, I put my head down and prepared to trudge a cheerless zig-zag route to our brand-new, modern home half a mile away.

On blowy days when I was younger, the blustery force channelled around the narrow streets, buffeting from the two-up, two-down houses with incredible energy. My exhilaration then was overwhelming. I danced madly in the back yard with the unseen sprites that skipped through my short hair as Mam clapped a flamenco rhythm from the kitchen doorway. Similarly, when Dad drove us the mile or so to Colwick Woods or on journeys into the countryside, I adored the sensation of breezy freedom, applauding the wind that twitched at the fresh spring leaves as if it had taken on a physical form and was determined to pluck them from the slender branches. And back in the city, when summer smeared into autumn, when leaves were whisked and whirled around the green metal stanchions of the swings on the park, I chased the brittle fallen foliage, throwing it into the air and shrieking with delicious joy when they gusted back in my face. Once, when Cyril the park keeper had amassed a substantial glowing mound of brown, yellow, and gold, I had dived into its crisp, crackly depths, ignoring his shouted warning: "You'll get all earwigs down your tabholes!" When I surfaced from this dry autumn ocean, he was leaning on his broom, laughing, telling Mam that I was a right little bogger.

The wind was my friend and playmate then. But now, with Mam dead and only a few buildings remaining to guide the flow, it was a miserable, untouchable enemy that thrust unhindered over the newly created wasteland.

I stopped and pulled up the hood of my parka, thus limiting my view as blinkers would restrict that of a dray horse, and I surveyed my surroundings. In the near distance, dark hills of jumbled bricks rose as if giant hands had effortlessly and indiscriminately toppled the sturdy Victorian walls. Closer, several empty dwellings defined the edges of the demolished streets with the bleak finality of gravestones. They marked the burial site of a unique community once resilient but rendered helpless against the plans of the city council and their onslaught of modernisation.

Denuded of bark, a tree trunk stood defiantly amidst the ruins of a back yard with a loop of knotted rope hanging from its single protruding branch. The stretched, rubbery black bicycle tyre attached to the rope evidenced its prolonged use as a swing and drooped from the bare tree trunk like a hangman's noose. I remembered my own swing, a luxurious creation that Dad made for me. He never did anything by halves and had bought lengths of hefty timber to construct an unmoveable frame he painted with white gloss, and it dazzled on even the dullest day. He purchased shiny heavyweight hooks and yacht-quality rope which he threaded through his precisely drilled holes in a block of mahogany that he stained to a rich hue. As the pièce de resistance, he'd upholstered it with a padded burgundy leather seat attached by gleaming bronze studs, and a frill of golden tassels dangled beneath it.

But now, our back yard lay smothered beneath a spoil heap. The physical proof of our family home had been so easily destroyed, along with everything that symbolised the happy, emotional security of my younger years. Of course, I had no idea what might rise from the destruction: houses, shops, maybe factories. But whatever form this urban regeneration took, it would never replace my wonderful life in our small house on Lamartine Street when Mam was alive. New buildings would eventually stand there, but I would forever be unable to ignore or refuse the magnetic attraction to where our mam had given birth to me.

But I still shouldn't have come this way. My weighty burden of sadness increased each time I approached the fragments of our shattered community and again, I'd fallen into a trap of my own making. Chrome lagoons of rainwater that had formed in the uneven toffee-coloured mud reflected the grey scudding clouds, and jagged pyramids of smashed floorboards rose skywards, interspersed with funeral pyres of splintered rafters and broken banisters, their charcoal smoke skewed and stretched by the changeable breeze. From within rust-edged oil drums, broken fingers of lathing ripped from walls now pointed to the tempestuous pig-iron sky, and I jumped when one length snapped, violently launching bright orange sparks into the miserable panorama.

A veil of melancholy draped me as the wind whistled mournfully around exposed living rooms, bedrooms, and kitchens. The first intimation of rain drummed an irregular beat on an intact window frame that lay like an enormous washboard, its wood-cased aperture covered with sheets of grey corrugated iron. The houses on this street had been taller than those on ours, and exposed chimney breasts as wide as ancient oak trees rose uninterrupted for three floors. Yawning fireplaces and ragged flags of wallpaper denoted each storey of the previously private rooms, now rudely open to public view should anyone travel through this lifeless setting where, hunched like napping cats, dormant bulldozers awaited the return of the workmen the next day.

I could no longer delude myself of my motive for choosing this route home. I succumbed to my craving as an alcoholic would reach for the bottle, and I turned back, desperate for my emotional fix. The wind pushed me towards the inevitable outcome. Once more, I stood at the top of what was our old street. A wooden toilet seat lay against the ridge of graphite-coloured kerb stones with the loneliness of a discarded lifebuoy on the deck of an abandoned ship. Closing my eyes, I relinquished the grip on my mental safety rails and submerged myself in the memory of one morning when I was off school, suffering with tonsillitis…

Mam was kneading dough on the floured bread board, and she paused when a vicious squall of rain lashed the small kitchen window with the ferocity of a raging sea storm against a porthole. A wispy cloud of flour puffed into the air when she clapped her hands before opening the back door. She looked at the deluge gushing from the broken guttering on the house next door and shook her head, then squeezed the bunch of seaweed dangling as a dark green epiglottis in the gaping mouth of the door frame. "Hmm. The Mablethorpe Forecaster tells me that this rain's set in for the day."

My heart quickstepped with excitement as I marvelled that Mam could tell the weather in this fashion.

She closed the back door against the downpour and returned to her bread-making. "I'm glad that your dad wore his galoshes this morning, otherwise his shoes would've been drenched by the time he got to work."

On this desolate day, I relished the temporary housebound cosiness of it being just Mam and me. The Dequadin lozenge I sucked on soothed my abrasive throat, its synthetic citrus flavour just like the exotic tangerine ice creams I'd loved on that summer holiday when I'd collected the seaweed Mam had just squeezed. I'd never been in a bungalow before, and after checking that there were no stairs hidden behind closed doors, I happily set off with Mam and Dad, my tiny hands locked tightly in theirs. I skipped and pranced between them as we headed to the beach on the first day, frustrated with their resistance to my tugging encouragement to hurry up.

 My motivation was their promised purchase of a new spade for me from the novelties emporium near the Louth Hotel on High Street. The cluttered capacity of the shop had been extended by a greenhouse-like canopy jutting out onto the pavement, an enthralling magnet for my impressionable mind. Within the elevated heat beneath the water-clear glass panes lay a panoply of delightful novelties: wobbly rubber snakes and paper flags of every nation attached to spaghetti-thin strips of wood; small, coloured pails and large plain buckets; striped cotton windbreaks and spotted plastic rain hats; shrimping nets and reels of orange crab lines armed with spiteful hooks. It would take a full day to explore the range of seaside miscellany in the shadowy depths of the shop but fortunately for me, the most enticing objects were displayed closer to the entrance. Spades sprouted from a battered bin, their shafts and handles bleached to the soft beige of the desert drifts on the pullover: that wide expanse of concrete where the infringement of wind-whipped sand tantalisingly advertised our proximity to the beach.

I was the proud owner of a new spade. I loved its discordant clanging as I dragged it behind me, the pointed red metal tip scraping along the promenade.

"Why don't you let your dad carry it, Son, or else the lovely paint will be chipped off before you've even begun digging."

I handed it over and happily swung my yellow bucket decorated with blue and green seahorses as Dad strode ahead to secure our traditional place on the stretch of broad steps leading to the sands. I remembered the family outrage two years earlier when someone else had set up camp in the place which, by unwritten rights, was ours. How dare they sit where we always sat? Perhaps Dad shared this memory, and it was that which powered the acceleration of his strong, assertive gait. His figure diminished as he lugged the holdall that bulged with towels, bathers, a flask of tea, aluminium-wrapped cheese and cress sandwiches, and the essential tub of Nivea cream in case the sun became too fierce.

I held Mam's hand for the rest of the walk until we reached our spot. As if he was a gold rush prospector, Dad had already staked our claim, and over the tubular handrails down to the beach hung the oil-stained tarpaulin he lay on when he worked beneath the car at home. Mam and I were impatient to paddle and set off across the damp sand. The tide was out, making the ocean a sparkling thread beneath several kites that rode the salty breeze like a flock of manufactured exotic birds with cloth plumage and tail feathers of coloured plastic ribbons. Here and there, mottled mussel shell castanets littered the smooth sand, interspersed with conical whorls of lugworm casts and five-star splats of grounded starfish.

All week, I'd loved exploring the shallow pools shining at the base of the sea defences that rose as man-made mangrove roots from the dank circles of saltwater. The rasp of my fingertips over the crusted embroidery of barnacles made me want to prize them from the slimy wood and somehow thread them into a necklace for Mam. It would be difficult to do, but Dad would help me if he thought that it was possible. I scooped up a pailful of tepid ocean, wrinkling my nose against the rank odour of aquatic decay. Earlier in the week it had smelled of the sun-kissed seaside, but now it had degenerated into a miserable reminder that it was the end of the holiday.

"Your gran reckons that's the best way to tell the weather by." Mam nodded at a glutinous, green-grey glove with its juicy bobbled fronds splayed wide. "Grab it for her. And while you're at it, find some for us to take home for above the kitchen door. I'm just going over there to look for some oyster shells to edge her back yard path."

With the seaweed submerged, I lifted the bucket from the sodden sand, leaving a harvest moon impression for brief seconds until it vanished. Shaded by the cooler stretch of darkness from the sea defence, a small silvery-blue crab lay dead, its broken legs pointing in multiple directions. I fumbled to gather it, dispelling minuscule black flies crawling on its underside, then tenderly lowered it into my bucket as if its microscopic heart still beat. It glowed against the seaweed like a pearl brooch on an emerald velvet cushion, surrounded by a cluster of pink shells the size of a new baby's toenails. Gulls screamed above me as I sat back on my haunches, delighted with the way the saltwater meniscus sparkled in a platinum halo framing my seaside scavenger hunt tableau.

I detected the slightest soft pad of footfall behind me, and a shadow extinguished the light as effectively as when Dad drew the blackout curtains of his photographic darkroom in the attic at home. I looked around. Mam was illuminated from behind and surrounded by an aura of golden light. I squinted and raised my hand to my forehead to shield my eyes. Her arms were tanned a light chestnut brown that contrasted with the yellow and white vertical stripes of her sleeveless frock. I could hardly discern her face as the wind plucked out strands of her tucked-up hair, whipping them into the snakes writhing around Medusa's head. But my beautiful mam was no gorgon. Her comforting voice rose above the mellow chimes of bells that gently swung from the necks of the donkeys as children rode upon their backs.

"Oh, that's pretty, Son."

I carefully adjusted the seaweed with my right forefinger. "I made it for Gran as a present. It's a living picture, but the crab is unfortunately dead."

Mam leaned over me and laid her hands on my bare shoulders that were misted with a gossamer sheen of spray blown from the ocean. "Oh, it's 'unfortunately dead', is it? Well, maybe you should just take Gran the shells for her garden and the seaweed for her to forecast the weather with."

"Do you think she'd like it, Mam?"

"I do, but I don't think she'd be too pleased with the dead crab."

I extracted a nearby half of a mussel shell from the sand and dug a shallow trough. I laid the crab in it and covered it, then pressed the shell into the sand to create a gravestone. "There, Mam. Now it can rest in peace."

The next morning as we packed in preparation for the drive home, Mam grabbed me as I ceremoniously paraded around the yard with my bucket as if it contained priceless bounty from a sunken Spanish galleon.

"You've not got that dead crab in there, have you?"

"No."

She peeped into the water. "Yes, you have then, you little sod! I thought you'd buried it yesterday."

"That was *that* crab, Mam. This is a different one. I found it up near the steps. So, I'm not really fibbing, am I?"

With the precision of a heron's dipping beak, she plucked out the crab, sniffed it, and grimaced. "Oh, Simon! This crab or that crab, or whichever crab it is, it pongs."

A deft flick of her wrist dispatched the crab over the constellation of yellow florets bursting from the black clouds of gorse that separated the bungalow from the disused railway tracks. With only the seaweed and shells remaining, I still insisted on transporting my aquatic bounty to Gran in genuine Mablethorpe sea water to keep it fresh. We were safely in the car when Nick elbowed me and snickered as Dad shut the doors.

"You're barmy. The sea is the same all over the world. It's not different bits of sea. It doesn't belong here or anywhere. It's just sea. Don't you know anything?"

The painted metal of the bucket was deliciously cool when I clamped it between the warmth of my bare, suntanned thighs. "It isn't then. It's real Mablethorpe sea, and Gran will know that. She'll be able to smell it."

"Huh. All she'll smell is rotten crab."

During the journey home, whenever the car tyres hit a pothole or juddered over a minor obstruction, the seawater slopped over the metal rim and trickled down my legs, making me squirm, though it wasn't a completely unpleasant sensation.

Weeks later, on that soggy afternoon when I was at home with my throat on fire, the glorious summer holiday was relegated to a different world, only recalled in the photographs that Dad had taken. Mam's seaweed forecast about the rain being set in was correct, and at my bedtime, I lay in the dark, wishing we were back at the coast in the sunshine. The soft indent in the feather pillow cradled my head as perfectly as an egg fitted an eggcup, and the gentle murmur of my parents' conversation downstairs mingled with the deluge gurgling through the iron fingers of the grate in the street.

And now here I was again, standing in front of that same grate that rainwater once splashed down and sometimes overflowed from, but which was now choked dry with dust and debris as I daydreamed of a golden, happy-go-lucky past. I'd covered the distance from the top of the street on autopilot, not needing to count my footsteps to know that I'd arrived at where number thirty once stood.

I scuffed the toe of my boot in the ochre brick dust that filled the gaps between the blue-grey cobbles, and I closed my eyes against the harsh reality, needing to go back, to recreate our street again. I gritted my teeth and clamped my lips together, and the chilled air enlivened my nostrils when I filled my lungs with a long, deep breath. Surrounded by a spattering of starbursts, houses shimmered against the cinema screen of my eyelids, quickly focusing my memories as they replayed, a jumble of lost voices chased around my head until they found the present day. Plunging deeper into my fantasy, it was easy to picture former neighbours, and when I cautiously moved my head from side to side, the images strengthened. Even the gloomy factory dominating the street opposite our house appeared, its blueberry shadow darkening the cobbles. Dad's amazing Alvis Firefly was there, the only vehicle on our street, and a black sit-up-and-beg bicycle rested against the wall of the corner shop.

A figure smeared the periphery of my fool's paradise, but I couldn't make out if it were male or female, no matter how much further I swivelled my head and scrunched my face in concentration. I was back in our thriving neighbourhood, a place filled with reliability and regularity. The memories became real, and I swayed as if in the ebb and flow of the crowd at Goose Fair. The bell on the corner shop pinged its single note as I giddily descended further into my phantasmagorical homecoming.

"Ragbo! Ragbo!"

The rag and bone man hollered his portmanteau job description above the clip-clop of his nag's shoes as the iron rimmed cartwheels trundled over uneven cobbles. Our white front door blossomed as a lily opening in time lapse, and behind it, Mam would be in the kitchen buttering bread for my tea of strawberry jam sandwiches. Dad would soon be home from work. He'd lug his black leather bag full of cameras onto the table, and Mam would light-heartedly chide him as she always did, "Oh, Sid, not on there, please."

My stomach rumbled as I reached for the red plastic doorknob, eager for my tea. A dog barked and like broken window blinds, my shuttered eyelids flew open onto the desolate scene. There was no white front door, no red plastic doorknob, no house, and no Mam making bread and jam sandwiches for my tea.

They were gone forever.

13

GOODBYE, YELLOW BRICK ROAD

Barbed-wire tears pricked my eyelids as I angrily cursed myself for again willingly breaking my resolve not to continue indulging in this sentimental diversion. Coming this way had been a stupid, and avoidable, mistake. Minutes earlier, when I passed through the school gates onto Bath Street, I should have walked the longer way along the more populated St. Ann's Well Road to our new house. Instead, I succumbed to the toxic lure of this threatening, alien area where I no longer belonged.

Random dollops of rain pattered, pockmarking the dusty paving slabs where ghostly grey doorsteps remained, covered with demolition dust. I scrunched my shoulders up to my ears. I must hurry back to the new house and wait for Dad's arrival from work so that I could show him the prize inside my parka.

I'd endured a week of gnawing impatience ever since I'd seen the notice outside the paper shop on the Robin Hood Chase precinct. The next edition of the girls' magazine *Jackie* would contain a "Super-Size Marc Bolan Pin-Up." Not just a pin-up, but a *super-size* one. The fifth of May couldn't come fast enough, and as the week dragged, its importance magnified and became my main topic of conversation, much to the irritation of my brothers.

"Will you give it a rest and stop going on about that pissing Marc Bolan poster."

"But I can't wait!" I pouted and tossed my head, making the crêpe paper corkscrew curls of my homemade wig-hat rustle. "And it's not a poster. It's a super-size Marc Bolan pin-up."

"Dad shouldn't be buying you girls' comics. People already think you're a puff. I mean, what other boy round here has *Petticoat*, *Jackie*, *Mirabelle*, and all that crap?" His recitation of the magazine names were bullets fired into my head. "What's up with yer? At the old house, me and Steve used to have *Hotspur* and *Eagle*. What did you have? Bleddy *Bunty*. I blame our mam for being so soft on you, letting you cut out that girl on the back page to dress up. No wonder everyone round here says you want looking at."

The long-awaited morning arrived, and I set off for school. But first, I had to exchange the shiny five pence piece burning a hole in the patchwork pocket of my purple bell-bottom trousers for the long-anticipated issue of *Jackie*. Although I couldn't run in the high heel boots that our Penny had given me, I succeeded in adapting my gait to a fast mince worthy of the speed-walkers that were occasionally shown on *World of Sport*. The doorway of the paper shop was my finishing line, and I staggered over it, scanning the shelves. Despite the previous week's advance notice, there was no trace of the magazine. My loud volley of exaggerated huffing drew the attention of the lady behind the counter.

"You sound all put out."

"I'm looking for the new *Jackie*, the one with the super-size Marc Bolan pin-up in the middle."

She wandered towards the back, indiscreetly calling out to an unseen colleague. "Sheila, it's that barmy lad in them women's boots again. No, stay there, he ant got the wig on. He wants the new Jackie. What… *already?*"

As she returned to the counter, the shrug of her shoulders combined with the verbal exchange told me it was bad news.

"I'm sorry, ducky. We did have it, but we're all sold out."

Every calamity on the BBC news couldn't compare with this announcement. "But you can't have. It's only half past eight. You can't have sold out."

"Well, we have."

"But you *can't* have."

"I just said we have, and we have, so be told, will you?"

"Could you please tell me if you'll get some more in later? It's especially important."

"I doubt it. When owt's gone, it's gone. We won't reorder unless it's summat special."

"It *is* something special."

"Well, it int really, is it? I mean, it's not like it's a royal wedding or a royal death, or war's been announced or owt like that, is it?" She began to unscrew the lid of a large glass jar full of brightly coloured sweets. "Now let me gerron with these midget gems."

I snorted and flounced towards the door with tears blurring my progress. This was dreadful. How could they have sold out? I'd throw myself under a bus. I'd just crossed the threshold with the busy main road in my sights when she called out.

"Oi, thingy! Hang on. I've got one." Her triumphant cry would have been worthy of her discovering the cure for blindness. "Sheila found it stuck in between *Reveille* and *Women's Realm*."

I paused outside the shop and luxuriated in a peep at the pin-up. Clad in a pink sparkly tailcoat, my pop hero sat astride a shiny silver toy tank surrounded by swirling smoke. This was perfect because Dad had bought me the latest T. Rex LP *Tanx* a few weeks earlier for my eleventh birthday present. The council house clock boomed a warning that it was a quarter to nine. I'd better hurry to school, but I couldn't arrive visibly bearing my treasure as much as I wanted to show it off. There'd been a plague of thefts from the cloakroom, and it would soon be nicked if anyone knew about it.

I removed my parka, and with the covert motions of a spy, I rolled the magazine into a loose tube and carefully slid it inside the right-hand sleeve until it buffeted against the elasticated wristband. Then, even more carefully, I slipped my arm into the hidden gauntlet and pulled on my parka. No one would ever guess.

Four o'clock arrived, and I set off for home. This time I wouldn't give in to the psychological command to revisit our old street. I'd go straight home and play *Tanx* for what must be the millionth time and contemplate where to put my fab new pin-up.

But at the school gates, as I tried not to jealously look at the knot of smiling mothers meeting their children, the grains of my promise not to return to Lamartine Street dissolved, and I set off across the park, reassuring myself that after just one more visit, I'd never ever do it again.

Standing amongst the drizzle and decay outside the phantom number thirty, I shook myself like a drenched dog, wishing that I could as easily discard the hypnotic reveries that only served to sadden me. Turning away and rejecting my scrutiny of the ruination, I forced myself to continue to our smart, bright new house. With my pictorial Bolan bounty safely wrapping my arm, I passed three vertical lines of a wicket daubed in white paint on a wall. Seagulls riding the breezes screamed in echoes of the excitable games once played when this served as a backstreet Trent

Bridge cricket ground. Mindful of Gran's opinion that severe weather was on the way when the gulls travelled inland from the coast, I shrugged my shoulders as if doing so would make my parka fit more snugly.

A clattering tin can rolled into my periscope vision at the end of the street. It was followed by two boys engrossed in tackling each other for control of the substitute football. They looked up and saw me. In a unified personality change from footballers to gunslingers, they swaggered towards me as if heading for a showdown on the parched main street of a Wild West township.

Obeying my primitive sense of danger, I crossed over to the other side of the street. The boys crossed over as well. The unyielding cobbles seemed to have been turned to jelly as I hastened back to the opposite pavement. The boys copied me once more, closing the gap between us. A lifetime ago, I'd hurried along this same street huddled with Mam beneath her brolly as we went to the Cavendish cinema to watch *The Wizard of Oz*. Shivering, I recalled the signposts in the dark, foreboding forest that warned Dorothy and her friends: *I'd go back if I were you.*

I glanced behind me along the street that stretched to a lonely vanishing point; it was too late to flee. Fear snapped at my ankles with the insistence of a yapping dog. I should try to run back towards school, but even if I fled in my women's boots, these boys would easily catch me. I moved my right arm closer to my torso, protecting my magazine, hoping that they hadn't noticed as they stood squarely before me. I guessed that we were about the same age, but that was where any similarity ended. One was heavier set, with a pudding basin cut of thick, oily hair that made him resemble the aptly named thug Bully Beef from the *Dandy* comic. The other was skinny and sallow-faced, with wispy straw-coloured hair falling over his forehead and ears in the style of the television wrestler, Catweazle. They both wore sturdy juvenile versions of my brother Tim's steel-toe capped boots.

Bully Beef glared with black button eyes and spat on the ground. His mouth moved but his words were muffled by my hood, so I slid it back. "I beg your pardon?"

"Do you go to Blue Bell Hill School?" His guttural tone was too deeply masculine for his age, and darkness shadowed his spotty top lip.

Dad would have brandish him a "lout." I shook my head. "No."

"Where d'ya go to then?"

Chucking Putty at the Queen

"Victoria Primary School on Bath Street."

Catweazle sniggered. "Are you one of the Bash Street Kids?"

It was the local nickname for my school, a tribute to the characters in *The Beano*. There was even an unofficial school anthem sung in the playground with a spirit that matched the rousing renditions of "Onward, Christian Soldiers" that the Salvation Army band sang on their Sunday morning street parades:

> *"We are the Bash Street Kids*
> *We fight with dustbin lids.*
> *We knock 'em out*
> *With Brussel sprouts*
> *We are the Bash Street Kids."*

The toughest lads at school ended this rallying call to arms by exploding into a brawl with no reason other than that they enjoyed scrapping. Their riotous playground free-for-alls terrified me, but at this moment on the forsaken street, I wished that I were as equally rough and ready, to be as hard as I instinctively knew that this confrontational duo were. But I wasn't tough. I didn't fight, or play football, or run around brandishing an imaginary Tommy gun, spraying schoolboy soldiers with make-believe bullets in a playground war where nobody really died. My reluctance to engage in such behaviour branded me a sissy. I was called "yellow belly" and "yitney," local slang for coward, when I ran to hide within a crowd of girls as soon as rowdy activities commenced.

Catweazle giggled and pointed at my feet. "What's them?"

That morning, buoyant on my wave of excitement of getting a new Marc Bolan pin-up, I'd swapped my usual olive-green fell boots for my two-inch high heeled boots. They were my favourite footwear, with silver zippers on the sides that ran in shiny train tracks through the black leather from ankle to knee. But even before lessons began, I'd had to surrender them to my incensed teacher and endured the rest of the day in smelly plimsolls from the emergency cupboard.

Catweazle leaned down and lifted a leg of my purple bell-bottoms. "He's got women's boots on!" He giggled again. "What you got them on for? You can't play football in *them*."

I wanted to show these oiks that I wasn't like them, that I stood separate from the masses whose lives were ruled by fervently supporting either of the two local teams as if nothing else in life mattered. "I don't intend to play football in them because I don't like football."

"Oo-er. Course you do. All boys like football."

"I'm not all boys." Even in this threatening situation, I couldn't restrain my prissiness.

"Who do you support: Forest or County?"

"Neither. I told you, I don't like football."

"Well, what *do* you like, then?"

"Skipping. I like skipping."

The seagulls mournfully shrieked as he stared at me.

"You don't like football, and you like skipping?"

The wind clanged a battered, rusty-edged metal advertisement that was half-secured to the wall. The trademark ragamuffin Bisto gravy kids depicted in chipped enamel paints perversely parodied the two boys in front of me. I hoped that they wouldn't notice my incremental shuffling away from them. "Yes. I much prefer skipping."

"You talk posh. You're not from round here, are ya?"

"Not anymore, although I was born here."

Catweazle's accusation reinforced the austere truth of the lonely landscape, and I sighed, waving my hand like a chiffon scarf lifted by the breeze. "I'm afraid that nobody lives here now."

Catweazle rested a hand on one hip and blew me a kiss. "You don't talk like you come from round here. You talk posh."

"There's nothing wrong with speaking correctly." This was one of Dad's favourite sayings.

"Ooh, la-de-da!" Catweazle doubled up, giggling, but Bully Beef just stared at me.

"Where do you live then? Buckingham Palace?"

Being uprooted from our old house was as devastating as the destruction that currently surrounded me but nevertheless, the jewelled novelty of our new house and its modern amenities had lost none of its lustre for me. The urgency to brag overrode the tingling itch creeping forwards from the back of my mind that something was very wrong. But I couldn't help myself. I just had to show off. "Oh, our house is over in the *new* St. Ann's. We've got an indoor bathroom with a toilet and *another* toilet downstairs as well." Their gawping spurred me on. "Actually, it's not

Chucking Putty at the Queen

just a toilet. It also has a corner hand basin, so I suppose you could say that it's more of a cloakroom." There were no expressions of admiration or even jealousy, so I upped my bragging. "*And* we've got a front garden, *and* a back garden with a shed in it. We're going to have a lawn and a pond with fish in it too." I failed to notice that my ostentation was tightening the noose around my neck. "And a greenhouse that we're going to grow tomatoes in."

Catweazle scratched his shaggy mane. "So how far is this house then?"

"Oh, *way* away. Right up off Sycamore Road. It's a considerable uphill walk but not too arduous, even in these heels."

Bully Beef snorted. "D'ya think you're summat special?"

I pulled away from the burst of stale breath. "No, I'm nothing special."

He twitched his shoulders and turned up the collar of his jacket and nudged Catweazle. "Say, pardner, I think this is the feller we want. Whaddya think?"

Catweazle nodded slowly. "Yup, I guess yer darned right."

Bully Beef stepped forwards. "You beat my little brother up."

"Pardon?"

"I said, you beat my little brother up."

"Me? No, I didn't."

"Yeah, you did. You beat him up last week. Right here after school. So, we come looking for yer." Bully Beef glared hatefully, the rain on his thick basin haircut making it as slick and shiny as a tar-covered motorbike helmet.

The council house clock boomed the half hour. If only I could wind its hands back by thirty minutes and be at the school gates. I would never have taken this stupid diversion just to look at where the old house was. "No, I didn't. It wasn't me, honest."

He turned to Catweazle. "He's the one, int he?"

"Yeah, it's him, all right."

"Honestly, it wasn't me. I don't know who your little brother is. I don't know who *you* are. I wasn't even here last week." Desperate to secure my safety, my thoughts raced as I hoped to placate them. "Tell you what, give me a description of who did it and if I see him, I'll come and tell you."

"Oh, okay then." Bully Beef raised his right hand. "He's about this big..."

I truly didn't see it coming. With my back against the broken pavement,

I stared up at the racing grey clouds as they squatted over me, rifling the outside pockets of my parka.

"Where's your dosh?"

After Mam died, Dad made sure that I had a duo of two pence coins for the public telephone in case I needed to ring him at work. They were alongside the one penny change from the magazine. I didn't believe in God but still made bargains with a non-existent force. Let them take my money, but please don't let them find *Jackie* with the super-sized Marc Bolan pin-up secreted within my sleeve. "Five pence. I've got five pence. I'll get it for you, but please don't hit me again."

My plea for clemency produced the opposite effect. A second and third punch to my face trebled the flashing in my eyes against the backdrop of the leaden sky. My attackers unzipped my parka and rummaged in the square patch pockets on the front of my trousers, easily extracting the coins and a small cellophane wrapped tube of small, lilac-coloured lozenges.

"Five lousy pence and some parma violets? They ain't proper tuffies. They're what girls have." Bully Beef chucked them down and ground them into the wet cobbles with the heel of his boot. "Ain't you got no Rolos, or Anglo bubbly, or owt like that? Why ant you got no proper sweets?"

I blubbed through the warm stickiness on my lips. "I like parma violets."

Bully Beef dropped back to his haunches, rested a hand on my chest, and leaned his broad, flat face near to mine. Ashtray-breath propelled his words. "What hand do you write with?"

"My right one." I was too dazed to understand. "Why?"

"Cos I'm gonna break your arm." When he grasped my right forearm, his eyes widened as the magazine inside my parka sleeve crumpled. "Hang on, hang on, what's this we got here then?"

They hauled me to my feet, wrestled me from my parka and tugged the magazine from its hiding place.

"*Jackie*? That's what girls have."

Another punch returned me to my prone position, and without the protection of my parka, my back was instantly soaked.

"Gerrum off him."

Their attention turned to my footwear, and their fumbling fingers yanked until the zips yielded. Within seconds, my boots were removed, and my assailants hurled them into the wasteland.

Chucking Putty at the Queen

Bully Beef slapped Catweazle on the back. "Time fer us to mosey on outta town, pardner."

His right boot connected with my ribs. Terror cemented me to the ground, and the rain moistened my burning, throbbing face. Only when I heard the distant, unmistakeable clanging of a tin can being kicked did I dare to turn my head. The street was as desolate as when I'd begun my now-regrettable journey. I wiped the back of my hand over my top lip and gasped at the scarlet that smeared my skin with the thickness of oil paint on a palette. My socks were soaked, and my trousers clung to my legs. I needed to retrieve my boots, but how? Broken glass and fragmented rubble littered the street. I was shivering not only from the cold but also from fear that they might return to finish me off.

Hardened mortar jabbed my palms as I struggled to a sitting position. A harsh bitter taste scoured the back of my throat, and my pulse thudded in my nose from the pain of their punches. At least my parka was within easy reach, and although wet on the outside, it was as welcome as a suit of armour. Resting at the edge of the ravaged landscape was a disembodied doll's head, pink plastic skin smeared with dirt, its unblinking glassy eyes the only witness to the terrifying assault.

My magazine lay face down in a shallow puddle, tinted lilac from the packet of pulverised parma violets that had dissolved into it. It was futile trying to peel it open it to the centre pages to look at the poster to check that it was okay, so I carefully rolled it into a soggy tube. Now that it was ruined, there was no point trying to hide it, but I still carefully slid it into the inside pocket of my parka, hoping that when I got home, it would miraculously be in a better condition. But what could I tell Dad? I couldn't throw it away. He'd been as excited as I was about it and would expect to see it. If I pretended that I hadn't bought it, he'd want the money back. All I could do was dry it out before he came home from work and somehow stop the pages from becoming wavy. But I wouldn't be going anywhere until I got my boots.

I found a broken length of wood with a rough V-shape cut into the end indicating its former use as a clothes prop. It now became an impromptu crutch that enabled me to pick my way over the waste ground as if it were a warzone, booby trapped with landmines. There was no one around to hear my anguished yelps when the soles of my feet were stabbed by the indiscriminate rubbish of demolition.

Eventually, I saw my boots. Astonishingly, they had landed upright but some twenty feet apart, giving the illusion of an invisible giant standing before me wearing them. Stumbling with the unsteady gait of a drunk, I wriggled my foot into my left boot and succeeded in zipping it. I hopped across the waste, retrieved my other boot, and once more fully shod, I staggered to the street, then down to the safety of the main road. None of the people that I passed gave me a second look. I was just another scruffy schoolboy to them, even if I was a scruffy schoolboy wearing soggy purple bell-bottoms and women's boots. I wanted to stop someone, anyone, and I searched their faces, desperately hoping to recognise one of Mam's friends so that I could blurt my misfortune, to tell them what the louts had done to me and my precious pin-up. But all were as expressionless as the dummies in the window of the dress shop that used to be here.

I slouched up the tree-lined avenue of Robin Hood Chase. The shops on the precinct shone with a strip-light glare through the fine rain that dripped from the fresh May leaves. It seemed that years instead of hours had passed since I'd emerged triumphantly clutching the pristine copy of *Jackie*. Now it was soaking wet inside my parka as my aching ribs and pounding head bore testimony to the beating I'd just suffered. I wilted against the solidity of a lamp post as a middle-aged woman emerged from the chemist's shop. She pulled something from her handbag which she shook until it metamorphosed into a plastic Pac-a-Mac. She slipped into its weatherproof protection and hurried towards me. At last, someone to help. She'd see my injury and take me to the nearby doctors' surgery.

I staggered towards her with my arms open and sobbed the definition I'd heard on the crime programme, *Police 5*, a few evenings earlier. "I've been mugged!"

But she nimbly side-stepped me. "I've got a bus to catch." She broke into a trot, urgently waving at the advancing dark green bulk of the number forty.

I had to get home, but my jelly legs seemed inadequate to support me. I passed no one else. Had the population been ordered to stay indoors, and I'd missed the message? I stopped to rest on one of the concrete benches whose utilitarian appearance perfectly indicated their uncomfortableness. Each dragging step had delivered me closer to the yawning mouth of the underpass, dark and foreboding on even the sunniest day. It had quickly gained a reputation for violence within its graffiti-splashed depths. The lights that studded the ceiling had only functioned for a few weeks before being vandalised and within hours of them being repaired by council workmen, they were smashed again. Illumination was the enemy of the shadowy knots of youths who blended with the dark jungle of evergreen bushes around the tunnel edges, waiting with weapons poised, ready to steal handbags and wallets from unsuspecting pedestrians.

There was no way I could risk further attack, so I circumnavigated to a walkway where, to my relief, I saw a friendly face. Valeria was a girl from our old way who was a couple of years older than me and now lived a short distance from our new house. Her fabulous name and her dusky, sultry glamour reminded me of Ayshea Brough from the teatime pop show *Lift Off With Ayshea*. Strolling on clunky platform shoes, she swung a knotted string bag bulging with cans, their metal edges protruding through the gaps. Momentarily, I ignored my trauma. I really coveted those bags and had seen them in MacFisheries on the Market Square, but they were out of Dad's price range. He chose to re-use plastic carrier bags, saying that they'd last for years if looked after.

"Ayup, Valeria!"

She spun around on her ungainly heels with the grace of a ballerina, not even stumbling. "Crikey, Simon, what's happened to you?"

"I've just been mugged." My hysterical wail soared to the rooftops.

"Who by?"

"Two youths got me round our old way. They punched me in the face and ruined my Marc Bolan pin-up."

"The bleeders. Come on, I'll walk you home. Will there be someone in?"

The house would be as cold and lifeless as the barren streets I'd just fled. Although we had instant heat by flicking a switch, it just wasn't the same as the coals glowing in the fireplace at the old house. "Nobody's there. Nick's doing football stuff, and Tim won't be in till half-five. And Dad won't be back from work till six."

"Oh, that's no good then." Valeria's thick eyebrows sagged as if forced downwards by a pair of thumbs. "And you haven't got a mam anymore, have you?"

Her unintentional indiscretion unleashed my reservoir of imprisoned tears. My anguished howls echoed from the rockface of concrete steps at the end of the narrow cut-through behind her house.

"Aw, Simon, come on. Don't cry like that." Valeria offered me one of the polished pine hoops threaded through the shopping bag as if it were a mystical cure-all. "Grab a handle, these tins weigh a ton. Tell you what, we'll go to my house. My mam's in. You know she's a nurse, don't you? She'll have a look at you, and you can wait till someone's at yours."

We covered the short distance holding the shopping bag between us as if we were taking an infant wearing a string vest for a stroll. Valeria's mam was visible through the gate, the motion of her shoulders indicating that she was washing up at the sink. The blue of her nurse's uniform was like a summer sky surrounded by the white frothy clouds of scalloped net curtains.

She looked up and stared, and then pulled the door open. "What on earth's going on here?"

I stepped into the kitchen. Instantly the comforting aroma of fried bacon wrapped around me. "I've been mugged, Mrs Melton." I was getting quite used to my dramatic statement.

She peeled off her yellow rubber gloves and laid them on the sparkling aluminium draining board. "You wait here a minute whilst I get my first aid kit."

Valeria opened the fridge door. "Do you fancy some pop? Or there's some strawberry Nesquik. I can make you one of them if you like."

"No, it's okay. A glass of pop would be lovely, ta."

There was a burst of white light when she pulled the fridge door fully open, illuminating a shelf laden with bottles that kissed with the tinkle of a rainbow-coloured xylophone. She recited their contents as if she were trying to sell them. "Today we have pineapple, lemonade, orange, lime and lemon, cherry soda, dandelion and burdock, ginger beer..."

"Ooh, yeah, ginger beer, please. It's my fave."

She reached into the icy whiteness. "Coming up. But you know what they say about it, don't you?"

"No, what?"

"Ginger beer makes you queer."

Rather than look at her, I surveyed the kitchen. Hanging from the wall above the cooker were an enormous wooden spoon and fork with *Porthcawl* carved into each wide handle. The dizzying wallpaper bore overlapping circles of lemon and turquoise, intersecting in regimented

Chucking Putty at the Queen

fresh lime ovals. I bet Marc Bolan's kitchen was groovy too and wished that the plain walls in our kitchen were so adventurous.

Valeria's mam returned, carrying a white metal box high in front of her as if it contained the crown jewels. "Who did this to you anyway?"

"A pair of muggers. I've never seen them before."

She gently examined my face, manoeuvring my head left and right, then up and down. I closed my eyelids against the discomforting glare of the faceted light fitting that sparkled as if full of diamonds.

"Is it broken? Will I end up looking like a fairground boxer?"

Valeria chuckled. "You do say some weird things, Simon."

Mrs Melton gently touched my nose. "No, don't be silly. It's not broken. Just a bit of blood, that's all."

"Will I need a transfusion?" There had been adverts on the telly requesting volunteers for the service, and already I could see myself lying on a hospital bed with a tube in my arm, being filled with someone else's blood.

"No, of course not. It's only a drop, and it's all dried now. I'll clean you up a bit." She stroked my nose with a small cloud of cotton wool. "Blood transfusions. I've never heard the like." She dribbled a pink, watery liquid onto the cotton wool and began to gently dab my nose. "I hate bullies and blame the parents. I don't mean *your* dad. He's a proper gentleman with nice, polite manners, and what he'll have to say about this to-do, I don't know."

That started me blubbing again. "And they ruined my *Jackie* with the super-sized pin-up of Marc Bolan. I've waited a lifetime for it."

But she wasn't interested in my poster and began to repack her first aid box. "There you are. You'll live."

I was a bit put out that she was indifferent to the soggy fate of my magazine. "Don't you want to see what they did to my *Jackie*?"

"You hang onto it until your dad can sort it out for you."

I couldn't wait to see Dad but doubted that even he could make the devastation right.

Valeria opened a circular metal tin. "Here's a Bar Six an' all."

I didn't eat chocolate much but welcomed this treat as she took my hand.

"Come through to the living room."

Although it was May, their heating was turned up high. Combined with the glow of the pink lampshades on the jazzy orange and yellow floral wallpaper, it was as if I'd entered a blast furnace. A shiny skin of transparent plastic protected their raspberry three-piece suite, and I was surprised that it didn't melt in the temperature of the room. The seat cushions were so low to the ground they could have been from a sports car, and when I lowered myself onto the shiny cover, a squishy, farting sound erupted.

"Ooh, pardon you!" Mrs Melton smiled as my face burned with both heat and embarrassment.

"Shall I take my boots off? I don't want to make a mess of your carpet." I hoisted my damp trousers up to my knees to display the splashes of demolition site mud spoiling the black leather. I didn't miss the wink that Mrs Melton gave to her daughter before smiling at me.

"They're nice boots."

"Thank you very much. They were my sister's."

"But you keep them on. I'll just give them a quick wipe over."

She returned from the kitchen shaking a tea towel, then held it up as if for my approval. It was horrible, printed with a grotesque, cross-eyed cartoon mouse wearing a red hat and lederhosen. Swirly letters within a bubble emerging from its disturbingly human mouth asked the question, "Fancy a cuppa?"

Mrs Melton shook her head. "And your lovely trousers are all soaked. Come over here and dry them by the heating."

The force from the dark grey metal grille was so ferociously high that my thin trousers first steamed, then quickly dried as my feet roasted in my boots. I checked the time on the clock on top of their white telly. A yellow plastic orb with red flip-over numbers, the timepiece was as glam as the rest of the décor. I watched, hypnotised, and counted the seconds in my head, then tried holding my breath, even though I still jumped when the digits changed. Being a year older, Valeria was already established at secondary school and chatted about how I would enjoy it because they had a big art department.

"There's two great big, massive classrooms, and one's even got a potter's wheel in it and a kiln. You'll love it."

Finally, the big red numbers on the white plastic panels flipped over to five-thirty. "Our Tim should be home by now." I was desperate to escape into the fresh air and his protection.

Chucking Putty at the Queen

"Come on then, I'll walk you home."

I was fearful that the louts had found out where I lived and would be waiting to jump me. There was no one outside, apart from Valeria's dad coming home from work.

"Oi, Val! Where you off to? It's teatime."

Valeria waved energetically. "Won't be a minute, Dad."

Tim was just putting his key into the front door and spun around at the sound of our approach. "Christ, what you been on with?"

"I've been mugged!"

I sobbed as Valeria explained, then patted my back. "You'll be all right now with your brother. Ta-ra."

Tim pushed the door open. "Come on, best get you inside. Tell me all about it. I'll find the bastards." In the kitchen, he shoved a packet of biscuits towards me. "Get one of these down yer neck. You'll feel better."

I nibbled as I relayed the events, pausing periodically to quell the horror that threatened to overwhelm me. I'd just reached the part where the youths threw my boots into the wasteland when our back gate latch clicked. I looked to the top of the yard. So engrossed in my woeful story, I hadn't detected the sound of Dad's car that I obsessively waited for every evening about this time.

"Ayup, Dad's back." Tim crammed two biscuits into his mouth. "I'll put these back or else he'll say I'll spoil me tea."

He'd just closed the cupboard door when Dad entered.

"There was hardly any traffic on University Boulevard and for a change, every traffic light was green... What the hell's been going on? Has Nick done this to you?"

"Some youths jumped him round the old way. He's been at that girl Valeria's house. Her mam's a nurse."

The front door slammed, and Nick entered, red-faced. The stench of cigarettes wrapped around him like a dirty grey blanket. He still thought that the rest of us didn't know he smoked. The kitchen was a claustrophobic cell imprisoning the four of us, and I instinctively stepped away from him until my shoulders pressed against the glass panel in the back door.

He scowled and dropped his school haversack to the floor with a thud. "What's up with him?"

"He got duffed up by two youths round the old way," Tim said.

"I wasn't duffed up; I was *mugged*. They took my money and ruined my new Marc Bolan pin-up."

"You were round the old way *again*? My mate Stephen told me he'd seen you there loads of times, just hanging around and talking to yourself."

The walls began to close in on me. "I haven't then."

"Yes, you have then. And guess what? Stephen told me that one day he asked you who you were talking to, and you said—"

"That's enough, Nick." Dad's warning sliced with the sharpness of the guillotine he used to trim photographs.

"Who?" Tim asked. "Who was he talking to?"

"Mam. He said he was talking to Mam." Triumph shone in Nick's eyes.

"Nick, that's *enough*!" Dad never raised his voice, or shouted at us, but his authority wasn't to be ignored. "Take your football stuff upstairs, please. The last thing I need is for you to be getting on at Simon again."

Nick dropped his eyes and tugged his haversack from the floor. "He asks for it anyway. Everybody hates him," he mumbled.

"I beg your pardon, Nicholas? If you have something to say, then I'd appreciate it if you enunciated correctly."

Nick's cheeks flared. "He probably did it himself anyway, just to get sympathy and attention." He clicked the door shut behind him, knowing better than to slam it.

Dad pressed the bridge of his nose between his forefinger and thumb, sighing so deeply that I feared his lungs would implode. "I try my best. This is all I need when I get home from work." He crooked his finger. "Come here, Son. Tell me exactly what happened, then I must go and thank your friend and her mother."

His tender examination was punctuated by my explanation of events gabbled through blubs and sobs as if I were aged five and not eleven. "And one of them punched me in the face, and then they nicked the four pence for the phone and the penny change from the paper shop and stamped on my parma violets and then pulled out my new *Jackie* and chucked it on the ground and stamped on it, and it's all wet and ruined."

"Take a breath, Son. I'm home now. It's all right."

"It's not all right, Dad. I loved getting that pin-up and now it's ruined forever, and it was the last one in the shop. I'll never get another one now. It's the end of the world."

Dad wiped my tears with his forefinger, then lifted his black leather work bag onto the draining board. "Open it, Son."

The zip growled as I parted the black leather flaps. Marc Bolan's face stared up at me from the new issue of *Jackie*. "*Dad!*"

"I'm no chump! I bought it in Beeston on my way to work, because I worried that Sharp's would have sold out, and I didn't want you to miss out on the poster."

I tenderly kissed the magazine. "I can't believe my eyes."

Dad chuckled and mussed my hair. "Come on then, tatty head. Let's get it up on the bedroom wall with all your others." He opened the door to the hall. "You see, Son, it's not the end of the world after all."

And as long as the world kept turning, I knew that my fantastic dad would always make everything all right.

14

LOUDMOUTH

"Don't look over your shoulder, but the Sex Pistols are coming."

The blistering heat of that *New Musical Express* report transformed the black print into glowing molten lava on a February morning in 1976. I devoured the short article several times, hardly able to comprehend it. Fronted by their singer, Johnny Rotten, the confrontational quartet boasted that they were not into music, but chaos. The pages scrunched as I gripped with increasing exhilaration. In a stagnant musical scene, this was just the excitement I'd been waiting for and from thereon, I scoured the music press hoping for news on this bizarrely appealing group. My inquisitiveness was temporarily satiated by a *Sounds* feature at the tail end of April, mentioning that they'd played in a Soho strip club. This boosted their allure to me and poured petrol onto my smouldering imagination. I needed more.

A few weeks later, I scuffed the soles of my clumpy platform shoes on the pavement outside school, disturbing the covering of cherry blossom. If only it would magically transform into a pinky-white glue that would halt my tortoise-like progress and prevent me re-entering the warzone in which I was the enemy. I had to quickly decide my survival tactics. If it were like any other day, I would have received a clout around my head from an unseen assailant before the first lesson began, though on the previous day, a cocky first-year squirt had been egged on by older boys to spit in my face and call me a queer. The best way to avoid further confrontation would be to lurk in the cathedral heights of the foyer until the bell rang to announce the commencement of lessons.

Deliberately being the last into school meant I'd avoid the jeers and shoves awaiting me on the stone steps up to the classroom. Then if I survived the morning break, at noon I'd be able to flee to the outside world and conceal myself in the hidey-hole I'd found behind the garage over the road. Otherwise, I'd resign myself to walking the streets again, wishing that I were anywhere else rather than return to school.

The sound of running footsteps made me instinctively tighten my back muscles, and I swivelled, fearful of another attack by those who continually hounded me. But it was only a girl in my class. Home economics was on the timetable that afternoon, and she carried a wicker basket hooked over the crook of her arm.

"Hey, wait a minute, Simon."

I was convinced that my heavy sigh of relief brought down more blossoms from the cherry trees. "Ayup. What's wrong?"

She slipped her hand into her basket. "Where's my English book gone?"

"Can't help you with that one, sorry."

"You remember our Graham taped you those LPs by Black Sabbath?"

"Uh, yeah." I couldn't forget how bored I'd been by the turgid dullness of *Sabbath Bloody Sabbath* and *Master of Reality* but hoped that my unenthusiastic response didn't make me sound ungrateful.

"Gotcha!" She tugged an exercise book from the wicker depths and waved it at me. "He wants to know if you've heard of a group called... Hang on, he wrote it on here." She frowned at the creased back of her book. "The Ram Ones."

"The Ram Ones?" The strobe light of a past *NME* feature flashed across my memory. "Do you mean The Ramones?"

"Yeah, that's it." She waved the book at me. "Graham's left-handed, and his writing's always a mess. The Ramones, you're right."

"Have I heard of them? You bet! I've read all about them. They've got this song called 'Now I Wanna Sniff Some Glue.' Why does he want to know?" Already I had my fingers crossed that another taping session was on the horizon.

"You know how I told you he's got a pen pal in New York? Well, he sent Graham their LP for his birthday. He reckons he's not heard anything to touch it and thinks you'd like it. Graham, I mean, not his pen pal."

"Hold up. You mean to say that his pen pal sent him an LP all the way from New York?"

She slid her exercise book back into her basket. "Yeah, it's barmy, isn't it? You'd have thought it'd get broken, wouldn't you? Fancy doing that: sending a record all that way. But the Yanks are like that. They're all loaded and can do such things. Not like over here. Anyway, Graham says if you give me a blank cassette, he'll tape it for you."

"I'll bring one in tomorrow." This was ace. Now I would hear what a music press article described as "a barrage of buzzsaw guitar." I bet nobody else in my school would have their LP. "What are they like? Have you heard them?"

The jailhouse clanging of the bell from the grim school block announced that nine o'clock was upon us.

"Yeah, I've heard it all right. He plays it in his room non-stop. It drives our mam crazy." She tugged the arm of my blazer. "Come on, quick. We're late."

We hastened up the wide steps leading to the foreboding tall doors, its windows reflecting the outside world. I'd soon be imprisoned away from it. I pulled at the heavy brass handle and held the door open. "What's it like then?"

She slipped through. "Well, it's not Abba."

Thus, within forty-eight hours my musical life was transformed by the high-octane, chainsaw guitar barrage of The Ramones, and I played the cassette so much that I worried the thin brown tape would stretch and snap. However, a couple of weeks later, those fears were soon wiped away by a stroke of luck that made the Agfa C-60 redundant.

It was Friday, and I couldn't wait for the respite that the weekend would provide. Despite the torment that I constantly endured in the playground, classrooms, and corridors, the idea of nicking off never occurred to me. The wind rolled an empty Winalot dog food tin across the dusty pavement, and as I followed its progress, my heart double skipped when I saw a pound note. Ace, what a find! I could buy a single. But it was only a discoloured receipt for Roses' shoe shop that stood here before redevelopment reduced the area to rubble. I never had any good luck.

The faded chitty evoked a late September afternoon laden with the spicy aromas of summer slipping away. I pranced alongside Mam as we went to collect the slip-ons that I was to wear as pageboy at Penny's wedding, and when the shop assistant laid them on the glass-topped counter, a punch to my stomach couldn't have left me more breathless. Such resplendent footwear was the stuff of fairy tales, and even the diminutive prick-eared helpers in *The Elves & The Shoemaker* couldn't have bettered these creations. The leather shone with an incandescent light as if polished by a thousand brush-wielding hands, and the gleaming silver buckles were surrounded by foamy hawthorn blossoms of gathered white and pink lace. My imagination sped ahead to the next day, picturing my ruffle-fronted platinum satin shirt tucked into the softness of the moss green velvet trousers that Penny made for me. I already knew how fabulous I'd look, but then I had an idea so absolutely brilliant that it made me giddy.

I sidled up to Mam and slipped my hand in hers. "Mam, may I wear your pearly earrings for the wedding?" I recalled an advertising headline in the newspaper that I'd memorised. "They'd be the *last* word in luxury."

"Hmm, I don't know about that." She shook her head. "Remember, a page boy mustn't upstage the bride."

In the morning, neighbours lined the street, eager to glimpse Penny as she floated on clouds of white into the waiting Rolls Royce. Never missing a chance to show off, I posed with my hands on my hips and pouted. Mam and Dad flanked me, magnificently attired, as if the luxurious car was going to sweep them to a function at Buckingham Palace instead of Tollerton village church.

A minor earthquake caused by a Wimpey Construction lorry thundering past pulverised the memories. Maybe there really was something mentally wrong with me for constantly wallowing in how things used to be before Mam died. The wedding, my amazing outfit, the shoe shop, and Mam only survived in my memory, and five years later, standing beside the few remaining bricks from the obliterated store, my teenage feet were clad not in frothy lace-bedecked leather but cumbersome dark tan platform shoes. I was no George Best, and my awkward kick sent the dog food tin on a rattling course until it butted against chunks of shattered masonry. Countless seed-denuded dandelions rose like monks' heads above the dainty blue speedwell, embroidering the pavement palette of weather-worn cigarette packets, green and ochre leaves of discarded bus tickets, and knife-blade slices of broken glass.

It was so easy to slide beneath the familiar security blanket of detachment. I descended from reality into daydreaming once more, and I floated, looking down on a Lilliputian world covered with Arctic drifts of paper scraps and cigarette nub ends flattened like stamped-on beetles. A wooden fork impaling a polystyrene chip tray became the mast of a ship grounded on a rocky shoreline, and someone had placed half a dozen empty Coca Cola cans in a regimented red line, reminding me of soldiers awaiting inspection from the queen at Trooping the Colour.

Chucking Putty at the Queen

The busy roar of the traffic mellowed into a comfortable hum as I allowed my mind to wander further. I was fooling myself that I could delay the progression to school. If I were brave, I'd just nick off for the day and spend my time leisurely exploring the canyons of books in the big library in town. If questioned by the snooty head librarian—who always looked at me as if I were trying to steal something—I could say that I was researching for an educational project, even though the only thing I'd accomplished at school was a perfect attendance record and never being late for register. I groaned, remembering when the teacher proudly informed my classmates that my one hundred per cent turnout was an exceptional achievement and something that they must endeavour to emulate. This gold star accolade only produced a black mark against me with the other pupils and an increase in hostilities. But no matter how bad the bullying became, I never resorted to truancy. There was no way in the world that I'd ever let Dad down.

I'd just resumed my progress to school when something caught my eye. A diamond dropped into a cow pat couldn't have gleamed more brightly. On the pavement lay a begrimed white card proclaiming *Record Token* in purple letters. I pounced on it like a cat on a cornered mouse, though I expected to find that the valid part had been removed. The inside was completely blank apart from an intact voucher for three pounds. Finally, my luck had changed. Chance had turned me into Dick Whittington, and the rubbish-strewn street was unexpectedly paved with gold. However, as quickly as my elation rose like a balloon, the darkness of my natural cynicism, suspicion, and paranoia caused it to crash in flames, burning like the Hindenburg airship. It was bound to be fake, part of an elaborate joke to make me look foolish. I was used to being the butt of pranks and practical jokes at school, and I looked around for laughing pupils to jump from behind the nearby advertising hoarding. But there was only me, the traffic, and the record token. With it safely slipped within the inside pocket of my blazer, I continued to school, my unimagined good fortune transforming my clumpy platform shoes into weightless pink satin ballet slippers.

At the end of the final lesson of the morning and having surrendered to guilt-by-association because of my brother Steve's history of criminal activities, I sheepishly approached my form teacher and held the record token before me as if it were a wallet full of twenty-pound notes that I'd pickpocketed. I explained my predicament. "So, you see, sir, if it were me who'd lost it, I'd go barmy. That's why I thought of taking it to the police station, so the real owner could claim it."

My teacher shook his head. "Well, now, Smalley. I know that logic is not your best friend, but let's look at the situation rationally. There's no name on it, so it could belong to anyone. It's grubby, so it could have been there for ages. If that's not enough to convince you to claim ownership, you know the saying, finders' keepers." He raised his eyebrows and grinned. "I suggest that you use it wisely. You could buy the new T. Rex album."

"Too late, sir. My dad already bought me *Futuristic Dragon* for my birthday, but if you're sure that it's okay to spend it, I know just what I'll get."

Five hours later, I'd been into town and exchanged my serendipitous booty for a vinyl copy of The Ramones album. There was no need to play the cassette again.

15

ANARCHY IN THE UK

THE BURGEONING NEW MUSIC scene spearheaded by the Sex Pistols flourished with bands bearing befittingly urgent names like The Clash, 999, Buzzcocks, Generation X, and the Vibrators. The music was attributed the name "punk rock," meaning that the musicians and fans were punk rockers. Without hearing a single note played or any lyrics sung by these bands, I was captivated. The table of youth culture was turned over, and the humdrum malaise of conformity crashed to the floor. Everything musically that went before was ripped up, matching the clothing of the punk rockers. Press reportage of their snotty, snarky attitude told of anti-fashion and of being as provocatively original as you wanted. More photos appeared in the music papers of the spike-haired punks dressed in black bin liners, their cheeks pierced with safety pins and necks adorned with studded dog collars, and the exotically named Siouxsie Sioux wearing a swastika armband whilst bearing her bosoms through a cutaway top.

My gauche attempt to gain punk credentials was accomplished when I wore my school blazer inside out, jabbed two safety pins through one lapel, and clipped ring pulls to the other one. Each year, my brother Tim and I painted my pushbike a new colour, and I liberated tins of vibrant Humbrol enamels from the shed at home. In those remnant blazes of pink, orange, yellow, and silver, I proclaimed my allegiance to these new (and still unheard by me) punk rock bands by aggressively daubing their names on the flap of the haversack that I stuffed my schoolbooks into. Once the paints dried, it resembled a scrap of the titular *Technicolour Dreamcoat* from the dreary musical featured in the school Christmas show two years earlier.

As well as their cheeks, the punk rockers had ears pierced by safety pins. Playground education taught me that if a man had his right ear pierced, it signalled that he was queer. This was deliciously confrontational, and when Tim, Nick, and Dad were out, I put The Ramones LP onto the stereo and selected a long needle from Mam's sewing tin. With an ice cube freezing my fingers as it melted and dribbled down my neck, I numbed my right earlobe and then with one of Dad's rough wine corks pressed behind it, I tried to shove the slender silver shaft through my unyielding flesh. It wasn't as easy as I'd anticipated, making me wonder what Mam would have thought if she could hear my squawks as I slowly thrust one of her needles into my skin. After fifteen minutes of fruitless jabbing, side one of the LP had finished, and my throbbing, bloody lobe resembled an overripe raspberry. I admitted defeat, and with a bobbin of black cotton at my side, I employed the needle for its intended purpose by altering my spare pair of school trousers from flares into straight legs.

The ticking punk timebomb exploded when during a live television interview, the Sex Pistols guitarist called the host, Bill Grundy, a "dirty fucker" and "a fucking rotter." The country's collective outrage erupted, and the ensuing tabloid frenzy included the report of a lorry driver kicking in the screen of his television in disgust at the swearing. Punk rock flared across the country and further scorched my imagination. But before I'd even had chance to hear them, the band were sacked by EMI records and their debut single, "Anarchy in the UK" was withdrawn from sale in a knee-jerk reaction to the adverse publicity. My immediate chance to experience this homegrown new music had passed.

A couple of days later I was in Woolworths, examining a box of singles discounted to fifteen pence. Breath knotted in my throat. There it was: the Sex Pistols disc. With trembling hands, I flipped it around. The B-side title, "I Wanna Be Me" gave a name to my searing teenage frustration. Immediately, every other record in my life became redundant, and ownership of this became as crucial to my existence as the blood speeding through my veins. But I had no money and knew not to ask Dad. He was aware of the group's notoriety via the sensational headlines on Tim's newspapers, and when he read about the swearing on television and learned that they wore spiked dog collars and swastika armbands, he'd become unusually angry, calling them "bladdy scruffy ignoramuses" before he embarked on a lecture about respect and manners. I had an idea of how to obtain the finance to ensure the record was mine but first, I had to make sure that nobody else bought it.

I stepped over to the counter where the assistant had her back to me. "Sorry to bother you, but could you reserve this for me until tomorrow, please?"

My spirits plummeted when she turned around. It was an older girl called Dorothy who used to live round our way. That was ages ago, and I really hoped that she'd not remember me.

It was not to be. Her jaw dropped, revealing a pink flash of bubble gum. "I know you."

"Do ya?"

"Yeah, you live up near me nanar's. I go up every Sunday for me tea."

"How nice for you."

She sniggered and popped the gum. "You used to have all sequins on your face and walked around in girls' boots."

"They were women's boots, *actually*."

Her eyes narrowed. "My nanar said you're Albert Brown's boyfriend."

"How refreshingly original. I've not heard that one before."

"Everyone calls you Peg Leg now."

"And they still call you Dot-to-Dot Dorothy 'cos of all the spots on your face." I checked myself. What on earth was I doing, bickering with a shopgirl? I held the record towards her and gave her what I hoped was a sweet smile. "I'd be eternally grateful if you'd put this to one side until tomorrow."

She blew a small cerise bubble and burst it between her teeth. "Ooo-er, hark at it. If you hadn't noticed, the sign over the door says Woolworths, not Central Library."

"*Please*. I'm sorry I called you Dot-to-Dot."

"I can't. It's more than me job's worth."

"It'll be worth even less if I tell that supervisor over there that you're chewing bubbly gum at the counter."

She stared but chewed less noticeably. "You wouldn't snitch on me, would you? I'm on two verbal warnings as it is."

"I won't say anything if you reserve this for me."

"I just told you, I *can't*."

"Aw, go on. Do me a favour."

"No. I'll tell you what, you do me a favour and get lost, Peg Leg. Coming in here talking all posh and threatening me." She blew an enormous bubble, and when it burst she manipulated the sticky mess with her fingers, stuffed it into her mouth, and turned towards a scowling lady who bore a startling resemblance to Annie Walker from *Coronation*

Street. "Yeah? Did you want somethink?"

The woman glared from beneath a green hat resembling a halved, hollowed-out watermelon. "Yes, I do want *somethink*." She snorted. "If you've quite finished chatting with your boyfriend, I'd like to purchase these." She struggled to lift a Kenwood Chefette food mixer, a box of wooden spatulas, and three baking trays onto the counter. "And if this were Jessops, young lady, there'd be someone here to assist me."

Grinning, I returned to the sale record rack, and with the slyness of a shoplifter, I scanned the other people in the store. No one was paying any attention to me, but why would they? I was just a boy in school uniform. But instead of secreting the record under my blazer and walking out of the store, I leaned over the box of singles and carefully hid it behind the thick white cardboard price sign at the back. Inflated with self-righteousness of not becoming a thief like my eldest brother, Steve, I floated past the shining wrappers of the Pick & Mix sweet counter and shoved open one of the plate glass doors, already wishing the next twenty-four hours away. I hurried home to find the money to buy the record. And I knew exactly where it was hidden.

Tim always wore a suit at weekends, and after pub closing time, he came home via the chippy with his supper, most often a double portion of chips and a king-sized saveloy in batter or half a deep-fried chicken, all drenched with glutinous curry sauce. He'd carefully drape his jacket over the back of the settee, then peel open the warm, soggy newspaper which wrapped his feast and, with both hands cradling the laden polystyrene tray, he'd drop backwards into his chair. As his bum went down and his knees went up, his pockets emptied like a jackpot win on a fruit machine, and his change slid down the side of the cushion into the void below. This minor inconvenience wouldn't stop the more important task of devouring his supper, and his curse was always the same: "Bollocks, I'll get it in the morning."

Yet I couldn't recall him ever retrieving those lost coins, which must surely have amassed into a king's ransom, or at very least, the fifteen pence that would buy me "Anarchy in the UK." I reassured myself that what I was about to engage in wasn't *real* theft. It was more of a recovery mission. With my breath trapped in my lungs as if I were a free diver searching for pearls beneath the turquoise ocean of taut polyester, I reached down and ignored the jagged complaints from my bad leg as my fingertips dredged the hessian seabed.

A tot up revealed a fortune of one pound, three-and-a-half pence of Tim's hard-earned cash, but the undertow beneath my wave of dishonesty dragged me into the murky depths of criminality inhabited by our Steve. I should return the bounty to its rightful owner, even though he'd no doubt say, "You keep it, buy yourself a single."

The reassurance of Tim's imagined reaction and the vision of the record waiting in Woolworths overrode any sense of honour and familial integrity. My scavenging had proved to be more productive than I'd hoped and after school the next day, it would allow me the luxury of riding on the bus into town to retrieve my hidden treasure.

The final lesson of the day was double geography, but there was a more urgent issue in my mind than the post-war economy of Guatemala. Each time Mr Davies turned his back to the class and wrote on the blackboard, I slipped another of my textbooks from the desk into my haversack until only my exercise pad lay before me. I loudly exhaled several times in rapid succession.

Mr Davis didn't look up from his notes. "Am I boring you, Mr Smalley?"

"No, sir."

"I wondered because of all of those puffs you're making."

"That's 'cos he's a puff, sir."

I glared at the smirking boy who sat a few desks away and wished that I had laser beam eyes so I could blow his head up.

"Enough of your incredible wit, Smith. I wasn't talking to you."

"But you got to admit it, sir. He *is* a puff."

This wasn't going how I wanted it to. My deathly moan successfully dragged the spotlight back to me.

"What *is* the matter with you, Smalley?"

"I don't feel right, sir. I think I'm going to be sick."

Mr Davis raised his arm and consulted his watch. "Can't you hang on for ten minutes?"

My answer was to introduce a volley of shoulder-jerking retches like next door's cat when it had a furball in its throat.

"Oh, no, not all over my desks, you don't. Go on, get to the toilet now."

This was my chance. When he resumed attacking the blackboard with vigorous white chalk marks, I slid my exercise book into my blazer pocket, grabbed the strap of my haversack, and five minutes later, I was on the bus into town.

    Woolworth's wasn't too busy, and imitating Roger Banister hurtling towards the four-minute-mile record, I clumsily raced to claim the winning prize of what was already *my* Sex Pistols record.

    But what was this? Someone was already standing at the box of singles. From beneath a headband of coloured beads, his untamed mousy hair blended with the shaggy fur trim of an Afghan coat. I stood as close as I dared, holding my breath rather than inhaling the cloying stench of patchouli oil. As he painstakingly flipped through the records with his dirty claws, my stinging impatience made me want to rip off his circular *Keep on Trucking* patch.

    Before learning of the Sex Pistols and their entourage, I would have loved his summer of love look with the pseudo-runic logos for the heavy rock group Led Zeppelin colourfully embroidered onto the greasy back panel. Now I hated his too-short patchwork bell-bottom jeans that dangled above dirty, sandal-clad feet with their revoltingly long, blackened toenails. This goat-faced hippy could do with a visit from a vet wielding a pair of hoof rot shears.

    And talk about a slowcoach. He was probably stoned or seeing things that weren't there because he was tripping on LSD. Just when I'd convinced myself that I could hear my own hair growing, he reached the last few discs. At last, he'd soon be out of my way. I'd retrieve my single, get home, and hear the songs that had had already become as essential to my existence as my thudding heart. But when he reached the last record, he yawned and moved his filthy fingers to the front of the selection and began slowly trawling through them again, nodding his head. The starter motor in the overhead light misfired with a maddening, repetitive click as it struggled to activate the misty neon tube. The hippy looked over his shoulder with poached egg eyes magnified by the thick lenses of his blue-tinted spectacles.

    "Oh, hi, man, I didn't know there was a queue. Are you waiting on me?"

    "No, no, there's no queue, just me, and you're quite all right." Despite my politely dishonest reply, I really wanted to elbow him out of the way. Eventually he reached the last single, which he extracted for examination then slowly returned it with a snail-like lack of speed. That's it, he'd inspected them all. Twice. Great. Go on, get lost. *Don't you dare start at the front again.*

He didn't. Instead, he slowly parted his curtain of hair, leaned forward, and peered at the cardboard notice as if, instead of the thick black letters proclaiming, *Sale Singles 15p,* the hallucinogenic drugs he was obviously on enabled him to see *Record hidden behind this sign.* With the soiled fingers that I now detested so much that I wanted to visit the nearby gardening department, grab an axe, and chop them off, he pulled the sign forward and lifted out the single I'd secreted there twenty-four hours earlier. The grumbling gurgle of my hungry stomach voiced the downward lunge of my horror when, instead of returning the disc ready for me to rightfully claim as my own, he shoved the long row of discounted records back into an upright position, patted them until they were level, and then loped towards the till holding my Sex Pistols single. I raised my face to the flashbulb flickers of the neon light and expelled my trapped breath in a defeated torrent. Like the athlete running close to Roger Bannister's heels, I'd been beaten in my attempt to claim the record.

16

NEW RELIGION

By the spring of 1977, punk rock was established as a disturbing, disruptive media sensation of outrage and disgust that rattled the nation's comatose complacency. My energization increased with the glam/punk collision of my musical hero Marc Bolan enlisting amphetamine punk rabble-rousers The Damned as the support act for his *Dandy In The Underworld* tour. I already knew how rambunctious they sounded because, following my defeat with the Sex Pistols single, I'd gone up to Goldsmith Street and bought The Damned's "New Rose" from Selectadisc.

One morning at the start of April, Tim swung his haversack onto his shoulder and opened the back door on his way to work. Behind him, yellow trumpets glowed against the lawn, and twisty lime sprouts bulged from the branches of the mountain ash growing outside the window.

"I didn't get you owt for your birthday, did I?"

"No, but it doesn't matter." It did, but I wasn't going to say so. Mam and Dad taught me that to ask for things was incredibly bad manners.

"I'm going down to Burton's on Saturday to get measured for a new suit. If you wanna come with me, I'll buy you an LP."

"Oh, wow, thanks, Tim." The Clash's debut album was firmly in my sights. I already had their ferociously raucous first single, "White Riot," which I'd obtained by saving the money Dad gave me for my weekly school dinners. The song on its flip side, "1977," proclaimed that this year was one of change. Appealing to my aspiration of being a graphic designer when I left school, the angular attributes of the repeated digits invigorated me into wielding my felt pens, pastels, and wax crayons to create jagged, energetic images incorporating the lines of the Union Flag and the triangularity of the digit seven. The Jamaican reggae trio, Culture, had released their album *Two Sevens Clash*, named after the prophecies of Marcus Garvey, who foretold the world would suffer cataclysmic chaos on the seventh of July 1977 when "the two sevens clash."

United with the unsettling atmosphere aroused by punk rock, a developing turbulence tormented me with swirling frustration, fear, and worry that amalgamated into a mental itch that I couldn't scratch. The bullying and physical attacks I was suffering at school created a paranoid apprehension which wasn't helped when a mad-eyed elderly Jamaican woman came to the door, a Bible in one hand and a blue and gold carpetbag in the other. I should have followed Dad's example in such situations by calmly telling her, "Not today, thank you" and shutting the door. Instead, I'd tried to argue my atheism against her evangelical determination.

She thrust her Bible towards me. "Be ready."

I stepped back and laughed. "For what?"

"Change coming soon."

"Thank you for letting me know. And talking of change, I must go now and get some for the milkman tomorrow." I shut the door. Talk about winning a losing battle. Religious nutters had no interest in the rational world, and I had a drawing of Joe Strummer to finish. But first, I'd have a cheese and pickle sarnie. I was halfway down the hall when I heard the unoiled letterbox opening.

"Be prepared. Change soon come."

I'd forgotten about the incident by Saturday evening. Tim had kept his promise and bought me The Clash's new album. Even though I was desperate to hear more by the band that I'd already determined was my crucial new favourite, instinct warned me not to play it until Dad was out of the house. He'd always taken an interest in my musical adventures but was lukewarm about my discovery of punk. Maybe sensing that he didn't need to hear this record, at eight o'clock he tightened the knot in his tie in preparation to saunter down to the Sycamore Inn for a pint. Like a runner poised in the blocks eagerly anticipating the explosion of the starting pistol, I hunched over the stereo with the stylus hovering above the vinyl rotating on the turntable, hating myself for wishing, for the first time in my life, that he wasn't there. But this was a pivotal point in my life moving forwards, and it had to be a private initiation. Punk wasn't as acceptable as the other bands I loved, like T. Rex, Be-Bop Deluxe, Roxy Music, or Sparks; it was as dangerous as a spitting cobra about to strike. And the ear-blistering track "What's My Name" perfectly exemplified my own paranoia, alienation, fear, and frustration. At last, someone else was speaking to me, and I was listening.

Chucking Putty at the Queen

As spring gave an early kickstart to summer, part of that year's Nottingham Festival was a rock and pop show held at Victoria Baths, close to where our old house once stood and where Pen and Marge had taught me to swim. Within the chlorine-saturated depths, I'd successfully completed my lifesaving exams and, before my leg injury, I'd represented the school in swimming galas, propelled to aquatic triumph by cheers and yells from teachers and spectators. Mam had always called me her water baby, and although I adored swirling beneath the surface with an instinctive seal-like fluidity, I already abhorred aggressive competition. Frequently, after powering the length of the exhibition pool, I reluctantly held the shining cup aloft amidst rapturous applause but did so without any sense of pride.

The revered building had undergone a makeover and was rebranded as a leisure centre. The advertising posters in the windows showed grinning, athletically trim people in overtight sportswear. With the flabby excess flesh on my chest a constant reminder of how miserable I was with my own body image, this only strengthened my resolve to never visit again. But when the unique oval-shaped pool was covered over and converted into a badminton court, the sense of historical loss was immense. After the earlier devastating demolition of St. Ann's, this further exemplified the city council riding roughshod over the feelings of the local populace.

Reneging on my promise to avoid this sports palace forever, I stepped into the brightly lit facility where the odour of chlorine still prevailed. My fickle about-face was because local punk band, Some Chicken, were appearing at the Radio Nottingham Extravaganza. As my first exposure to real punks, a fantastically memorable part of their appearance was when the guitarist produced a vibrator and buzzed it against the strings of his guitar instead of using a plectrum.

Then, on an already sultry Tuesday evening at the end of May, the red line in my punk thermometer soared when Captain Sensible and Rat Scabies of The Damned appeared as part of the festival in the Old Market Square. Having only seen a provincial punk group so far, I was frantic to see my first authentic London punk rockers. With my hair satisfactorily tousled and messed, I shrugged my inside-out school blazer over my lemon-yellow Marc Bolan top, recalling his rationale for inviting The Damned to tour with him. He'd seen a photo of the band and said, "One of them had the good taste to wear a Marc Bolan T-shirt." I cockily rolled my shoulders to ensure that the safety pins I'd speared into the black cloth glittered in the spring sunshine and departed for town.

For almost half a century, the Council House had dominated Old Market Square, but attention to its stoic bulk was temporarily relegated to second place by an enormous futuristic canopy of scarlet synthetic material. Tethered to the ground by skeletal metal uprights, it stretched into taut geometric angles that covered the stage where the DJ manned the record decks. Every tacky, crummy Saturday night variety show seemed condensed into what was locally known as Slab Square, where a couple of hundred people conglomerated, listening to the DJ play singles by Brotherhood of Man, David Soul, and the eternally depressing "If You Leave Me Now" by Chicago. Perhaps the story of the two members of The Damned coming was just that: a story. However, my drop into despondency immediately changed when the DJ called an alert.

"All right, you 'orrible lot. Who's heard of The Sex Pistols?"

A couple of cheers of assertion popped from the crowd, and a few hands stretched up as if kids at school were being asked a question.

"You all know that they're naughty boys."

A dull murmur rippled through the gathering.

"Do you want to hear 'God Save The Queen?'"

A few enthusiastic voices, including mine, yelled confirmation.

"Well, you can't."

An empty Coca Cola can rose in a shiny red arc and clattered on the edge of the stage. A policeman moved to the back of the crowd to presumably find the culprit as the DJ continued his patter.

"We can't play it by law; it's banned. But you can hear the other side!"

Irritatingly, he maintained his inane chatter over the single's flip, "Did You No Wrong."

"And we're just waiting for our guests of honour, Captain Sensible and Rat Scabies, those terrorizing punk rockers from The Damned!"

Pissed off at his trivialization of something so important to me, I cupped my hands around my mouth. "Get on with it, grandad!"

As if time were going backwards instead of forwards, the next vinyl platter served was the novelty hit from a couple of years ago, "The Bump" by Kenny. A gaggle of girls wearing matching cardigans and with their heads covered by free Radio Nottingham cardboard sun hats began the accompanying dance, bumping their hips and backsides together to the lyrically unchallenging, foot-stomping sound, grinning as they claimed their Warholian five minutes of fame. Just when I thought that it couldn't get worse, my heart sank further with the appearance of a group of older men wearing Teddy Boy regalia, their pomaded quiffs and heavy sideburns signposting to the past. They swaggered down the wide steps with their arms around much younger girls in tight, low-cut T-shirts, and skirts puffed out by frothing white petticoats beneath. I groaned inwardly. How I despised the mawkish obsession with the nineteen fifties and the national preoccupation with Americana that was evidenced by imported television shows such as *Happy Days* and the film *American Graffiti* that perpetuated the cosy, idealized post-war US dream. It was tragically jaded and made me sick. I wanted to see and hear something from right now that exemplified my frustration and would liberate me from the stagnant mental pool that I was drowning in. I *needed* to see the real London punk rockers who had just toured with T. Rex. To my delight, Some Chicken represented our homegrown punk talent, and after an interview with them, the DJ tapped the microphone and winced at the shrill screech of feedback. "It seems our guests of honour are drinking cider in the Flying Horse." His attempt at sounding nonchalant only made him sound pissed off and prissy. "So, we're sending over for them."

A man was dispatched to the pub to retrieve the errant punks, but he returned alone, bearing the news that they'd be over when they'd finished their pints of cider.

"Don't hold your breath, 'cos they're drunk," a St. John's ambulance man called.

But within a minute, the duo stumbled onto the set, shoving each other and pretending to trip over cables and wires that weren't properly taped to the stage. Captain Sensible belched into the microphone and after a few words with the DJ, the pair lurched past him and grabbed a handful of singles from a unit at the side of the record decks.

The captain grabbed the microphone and faced the crowd. "Who wants a free record then?"

Audience hands thrust forwards with fingers twitching in encouragement as if they'd not eaten for weeks and he was distributing sandwiches. I wouldn't show myself up by being so desperate, so attempted to look cool and punky by scrabbling at my hair with my fingertips and chewing an old bus ticket I'd found in my pocket. I never had real gum because Dad said that chewing it was "loutish and uncouth" and "symbolic of a vacuous mind." A thousand silver punk rock safety pins stuck in my heart when Captain Sensible leaned forwards and pointed at me, and I gulped the saliva-wetted nub of masticated bus ticket down my throat. I spluttered and stared up, seeing two stretched reflections of me in his wraparound shades. I was terrified that this ripped and torn vagabond was about to make fun of my gauche attempt at punk couture.

"'Ere—you got good taste, young sir. We just finished a tour with Marc."

Captain Sensible was speaking to me! "I know." I pushed my chest forward just enough to proudly expose my T-shirt, but not reveal my pappy chest beneath. The bassist raucously emitted another belch like a crow's call. Dad would really hate him.

"Marc's a lovely geezer. The best. Have some singles." He examined the discs. "Oh, fuck that one; it's shit." He tossed it to the floor and raised the next one. "Gorblimey, it's Aunty Cliff." He lifted his shades. "*You* don't like Cliff Richard, do ya?"

It was an accolade rather than a question, and my head swelled as he skimmed the record to Rat Scabies who, after a grimacing effort, snapped it in half.

"'Ere we go, you'll like this one."

Captain handed me "Chinese Rocks" by The Heartbreakers. This was an unprecedented moment in my life. I'd known from the music papers that they'd risen from the druggy ashes of the New York Dolls and were led by the fabulously named Johnny Thunders, whom I guessed took the appellation from the old Kinks song.

"And this lot, they're good but a bit art school poncey." He flapped his wrist.

I grabbed "Young Savage" by Ultravox! The urgent exclamation mark at the end of their name mirrored my disbelief at this amazing encounter.

"And these are ace, cobber."

With trembling fingers, I grasped "Erotic Neurotic" by Brisbane four-piece, The Saints, and a fantastic seven-inch sticker bearing their dripping paint logo and *(I'm) Stranded*, the title of their LP. This was wild! I'd couldn't wait to write to tell Marge in Australia.

The Damned's bassist belched again, then stuck his tongue out. "Ugh, you'll hate this one. It's utter shit." He shoved a disc by Tom Petty at me.

Chucking Putty at the Queen

    The scowling DJ put an end to this unofficial giveaway jamboree, and after answering his perfunctory questions, the punks returned to the Flying Horse, their raucous demands for more cider diminishing beneath the volume of "There's A Whole Lot of Loving" by Guys & Dolls. Their exit and the start of the schmaltzy sentimentality signalled the end of the evening's event for me.

    At home, the urge to document my outrageous experience invigorated me into hauling my typewriter onto the table. Ages ago, Dad had presented me with a green celluloid visor of the type worn by newspaper editors in old films. I pulled it down until the emerald crescent rested above my eyebrows. With my new singles stacked on the stereo auto-changer, I slid the sheet of A4 into my Smith Corona. The spiked urgency of the records blazing from the stereo stoked the furnace of my enthusiasm. I hunched over my machine and set about creating my first punk fanzine that I'd already decided to call *Sniper*. My machine gun reportage shot black typeface bullets onto the white paper target as I quickly developed my own spitfire syntax. Obeying the compelling command to verbalize my frustrated excitement, ripped phrases zipped across my mind as I reviewed the energetic new sounds with desperate alacrity. "Born To Lose" was the last record on the autochanger, and the stylus lifted just as I stabbed down the final full stop, whipped out the paper, and threw my head back, exhausted. I rapped a satisfied staccato tattoo onto the table with my fingertips and grinned at my musical appraisals. My punk prose gushed in excitable praise of each single apart from one, because my new best mate, Captain Sensible, had been completely right about the Tom Petty song.

17

THE MAD PARADE

The fermenting fervour of the queen's silver jubilee celebrations was intolerable. It was as if nothing else mattered. For weeks, the mouth of the British bulldog had frothed in a rabid frenzy of patriotism, and no object or person seemed to be excluded from being covered in red, white, and blue. The obligatory, insincere bonhomie turned my stomach. It was all so fake, and I wanted no part in it. Street parties were organized, and the choking, overwhelming atmosphere was that of a ghastly, exaggerated version of Christmas when everyone pretended to be best friends and proclaim that the world was a wonderful place. I knew full well that it wasn't.

Nottingham was covered in a suffocating blanket of toxic artificiality. I believed the royals were contemptuous and patronizing after I'd read that Queen Elizabeth (who was now the Queen Mother) stated, "Now we can look the East End in the eye" after Buckingham Palace suffered bomb damage in World War Two. What was she on about? She had dozens of rooms in which to live, and *she* didn't have a bucket inside a backyard Anderson shelter for a toilet. Nor had she cowered in the Underground until the all-clear siren sounded, only to discover that not only her house was no longer there, but also that everyone and everything in streets surrounding it were annihilated by Luftwaffe bombs. The royal family had supreme wealth and countless sycophantic minions, and there would have been no difficulties in financing and undertaking repairs to the palace.

The trouble was that Dad was a staunch royalist and was irritated that his busy work schedule precluded him from taking the afternoon off when the queen visited Nottingham.

"You'll have to go for me, Son. We can't let the side down, and I'm counting on you for a detailed report." About to drive to work, he paused with the car door open. "And if you have to push to the front of the crowd to get a good place, then bladdy do so. It will be your chance of a lifetime to be so close to the queen."

I prepared for my jubilee mission, still buzzing after seeing the video of the Sex Pistols' third single, "Pretty Vacant" on *Top Of The Pops* seven days earlier. My magpie mind had noted every detail, particularly Johnny Rotten's attire. As the band boorishly filled the screen, he sneered into the camera, wrapped in a bedraggled white muslin shirt with "Destroy" emblazoned in blood red above a swastika and an inverted image of Jesus on the cross. I'd already fashioned my own approximation of the remarkable garment. On the front of a baggy old white shirt I'd created a rough Union Flag and replicated the ragged-edged moniker. Beneath that was my reproduction of the already-infamous Jamie Reid graphic for the antagonistic "God Save The Queen" single.

My legs were wrapped in a cut-down pair of green bib-and-brace overalls that I'd salvaged after my brother Nick's apathetic and fleeting tenure at the city council parks and gardens department. I'd cut off the shoulder straps and stitched them so that they hung between my legs a la the McLaren & Westwood bondage trousers, and black and white baseball boots shod my feet. I had no access to hair dye, so I improvised with a paste of Vaseline and curry powder. When I'd spread the foul-smelling concoction onto my hair, it didn't make it spiky. Indirectly, Mam provided the answer. I tugged on the woollen bobble hat she'd knitted for me and using her crochet hook, fished out clumps of hair through the weave. When I removed the hat, the resultant upright rats' tails looked completely punky. But they stank, and my scalp itched like crazy. Crowning it all, in homage to the Sex Pistols' guitarist Steve Jones, I carefully positioned a ripped Union Flag carrier bag with knotted corners onto my messy hair. I was ready.

I limped into town, sweating in the clammy July heat. I cursed my bad leg, a constant reminder that my appointment with an orthopaedic surgeon grew closer with each page torn daily from the kitchen calendar. Soon the countdown would be in single figures. The injury to my leg was serious, but I refused to think about it. Something far more urgent occupied my mind. I worried that my fingerprints would be damning evidence on the ball of putty in my pocket, but I shucked off the spineless concern. I was powered by the courage of my convictions. After my mission was completed, there was no way I'd flee—not that I was physically able to run off anyway.

Chucking Putty at the Queen

    Unable to resist the fierce urge to parade my homemade regalia to others who would appreciate my anti-establishment creativity, I'd set my sights on the Virgin records shop on King Street, but I had underestimated the fevered royal fan club contained by steel barriers like the unimaginative sheep they were. It would take me ages to get down to the Market Square where only a few weeks earlier I'd met Rat Scabies and Captain Sensible.
    I made an about-turn and trudged back up Mansfield Road. I must have cut a curious figure as I hobbled along, ignoring the bemused stares of adults and giggles from children. The nagging ache in my bad leg transformed into electrical jolts. It would probably be better to go home and rest, but I couldn't. There was something that I had to do.
    Persevering, I squeezed through the multitudes who waved Union Flags. I ducked and dived to avoid the spokes protruding from energetically rotated commemorative umbrellas of red, white, and blue panels. Countless windmills whirred as I shoved through unimaginative human cattle adorned in red, white, and blue knitted berets, crocheted tams, straw boaters, plastic toppers, and cardboard bowlers. Ugh, endless homemade or mass-produced shop-bought tat. Poison curdled in my guts. Everything in the UK flag colours. How I hated the fawning social compliancy they represented. It was as if the rest of the spectrum wasn't allowed to invade this most imperial of days.
    The junction of Mansfield Road and Woodborough Road would be the perfect place to become immersed within the jubilant crowd, even with my appearance being more outré than the crowd of thousands whose excitement I was already suffocating within. I threaded my way through the toxic atmosphere of over-enthusiastically applied perfumes and aftershaves and took up position behind the mass of a burly, balding middle-aged man, his moist scalp the same texture as a withered mushroom that I'd once found in the bottom of our fridge. Damp tendrils of wispy hair dribbled down his sweaty neck and crept over the greasy collar of the thin white nylon shirt that strained to contain his torso, and the hair on his back was trapped under the diaphanous threads like tiny black slugs beneath a misted pane of glass. He thrust his hirsute arm aloft, brandishing a portable cassette player. The raw, tinny volume from its single speaker blasted the national anthem, multiplying my sense of sinking in a tri-coloured swamp of conformity. It was all so predictable,

the blind devotion to being a part of a fearsomely traditionalist entity. The cloying mob reminded me of the misery I'd endured when my brother Nick bullied me into going to football matches years earlier.

The powerful statement that I'd stencilled in pink enamel paint on the rear of my shirt, *Don't be told what you want. Don't be told what you need* seemed to burn into the skin of my back, and I hoped that the chemical words would adhere to my flesh permanently like a Maori tattoo. It would indelibly proclaim my allegiance to the revolution I'd been instinctively drawn to: the furious flame of punk rock.

A woman pressed at the side of the big man sniffed the air and wafted her flag under her nose. "Bleddy hell, Maurice, have you farted? It smells like that curry sauce from the chippy."

"Cheeky cow. Course I ant."

"Well, someone round here has." She turned around and stared. "Ooh-er, what you come as?"

"Me."

"Did you just fart?"

"No, it was Maurice."

"You bleddy cheeky bogger."

The ripples of anticipation swelled into an inescapable tidal wave flowing towards me. Flags fluttered frantically and the cheers and clapping magnified in volume and hysteria, marking the approach of the royal vehicle. Over the road, the crowd that thronged the pavement outside the International Community Centre surged forwards. The metal barriers swayed but didn't collapse.

The woman in front screamed, "She's here, she's here! I don't believe it!" and cheers blasted like corks flying from champagne bottles.

The royal vehicle's transparent panoramic canopy glinted between the heads of restless pennants that blurred into one, compounding the celebratory claustrophobia that crushed my whole being. I was wedged in on all sides, and when flag-holding hands stretched to the sky as if a gunman had shouted, "Stick 'em up," the bitter, smothering stench of stale body odour from dozens of sweaty armpits made me retch. I was sinking in an oppressive ocean of mandatory jubilee happiness. I fought for breath, my mouth and nose blocked just like when I'd pulled a polythene bag over my head earlier in the year to escape the school bullies forever. Noxious needles stabbed my scalp as my curry and Vaseline hair pomade fizzed in captivity beneath the knotted Union Flag plastic bag, creating a ghastly wetness that trickled down the back of my hot neck. What was I doing here? Yes, of course, I knew why I'd fought through the crowds to reach my position.

The alienation and paranoia that had imprisoned me for uncountable months whirled in a vortex, sucking me down, replaying the dizzying litany of taunts from the local kids that followed my lurching progress wherever I went.

"Peg leg, I've lost my leg, I don't know where to find it."

"Here's that queer."

"Oi, Smalley, you bummer."

I saw my towel on the floor of the gym changing room, soaked after the other boys urinated on it, and felt the unstoppable hate-powered punches smashing into my face when the bullies beat me up again and again.

The crowd behind pushed, and a shove to the middle of my back forced my eyelids apart. Amassed within the fluttering leaves of the trees lining Mansfield Road for as far as I could see, the grotesque, blue-faced winged monkeys from *The Wizard Of Oz* grunted unintelligible threats. My skull seemed to simultaneously shrink and expand and crackle as if about to shatter. On the other side of the wide road, the face-splitting, ecstatic grins exploded into crystalized fragments and reformed into the grimaces of those who vowed to kill me as I lay on my back in the school corridor, trying to protect my head from their kicking feet as my futile screams for help reverberated against the dark walls. I sucked in diesel-tainted, perfume-swamped, stale sweat-saturated air, and all the time, a pneumatic drill tried to escape through my ribcage. My pulse punched my ears, and the steely sky lowered until I was sure it would crush me and burst my head apart. Jostled and elbowed on all sides, a stifling, dissociative panic once more returned me to when Mam died. I would never escape that exhausting, domineering pain. Over the funereal black river of asphalt, the faces from the school corridor glared at me from the shadows at the back of the crowd, dragging their fingers across their necks in a cut-throat action, and behind me a dark voice promised, "You're fucking dead, Smalley, you queer."

Instantly, I saw my history as a completed jigsaw that someone had tipped over and chaotically reassembled, displaying my impotent inability to retaliate against those who'd made my life unbearable and my inadequacy to resist their sustained bullying that had prompted my suicide attempt. My shame and disgust at the excess flesh on my chest coalesced with fear and hatred, and Mam's death was the hardest, most vicious flashback of all.

And still, all around me the crowd pushed, shoved, and cheered with delight at the lovely shining world as I silently screamed, *let me out, let me out, let me out* until my simmering hatred reached boiling point, sizzling and sputtering resentment and paranoia.

In my trousers pocket was a tennis ball-sized lump of putty that I'd taken from Tim's donkey jacket before I'd left home. The gummy adhesive was my solution, my way to fight back against everything. For once I'd be the winner, and everyone would fuck off and leave me alone. This was a riot of my own. I squeezed off a piece of putty, so beautifully soothing and calming as I rolled it into a smooth orb between my sticky palms. I shoved forward through the clamouring bodies and hurled my missile at the polished blackness of the queen's Rolls Royce.

"No future! Anarchy in the UK!" My second putty grenade arced over the sea of waving flags. "You're a redundant concept! It's a fascist regime!" The gloriously liberating third putty bomb soared skywards in an arc of freedom. "No future for you! There's no fut—"

Powerful hands grabbed my shoulders from each side. The heels of my baseball boots juddered over the uneven tarmac as two policemen dragged me backwards and slammed me against a wall. Brickwork connected with the back of my skull and a hot, thick hand wrapped around my neck.

"Drop it, you fucking piece of shit!"

Forceful fingers unfurled my right hand, and the last of the putty dropped to the ground. A punch to my gut thrust out the contents of my lungs, and twinkling stars overlaid the hazy, patriotic melee from where furious condemnation clamoured. The crowd parted as a third officer appeared with a silver-topped swagger stick tucked in military-style beneath his arm. The ornate crescent embellishing the shining black peak of his cap proclaimed his senior rank. Wire-rimmed spectacles shone as bright as the glare from behind the lenses as he put the silver tip beneath my nose. I registered the cold of the metal before he viciously thrust it upwards, forcing my head back against the wall.

"Not so bloody clever now, are we, sonny? What the fuck do you think you're playing at?"

A second silver-topped thrust electrified my head, and I cried out again, tears streaming down my furnace cheeks.

"Answer me when I ask you a question!"

The third, most violent jab made my head burst at the same time as the other officers forced my arms so far up my back that I was certain my joints would dislocate. I tried to escape the pain by rising onto tiptoe while the world undulated through my streaming eyes.

The senior officer leaned forwards, his breath hot and minty. An angry red nick on his swarthy chin showed where he'd cut himself shaving. "Look at me when I'm talking to you, you little bastard." Without moving his eyes from mine, he barked at the two officers, "All right, take him round there."

The crowd parted as they frogmarched me to a calm oasis outside a car repair garage. Covered in dark blue greasy overalls, a mechanic with a black Zapata moustache emerged from the gaping open mouth of a car bonnet, grabbed a grubby rag from the top of the radiator, and rubbed his oily hands.

"What's he been up to then, mate?"

The coppers ignored him and subjected me to a barrage of rapid-fire questions, my answers noted in a black notebook. Name. Date of birth. Address. School.

"Who's at home?"

"Nobody. My dad doesn't get in from work till six."

"Mother? I suppose she's at work as well?"

The mechanic withdrew a dipstick from the car engine, examined it, then winked at me as he stuck two fingers up behind the policemen.

"Well? Is she? Is she out at work as well?"

I stared at my baseball boots. The rubber edging had perished and was separating from the black canvas. I'd have to get Dad to put some Evo-Stik onto it when I got home. He'd moved it from the shed and hidden it shortly after he walked in on me playing The Ramones song, "Now I Wanna Sniff Some Glue."

"Answer me!"

"She's not there. She's nowhere. She died when I was eight, okay?"

The festering, filthy abscess trapping six years of black, corroding poison finally burst, spurting a torrent of furious resentment. "She had breast cancer, and it ate her up, and she had to have her tits chopped off to make her better, but she still died, okay? She still fucking *DIED*."

I despised the stupid tears that rolled down my face and the sobs that contorted my body. But most of all I loathed myself for using such disgustingly crude words about my beautiful mam. But what she had endured in hospital turned her lovely life ugly and rotten, and it shouldn't have happened to her. Not to my mam. And for me, there was no ultimate release, no liberating sensation from my filthy verbal tantrum. Instead, shame shrouded my being for so viciously vocalizing the hateful truth through a mouthful of metaphorical broken glass. But I needed my pain to be someone else's responsibility, for it not to be mine anymore, for it not to be in my head every waking hour, forever tormenting me with its suffocating misery and always haunting my sleep.

"Oi!"

The taller policeman shoved my shoulder, and I stumbled backwards. My clammy palms connected with the side of a red Ford Cortina. The bonnet was open, and its engine, carburettor, and assorted wires lay on the tarmac like the greasy, eviscerated guts of a mechanical beast.

"Shut it, little boy. Just don't swear again. You're not big, you're not clever, and you're in enough trouble as it is."

He growled into the radio clipped to the front of his tunic and within a minute, a police car pulled up, its blue light flashing but no two-note sirens to draw further attention to my predicament. I was bundled into the back next to another officer as his companion slid into the front passenger seat. I stared at the back of his head, noting how his straight black hair fell over his collar. Dad wouldn't approve of that. Thank god he was at work.

The jab of a black serge-covered elbow in my neck jerked me back. "Do you realise just what you've done?"

I shrugged and blew out my disregard in a loud puff of bored bravado.

"You need to buck your ideas up, lad."

Through the window, puddles in the uneven ground were stained with oily spectrum swirls. The engine idled as they conferred with the control room via walkie talkie. The queen's visit had exceeded the anticipated disruption to the normal smooth running of the city; it would be a waste of manpower taking me to the police station. The final crackling message announced how I'd been let off the hook—for now.

Chucking Putty at the Queen

"We need all available officers on the street. Just take him home and leave a card for the parents. Someone will call round tomorrow evening to see them."

Them. There is no *them*. Weren't they listening? Or were they just trying to get a reaction so that they could punch me in the gut again?

The crowds lining the main road dissolved, returning home now that they'd had the thrill of their lifetime: a fleeting, tenuous connection with royalty. They gawped at the additional minor excitement of seeing the police car pull away from the small garage forecourt. When the driver shifted gears with a tortuous grating sound, my thoughts were already in overdrive. If the coppers wouldn't be able to see Dad until tomorrow, then I would have enough time to broach the subject with him, although what the hell I was going to tell him was a mystery as secure as the crown jewels were in the Tower of London.

The police car tyres screeched with the urgency of a chase from the television detective series *The Sweeney*, and we set off up the hill. The ear-popping ascent reminded me of when Dad took Nick and me to Blackpool for a week in August 1972. The afternoon sun blazed on the towering wooden structure of the Pleasure Beach rollercoaster, creating stark contrasts inside the latticework of vintage timber that creaked and groaned from the motion of the hurtling carriages. The screams of delighted terror from its passengers were enough to convince us that riding it was not for us. Instead, Dad suggested that we have a go on the more genteel log flume.

I tugged Dad's arm. "Bags me the back seat."

"Are you sure, Son? Wouldn't you rather sit at the front? You'll get a much better view."

"Oh, yeah. Okay, Dad."

We crammed into a hollow fibreglass tree trunk like the three bears: Dad at the back, Nick in the middle, and me at the front. Powered by a clunking, clanking mechanism, the imitation tree trunk struggled to the pinnacle. The screams from the nearby rollercoaster overpowered my own shrill squeal as we plunged freefall down the other side and through a pool of water, soaking me as thoroughly as Dad and Nick's laughter.

But now, as the police car reached the top of the hill and swooped down to the row of houses, laughter was the furthest thing from my mind.

Dad's car was parked in its usual place outside our back gate.

18

NO PITY

"Get out."

Rubber replaced my leg muscles as I struggled from the police car, watched by two young boys sitting on the kerb.

"Is he in trouble, mister?"

The policemen ignored them and shoved me towards the gate. I could see Dad framed in the kitchen window, his tie thrown over his shoulder as he looked down, engrossed in activity. I bet he was washing soil from the new spuds from Tim's allotment or maybe top-and-tailing the young kidney beans that grew up the side of the shed. Or he could be shelling the peas we'd bought on the market, even though that was my job. At the old house on a Sunday morning, my backside became numb as I sat on the kitchen doorstep with Mam above me, perched on a stool, shelling peas together whilst she hummed an old tune. She'd always laugh and tell me that I was eating more peas than I was putting into the colander, and our session wouldn't be complete without her telling me to open my mouth before she attempted to toss a pea in from her elevated position. I'd give anything for that happiness to be my reality now, but I couldn't undo what I'd just done. I bit my bottom lip between my teeth until I tasted blood and kept my eyelids stretched wide. Just one blink would release the pressure of the tears that threatened to pop my eyeballs from their sockets.

The latch clunked, and Dad raised his head. I kept my vision adhered to the cement path as I was jostled down the yard.

"What the bladdy hell's going on?"

I looked up. Bordered by the white frame of the open door in a snapshot of outrage and confusion, Dad flipped his tie from his shoulder and tightened the knot.

One of the policemen cleared his throat. "Is this boy your son, sir?"

"Yes, of course he's my son. What's happened?"

A hand tightened on my bicep, and the gentle scent of the sweet peas that wove through the slatted fence couldn't beautify this ugly moment in my life. My misdemeanour had brought an anarchy which violated the slow tempo of the afternoon. The goldfish swam aimlessly in the tranquil pond beneath the luscious green leaves of what Dad had named the "Minor Oak" that we'd grown from the acorn that Mam and I collected in the woods. My tortoise, Oscar, munched on the remnants of a slice of melon that Tim put down for him a couple of days earlier. I was a stranger intruding into this tableau of comforting normality and couldn't bear to look at Dad.

The grip tightened on my arm. "Explain to your father just what you've been up to this afternoon."

"What are you doing home?" I asked.

"It's a good job I am. What's going on?"

"Be a good little boy and tell Daddy what game you've been playing." The policeman squeezed ever more forcefully.

"I chucked putty at the queen," I mumbled, too quietly for anyone to hear.

"Look your father in the eye and tell him."

"I chucked putty at the queen."

Dad's face coloured the deep elderberry of the wine fermenting in a demijohn on the kitchen windowsill. "You did *what?*"

The pressure of the copper's grip increased. "Louder!"

"I chucked putty at the queen, okay?" The confrontational tone of my confession was followed by my gabbled justification. "But at least I'm not like Nick and Steve, drinking and smoking and gambling and stealing from people."

Dad churned his mouth as if he were trying to shift an obstruction in his teeth. "You chucked putty at the queen."

His calmness was unnerving. He might as well have suggested us having a nice cup of tea. I remembered him telling me of the night Mam died. He stayed up by the coal fire, with a glass of beer and a bowl of peanuts at his side as he waited for the inevitable knock on the door. When it happened—he described it as if the person on the other side of the door didn't want to announce their presence to the rest of Lamartine Street—he still jumped. He opened the door to a fresh-faced rookie constable who announced that he had very bad news, and his pale cheeks flushed when he awkwardly revealed that it was the first time he'd undertaken this duty.

Chucking Putty at the Queen

Dad invited him in and poured him a glass of his homemade beer. The new officer at first hesitated to accept the offer, but Dad reassured him that he was friendly with the sergeant at the small police station on the edge of the park, and he knew that he wouldn't mind just this once. When the young officer had finished his drink and was leaving, he shook Dad's hand and thanked him for making a procedure he'd been dreading into an easier experience. Had Dad faced other traumatic events with such composure? It wouldn't have surprised me because he never raised his voice in anger, and he'd never lifted his hand to any of us in violence. But when I looked up at him, his eyes glared his displeasure.

"Yeah, but *they* punched me in the stomach." My head jerked sideways, almost dislodging my plastic bag Union Jack headwear. "And they swore; they used the F word."

"Why the hell would you do such a disgraceful thing? This is not how I've brought you up."

"Because there's no future. It's a fascist regime," I said, trying to maintain my punk-influenced bravado. The last time I'd seen Dad's face resemble one of the monumental stone heads on Easter Island was in the headmaster's study at school when he'd warned that he'd go to the police unless the bullying campaign against me was stopped. Now, the usual twinkle in his eyes was gone when he turned a frightening granite glare upon me.

"And what do *you* know about fascism, Son? I fought the Nazis when I was a tail gunner in the RAF. I was shot down and still returned to fight as soon as I was able. Don't you *dare* to try and tell *me* about fascism. You're only fifteen. You don't know anything about it. Do not have the audacity to insult me nor the millions of innocent people who died and those who fought to give you the freedoms you enjoy by telling me that it's a fascist regime. I've never heard such utter bullshit."

He threw his head back and fiercely blew through his pursed lips. When he looked at me again I knew that for as long as I lived, I'd never be able to unsee his expression.

"And from *you* of all people. I thought that you had more common sense than to engage is such bladdy tomfoolery. What the hell do you think you're playing at? God knows I've tried my best since your mother died. That chump in the pub told me, 'You're brave, Sid, keeping that youngest. I'd have put him into a care home.' Well, I'm not brave. I love you, and I've tried my hardest to raise you how your mother and I decided was the right way."

I couldn't bear it. "Please, Dad, stop." He'd never told me off like this before, and my humiliating, bitter tears ran freely. I was eight again and needed him to hug me, to reassure me that everything was all right, just as he had when Mam died. The steel bands of police fingers on my arm relaxed, and I stepped forwards to Dad, desperate for him to wrap his arms around me.

"Don't."

I stopped dead in my tracks, and my mind again whiplashed back to that hateful Sunday morning when he spurned Steve's insincere, open-armed advance. His same one-word rebuke was a bullet to my chest. If only it had been a genuine gunshot to end my gut-wrenching misery. He'd just rejected me for the first time in my life. "Dad..."

"What happens now?"

"Fortunately, sir, there was no damage done. We intercepted and restrained him before Her Majesty was within his range." His grip tightened on my bicep once more. "He's not a very good thrower."

"I hate sports," I mumbled.

The officer shoved my shoulder. "He hasn't been arrested, and the superintendent says there will be no charges pressed. It will just be a caution. But I suggest that you have a serious word with your son about his attitude and all of this rubbish." He flicked my homemade shirt.

"Simon. Apologise."

"I'm sorry." I mournfully stared once more at the orange fish swimming languorously in the pond where, in the oppressive late-night heat of the previous summer, Dad and I had sat side by side in our pyjamas on the dining chairs we'd taken outside, him with a glass of beer and me with a glass of pop, and enjoyed the silence as we cooled our feet in the soothing water. I would've done anything to turn back the clock to the innocence of that heavenly night.

"Simon. You're apologising to the goldfish. Look the officers in the eyes and apologise properly."

The crystal pool sparkled, multiplying through my tears. "I'm sorry."

"Apology *not* accepted. You need to have a long hard look at yourself, young man, or you'll end up in big trouble. How does a spell in Borstal sound?"

Chucking Putty at the Queen

I'd really messed up, but it was going to get worse.

Dad stood to one side. "Simon. Inside. Now."

When I made an ungainly attempt to slip past him, he cuffed the top of my head with the tips of his fingers, causing the knotted Union Jack polythene bag to slip from my head. My wonderful Dad had never hit me before. My world was ending. Clutching the artificial handkerchief, I was two steps away from the door into the hall before Dad put the brakes on my progress.

"Stop! What the bladdy hell have you got on your hair?"

"Um, Vaseline and curry powder."

"Vaseline and curry powder!"

"Yeah, I wanted orange hair like Johnny Rotten, and I knew you wouldn't let me dye it, so I used that curry powder Tim bought on the market. I thought it'd work."

He gestured to my old bobble hat which lay sodden on the draining board, copper-tinged suds glistening in the threads. "I found this in the bathroom. Has it got anything to do with it?"

Recklessly pleased with my coiffure innovation, I said, "Oh, yeah! I covered my hair with curry powder and Vaseline and put the hat on and pulled my hair through the weave, then when I tugged it off, my hair went all spiky just like Johnny Rotten's."

Dad's hands flew towards the ceiling. "You used curry powder to colour your hair orange because you wanted to look like Johnny bladdy Rotten?" His sigh seemed as if he'd bottled it up for years. "You know, son, I preferred it when you made crêpe paper wigs because you wanted to look like Marc Bolan."

I hoped that his wry remark was a signal of his forgiveness.

He squeezed the bridge of his nose and sighed. "Your mother knitted that hat for you; it was the last thing she knitted before she became ill. She'd be heartbroken if she were alive to see you using it so disrespectfully."

The words crumpled my insides as surely as if he'd punched me in the guts.

"I'll talk to you later but first, go and wash that muck off." He rubbed his temples with the forefingers of each hand and shook his head. "Bladdy Vaseline and curry powder."

Standing in the kitchen, with his crisp shirt starkly white against the black police uniforms, I was overwhelmed again by the terrifying sensation of not being there, of being disconnected and floating, of observing instead of being involved. My lungs strained with a similar tension to the first time I'd dropped from the highest diving board at Carrington Lido when I was younger. I'd plummeted deeper and deeper, holding my breath, and fearing that I would never rise to the surface.

Dad's words excavated memories that were never totally buried. Mam had taken me to the barber Edgar Wood for my regular short back and sides. The jovial haircutter had slicked my cut with Brylcreem, but as soon as we'd returned home, Mam told me she was going to "wash that muck off" and vigorously cleaned the greasy hair preparation from my smart coiffure.

But whatever was going to happen now, Dad had still called me son. I clasped that one word as if it were an olive branch indicating that he still loved me, and I hoped that I'd not completely blown it by rewarding his love and compassion with bad behaviour. My quivering contrition told me that I couldn't be a particularly good punk rocker if I allowed myself to be so emotionally devastated.

To my surprise, the open living room door showed the table laid with two plates of artfully arranged triangular sandwiches. The faceted points of the cut glass jug glowed pineapple yellow beside a Victoria sponge. The sugared fruit on top glittered like the sequins I'd sewn and stuck to create my glamorous couture before punk rock relegated it to the sartorial history bin. What was going on? And why was Dad home from work early?

In the bathroom, I leaned towards the open window. The blackbird that Dad always called "our blackbird" sang deliciously fluid notes from the top of the shed as the voices beneath me easily carried upwards with the intoxicating fragrance of early honeysuckle and sweet peas.

"Is that your vehicle parked outside, sir?"

Oh god, what now? Were they going to do Dad for a car-related crime? But instead, they started discussing Dad's Rover as if they were old friends from a car appreciation society. When Dad proudly introduced the subject of his prized Alvis Firefly, I knew that he'd pulled his wallet from his back pocket and was showing them the photograph of him standing beside it in a country lane. I wouldn't have been surprised to hear their jaws hitting the floor with awe.

"I'm very sorry for all the trouble Simon has caused and appreciate your lenient approach." Dad's tone was apologetic but not weak.

One of the policemen cleared his throat. "We understand that there are exceptional circumstances. When we questioned him, he became very agitated and said that his mother died some years ago."

"Yes, six years ago. Simon was eight."

"That must have been difficult for both you and him."

Hang on a minute. Was this the copper that only half an hour earlier had called me a fucking piece of shit? Or was it his comrade who'd punched me in the gut? I pressed closer to the gap to hear Dad's reply.

"I don't understand it. He's never given me any trouble until this. He's not like other boys and doesn't rag around the streets causing trouble. He's a real home bird: mad about music, writing, reading, and art. He's highly creative and designs his own gear... But as you can see, he's become terribly crippled. We have an appointment in a few days to see an orthopaedic consultant at the General Hospital."

"With respect, sir, that's no excuse for his actions."

"I'm not making excuses, merely trying to explain that there has been a lot of mental disruption for Simon since his mother died. I only very recently learned that he's been the victim of a sustained and prolonged campaign of bullying at school."

The officer gave a sardonic chuckle. "Looking at his appearance, is he very impressionable? My uncle was a Teddy Boy; he's often told me about them slashing the seats when *Rock Around The Clock* was on at the pictures."

Dad gave one of his snorts. "Teddy Boys. Uncouth rabble. I suppose punk rock is just the modern equivalent for Simon."

They were becoming so pally that I half expected Dad to invite them in for a cup of tea and some of the cake and sandwiches on the table downstairs.

The policeman gave a discreet cough as if he were about to give evidence in court. "You know, sir, there are professional organisations who can help you if you're finding things too hard to cope with."

"Certainly not. I won't have a do-gooder poking their nose in. He's sixteen next year. I've managed since he was eight, and I'm buggered if I'm going to give up on him now."

Although I couldn't see it, I knew that his shoulders would be back, his chest thrust forwards, and he would be twisting the ends of his handlebar

moustache.
"Well, just keep an eye on him, sir. He's incredibly lucky that he's only had a warning."
"Thank you. I'll ensure that nothing of this nature happens again."
"Then in that case, we'll bid you good afternoon."
The back gate latch clicked, the police car doors slammed, and by moving my head as low as I could and slightly to the left, I saw the inevitable gaggle of local women standing in their slippers, arms folded, watching intently as the police car drove away.
I twisted the hot tap. Steaming water splurged into the sink as I grabbed Tim's Vosene and shampooed away the sticky, smelly gunk coating my hair, relieved to be free from the itching that my dubiously inventive hair colourant had provoked. Whilst the turmeric liquid spiralled down the drain, I towelled my hair with the cloth Dad used for mopping the tiles around the toilet pedestal, as Tim and Nick frequently missed the bowl when they'd been out on the beer. I didn't deserve a nice clean towel. A disgusting old rag would be my punishment for subjecting Dad to such embarrassment.

19

CRY LIKE A BABY

As I had back in March, I sat on the edge of my bed and stared out of the window. Dad entered and sat next to me. "Sorry, Dad."

He'd never been really cross with me before, only mildly irked. He never hit or used his leather belt on any of us, nor did he rant and rave in anger. In return, we respected him and didn't overstep the unseen, yet understood, mark. Apart from Steve, whose teenage criminal career was a different kettle of fish. Although my performance earlier was in a superbly different league to any of my previous misdemeanours—for example, my attempt to jump down the stairs from top to bottom at the old house, or falling into the clay-lined, water-filled gully in the woods after he'd specifically told me not to play there—Dad always chose diplomacy and gentle debate over violence.

He leaned forwards and slid a hardback from the bookshelf that Tim made to fit under the window. It was a cherished book from my younger years, which I'd heard narrated on the children's BBC story-telling program, *Jackanory*. As always, it was effortless to change my mental gears and reverse a few years. I closed my eyes. The weight on the bed next to me wasn't Dad, but Mam. I sat beside her on the old settee after she'd collected me from school, and together we ate blackberry jam sandwiches as we listened to that day's instalment of the charming tale.

"*The Hartwarp Light Railway.*"

Dad's words forced my eyelids apart, just as a puff from his pursed lips dispatched millions of dust sprites from the top of the book, churning like the smoke from the railway engine in the story. He sighed. "It seems a long time since we bought this, Son. Do you remember that village fete?"

Of course I remembered the sun-kissed afternoon in that emotionally tumultuous summer the year Mam died, when it was just Dad and I meandering around the Lincolnshire countryside in his dependable black Rover. We'd spied the hand painted sign at the same time: *Village Fete. Church Field. 2 p.m.*

Dad bumped the car onto the shaggy green verge outside the Crown & Mitre pub opposite the church, instantly releasing the fragrance of bruised grass into the hot air. The jolly activities were well under way in the lush paddock, its boundaries bedecked with waves of dangling triangular flags made of what appeared to be scraps of old floral frocks. A gentle breeze undulated the flap of a white canvas marquee, outside which a donkey was tethered to a wooden post, its erect hairy ears spiking through holes made in a dishevelled straw hat adorned with pink dog roses. Nearby, a sign advertised the location of the cream teas that, despite the country now being in the modern age of monetary decimalization, quaintly cost one shilling instead of five new pence, with all proceeds in aid of the church spire repair fund. I smiled and was about to comment on the refusal to embrace progression when my eyes alighted on a decorating table laden with paperbacks and hardbacks. Another notice advised that the income generated from their sale was also to benefit the spire repair fund.

"Look, Dad: a book sale!" I began to scrutinize the titles. To my incredulity, amongst them was *The Hartwarp Light Railway*, the story that Mam and I had listened to on *Jackanory*. With the volume firmly in my grasp, creating a connection between Mam and the present moment, I revelled in the serenity of this countryside world that was straight from the pages of one of my Enid Blyton books and as far away from our busy, factory smoke-choked city environment as the earth was from the moon. I wouldn't have been at all shocked to see the *Five Find-Outers and Dog* sitting with a picnic hamper in the shade of the magnificent horse chestnut tree.

A lugubrious vicar left a gaggle of women and reverentially approached Dad.

"Excuse me, sir." He doffed his cream-coloured Panama hat. "I wonder if you would do us the honour of judging the Dog with The Waggiest Tail competition?"

With his handlebar moustache and dressed in a dark green tweed hacking jacket, charcoal grey trousers, and sturdy brown brogues, Dad looked more like the local squire than a man born and raised in the tough two-up, two-down environs of St. Ann's. Succumbing to the blissful escapism of the afternoon, I tucked my book under my arm and laughed and clapped when he presented first prize of an enormous bone wrapped with a red ribbon to an overweight dachshund. Dad was always sketching and upon our return home, the point of his pencil flew across a folded sheet of white paper as he captured the encounter for me, and later, I pinned it to the side of the bed.

Six years on from that magical day, Dad returned the tatty hardback to the bookshelf. "It was a lovely afternoon, wasn't it, Son? I know it's a cliché, but it was so quintessentially English."

Enmeshed in mellow reminiscing, I lost my caution. "Yeah, it was very posh. I half expected to see a horse-drawn golden carriage arrive carrying the queen—" Too late. In an unconscious act of self-sabotage, I'd conveniently handed Dad his opening.

"Yes, Son. The queen. I don't know what the bladdy hell you were thinking about. The thing is that if you do away with the royal family and standards, what do you replace them with? You've stencilled 'chaos' and 'anarchy' on the arms of your shirt, but your own life has been chaotic ever since your mother died." He looked down at his watch and fiddled with the metallic expandable strap. "Now you're suffering with your leg injury, and believe me, Son, if I could take that from you and have it myself, I'd do it like a shot. Then there's the bullying you've endured at school. Don't you think that there's been enough anarchy and chaos in your life already? Wouldn't you prefer a calmer one?"

I hoped that his reasonable words indicated the end of this speech and I'd be able to release my tensed muscles. Despite him telling me how angry he was, he laid his arm across my shoulders just as he had when I'd arrived home from school earlier in the year, bloodied and bruised after being beaten up again. The memories of what we'd been through together raced through my mind, making my wretchedness lump in my throat.

"I know how utterly unbearable the past few years have been for you, and that you're growing up, Son, and finding your own feet. That's understandable. And natural. I've tried my best ever since your mother's death." He paused as if uncertain whether to continue and reached forward with his left forefinger to press the spine of the book until it was neatly aligned with its companions. "You don't know how much I wish that she was here to share watching you grow up."

I didn't dare to look at him.

"You know that I work every day. I go in from seven until ten each

Saturday and Sunday to earn the overtime. Sometimes I accept it in my wage packet to pay the bills and run the car, and other times I let it accrue so that I can have the odd day off to spend with you in the school holidays and take you out to the countryside. I managed to come home early as a surprise for you. Apart from Jacqui, you haven't really got any pals. You're having a rotten time with your leg, and I know that you're worrying about seeing the consultant. I thought it would be nice to make you a lovely silver Jubilee tea." He removed his arm from my shoulder. "And now you've ruined it."

He stood up and with his weight removed, my part of the mattress lowered.

"You know that unlike a lot of fathers, I never hit or shouted at any of you, and I'm not about to start now." He tugged his neatly folded handkerchief from his pocket and handed it to me. "Come on, Son. Wipe your tears, and let's have some tea."

His emotionless tone was more disconcerting than if it was loaded with anger. We had a unique bond, and I adored our unshakeable closeness, but he'd never been so remote with me before, and I was terrified that our relationship was irrevocably altered. I remembered a face distorted with religious fervour. "Change coming soon." Could Dad's detachment be the change that the crazy woman at the door prophesied? I dabbed my hot face, soothed by the condensed smell of him trapped in the soft cotton, and reluctantly handed it back, even though I wanted to keep it so that his essence would be easy to access when he wasn't there.

At the door, he stopped but didn't turn around. He tapped the poster of a leering Johnny Rotten that covered most of the dark, laminated wood, and harrumphed. "We shall say no more about your egregious behaviour but know that I expected better from you of all people."

It was then that he turned around. His anguished expression made me wish that he hadn't because it told me that, for the first time, Dad wasn't on my side.

"For Christ's sake, you could have been arrested and tried for treason! You've let me down, Son."

His words made me wish I'd succeeded in suffocating myself back in March.

Although he was no great drinker, Dad went to the pub earlier than usual that evening, which I knew was an indication of his annoyance with me. To try and fool myself that I wasn't really bothered, I acted on my urgency to create a commemorative royal visit edition of *Sniper*. The barrel of my typewriter was soon wrapped with a new sheet of paper, and the stereo loaded with some of my growing collection of punk singles.

Yet something was wrong. I rested my hands on the table and stared out into the garden. During the past half an hour, a gentle breeze had gradually dispersed the metallic sheets of cloud that clamped down the oppressive stickiness of the day, revealing the descending twilight in a celestial palette spectacularly streaked with amber, lilac, and violet. I leaned forward and peered through the lower branches of the mountain ash, already blackened by their own shadows, my strained senses fragrantly soothed by the delicate scent of the tobacco plants whose buttery trumpets nodded gently beneath the open window. My tortoise pottered towards the small wooden shack that Tim had built for him and placed beneath the marrow leaves that were already the size of elephant ears. Oscar had finished feasting upon the coral pink melon flesh and now all that remained was the white rind in a luminous Cheshire cat grin against the sage shadows.

In our first spring here at the new house, Dad had paid for a lawn to be laid, but when the men left in their ten-ton wagon, an ugly manhole cover remained visible in its square concrete surround. He hated this unsightly blemish, and with the help of one of Tim's mates who worked on the roads, he obtained foot-long lengths of kerb edging. Following judicious chipping with his mortar chisel, Dad created what he called "Simon's Fairy Steps." These camouflaged the manhole cover and forged a link from the grassed strip beneath the back window to the small lawn. Above those grey stony lengths, the white blooms of the Iceberg rose bush floated, and through their prickly stalks, the nearby stretched squares of celluloid that Dad had substituted for glass on the greenhouse reflected me in a gallery of distorted, grotesque portraits. I glanced over at the square Art Deco mirror which gave a true reflection of my unblemished fifteen-year-old face. I'd recently read Oscar Wilde's *The Picture of Dorian Gray* and ridiculously imagined my insubordinate actions being supernaturally transposed onto the panes of the greenhouse. Drowning in my fanciful contemplation, I recoiled when a furry brown moth fluttered against the windowpane, drawn to the glow that pooled upon my typewriter from beneath the velvet shade of a standard lamp, its frilled ornamentation hanging in a circle of cerise thistle flowers.

In an attempt to dispel my despondency and to fortify the dam restraining my tears, I swigged from a bottle of pineapple pop, pretending that it was the cider that the London punks got drunk on, and revisited my afternoon. Come on! I'd chucked putty at the queen and been taken home in a police car. That really was a headline worthy of the Sex Pistols.

The last record slid down the silver metal spindle. Appropriately it was "God Save The Queen," the official anthem to my afternoon of delinquency. I joined in with Johnny Rotten's final, desperate howl that there was no future, the very assertion that I'd furiously yelled a few hours earlier. But when I tentatively walked my fingertips across the bump on the back of my head from where the copper had bashed it against the wall, the memory of Dad's expression when I walked down the yard rendered my punk demonstration as worthless as a bunch of flowers in a dustbin. What I'd done wouldn't bring Mam back or cure my leg injury, nor would it stop me being bullied at school.

The strength of my remorse was brutal and unforgiving. I buried my burning face in my hands and sobbed. Dad had done everything possible to make me happy after Mam's death, and his judgement that afternoon tore my heart apart as ferociously as the rips I'd deliberately made in my shirt.

"You let me down, Son."

I'd never forgive myself.

20

YOU CAN'T PUT YOUR ARMS AROUND A MEMORY

THE FREQUENTLY UNRELIABLE WEATHER forecasters were finally vindicated for the final New Year's Eve of the 1970s. Borne of freezing, mournfully whistling northerly winds, sleet covered the roofs of the houses opposite ours in the wrinkled lines of an old man's forehead. Beneath them, necklaces of sparkling icicles dangled from grey plastic guttering. Unlike the narrow Victorian casement windows of the back-to-back houses round our old way, the spacious new homes boasted five feet square panes of gin-clear, beautifully unrippled glass. As Christmas approached, householders used lengths of masking tape to dissect these into smaller portions, then sprayed the corners with swathes of aerosol snow, instantly transforming the rows of modern houses into a simulated wintery Dickensian scene.

Within the fuzzy bloom from the sodium streetlight, snowflakes turned into billions of orange nasturtium petals falling onto two figures as they navigated the slippery path with the cautiousness of tightrope walkers. In these challenging conditions, the slope outside our house was an irresistible attraction to local kids who created a perilous slide from top to bottom. Screams and yells split the freezing air as they whizzed past, their backsides protected by ripped rectangles of old lino or squares of flattened cardboard boxes. Eventually these impromptu sledges compressed the snow until it was as treacherous as a bobsleigh run. Unkempt tussocks of grass at the edge of a lawn looked like a procession of albino hedgehogs, and the heels of a woman's black stilettoes disappeared amongst them as she tried to avoid stepping on the slide. I watched her struggle for balance as she negotiated the serpentine lower part of the walkway, her snow-laden brolly resembling a huge coconut macaroon. I'd have to confront this wintry assault course if I went down to the pub later for the celebrations. Such doleful conditions were an appropriate way to end a decade that had begun so tragically for our family when cerebral haemorrhage delivered my paternal grandmother to her grave.

My mind easily slid back to that dry Wednesday afternoon in September 1970. The earthy sweetness of autumn was detectable on the soft breeze flapping the sheets that Mam pegged out in our narrow back yard. Monday was traditionally her washing day, but when we'd parted at the school gates that morning, the fatigue that had recently added shadows beneath her eyes, and a dryness to her soft cheeks was replaced with an optimistic smile as she sniffed the air.

"I'll pull the dolly tub out and get a wash done. It's such a lovely drying day."

Our weekday routine was reassuringly changeless. At midday, Mam met me at school and walked me home for my dinner. Sitting at the table, the scent of carbolic soap rose from my freshly washed hands as she ladled chunks of kidneys and beef onto my plate from the casserole pot. Movement beyond the net curtains caught my eye. The chair's aged wooden joints creaked when I pivoted backwards on two legs to better see the billowing sails of a seafaring galleon down the yard. I loved this unexpected extra laundry day and couldn't wait for bedtime, with its fragrance of boil-washed bedding brought in from the line and aired over the clothes horse in front of the coal fire. When I leaned back even further, Mam hovered the ladle over the casserole pot, droplets of glutinous gravy plopping back into its depths.

"All four feet of the chair on the floor, please."

"Sorry, Mam." I knew that she wasn't really cross with me when she gave me one of her comedy looks of reproach, the one where her eyebrows almost vanished into her hairline, and her eyes resembled gobstoppers.

After my pudding of apple pie with custard—made nice and thick just how I loved it—Mam stood at the bottom of the stairs swinging my duffel coat by its hood like a pendulum marking the seconds until I had to return to school.

"Aw, Mam, do I have to? I can't move, I'm podged." As always, going back to lessons was exasperating, because I was cosy at home with her. However, my protestations were half-hearted. On this day, the afternoon curriculum was my favourite: reading aloud, followed by painting. When Mam waved me goodbye from the black-glossed gates, I pranced up the steps in anticipation of dipping my brush into the bright, primary-coloured powder paints, and then transferring them onto the pastures of green, brown, and ochre sugar paper. When Mam returned at four

Chucking Putty at the Queen

o'clock, I presented her with my still-moist vivid daubs that depicted her surrounded by fantastical red tulips as she hung out the washing, bathed in dazzling canary yellow sunshine.

"There's more paint on you than on the paper." Mam chuckled and winked at my class teacher, Mrs Kirby, who stood at the gates.

"I managed to get as much as I could from his hair and jumper, Mrs Smalley. Simon's a very energetic painter."

With Mam carefully carrying my artwork as if it were an undiscovered Rembrandt, we walked homewards through the park beneath trees already blemished with the first autumnal hues of oxidised iron. Unexpectedly, she suggested that we sit for a minute on one of the low wooden benches painted in council green and scarred with gouged initials and love hearts speared by arrows. What was up? We never sat on our way home, not ever, because I was always in a hurry to get to my sandwiches and glass of milk. As we rested beneath the towering limes and sycamores, it was obvious that tiredness had replaced her exuberance of the morning. A trio of yelling boys hurtled down the path leading towards the iron dome of the drinking fountain.

Mam rested my painting across her lap and pulled me close to her. "You know how your gran's been poorly since she had her falls, and you remember when your dad and Uncle Bill had to move her bed downstairs."

She was telling me rather than asking me, but how could I forget the great adventure when Gran's new, unusual sleeping arrangement happened. Dad and my uncle struggled down the narrow staircase with the mattress and components of the dismantled Victorian iron bed.

Dad missed a step, and the bed frame shuddered. "Hold on, Bill, my fingers are trapped."

With a shaky hand, Gran removed her tortoiseshell-framed spectacles and clamped the other hand over her eyes, complaining that it was a right palaver. I cheekily sang the opening verse of Bernard Cribbins's novelty song "Right Said Fred," one of my favourites on *Junior Choice*, the weekend radio program hosted by Ed "Stewpot" Stewart.

"Oh, you are a torment," Gran moaned, not for the first time. "If you don't give over, I'll lock you in the coalhole with Jimmy."

She turned and shuffled carefully into her back parlour as I froze, once more instantly terrified of her never seen underground prisoner.

Sitting with Mam on the park bench, I watched the progress of a magnificently craggy mountain range of cloud as it slowly obscured the sun and robbed the air of warmth. Across the park, through the gnarly tree trunks and skeletal metal posts supporting the swing boats, my school was a foreboding silhouette.

Mam sniffed the air just as she had that morning at the school gates. "It's getting very Goose Fair-ish."

Her use of the local vernacular was a definite sign of the year advancing, when the vibrantly ornamented fairground rides and sideshows congregated on Nottingham for the first Thursday, Friday, and Saturday of October.

With a violent trumpeting, she blew her nose into a tissue, scrunched it into a snowball, and dropped it into the wire waste bin next to the bench. "I'm sorry, my lad, there's no easy way to tell you this, but you see..." She breathed in deeply as if she were about to sneeze. "Your gran died today."

Minuscule whirlwinds of dry grey powder swirled around the paths, and I thought of the framed photo of the grandad I'd never known that stood on the mantlepiece in Gran's darkened front room. She'd always kept the heavy aubergine velvet curtains half-closed as a mark of respect and to demonstrate her devoted mourning. The majestic cloud had continued its course, gradually revealing the sun which pushed the charcoal shadows of the trees further towards us over the dry, cropped grass, almost reaching the toes of my shoes that once belonged to Florrie Dewhurst's grandson. When I inherited the smart footwear, Nick gleefully told me that I was wearing "dead boy shoes" as the lad had been run over by a lorry, which I soon learned was an untruth. Recently, next door's ancient ginger tom was found dead behind a dustbin in the back entry, and two of Gran's oldest friends, Elsie and Martha, had died within a week of each other. Mam just told me that Gran was also dead. I wriggled with discomfort not only from the hardness of the wooden seat but also from the melodramatic thought that the shadow of death was encroaching into my life as quickly as the shadows of the trees. "But–"

"Yes?"

I scratched my scalp as the three noisy boys charged from the water fountain towards the swings. "Gran was Dad's mam, so does this make him an orphan?"

Mam smoothed my hair with the palm of her hand. "That's an odd

Chucking Putty at the Queen

thing to say, but yes, I suppose he is."

I noticed that the toes of my shoes were scuffed, so tucked my feet beneath the seat. I didn't want Mam to see them and tell me off. "Poor Dad, not having a mam."

When she kissed the top of my head, I thought how lucky I was to have such a loving mother.

"Come on, it's teatime. I've made you and Nick a special treat."

I daintily nibbled all the crusts from my fish paste and cucumber sandwiches and thought about Gran's death. Mam and Dad weren't religious and wouldn't disguise the truth with nonsensical stories about her going to meet Jesus. Nor would they tell us that she was now an angel living on a cloud in heaven. I reached across the table to the plate laden with slices of moist malt loaf so dark that the butter on top glowed like strips of gold leaf. The net curtain darkened as thunder rumbled. I tensed as many muscles in my body as I could in delicious anticipation of a storm and flashed a look at Nick who was, as usual, gobbling his tea.

Despite the solemnity of Mam's news, I still giggled when I remembered how in a thunderstorm, Gran would urgently turn all her pictures and mirrors to face the wall, scared that lightning would come through the window, ricochet from the glass, and strike her dead. Once, she'd been so frightened during a ferocious tempest that I'd sat with her beneath the table in her parlour. She pulled the white linen cloth until it almost touched the carpet and in the makeshift shelter, I held her trembling hand as she whimpered that the weather would kill her. Now she really was dead.

Nick had wolfed his tea and leaned forward, eyeing my remaining malt loaf.

"Get lost." I quickly squished it, crammed it into my mouth, and breathed noisily through my nostrils, struggling for air as I chewed the succulent slice.

He slapped the back of my head. "Mam, can I get down from the table?"

She was washing up with her back turned to us. "Yes," she called without looking round. "And it's '*may* I get down,' not '*can* I get down.' You're the boy at grammar school, you should know that."

Nick stuck out his tongue, then stepped over to her chair under the window. For a few seconds, he knelt on the saggy cushion and peered through a gap where the net curtain didn't quite meet the turquoise window frame. His knees left a deep imprint in the cushion when he got off and moved to the kitchen doorway.

"Mam, do me a favour."

"Do you a favour? What's that then?"

"Can I tell Dad that Gran's dead?"

Mam came to the door, wiping her hands on a tea towel. "I don't believe you. Can you tell your father that his mother has died? Certainly not. *I'll* be the one to tell him, not you."

Nick scratched at the paint around the slim panel of aluminium Dad had screwed to the door to prevent grubby fingerprints discolouring the area around the handle. "Do you think he'll be upset?"

"Do I think he'll be upset? For Christ's sake, she was his mother. What do you think?" She swatted his hand away from the door. "And don't pick at that; your dad's just painted it."

Nick frowned. "Do you think he'll cry?"

Mam shook her head. "Sometimes I wonder about you, I really do. Will *you* cry when *I'm* gone?"

I clumsily slid from my seat and threw my arms around her waist. "Don't say that, Mam, please! You mustn't."

She squeezed me tightly. "Shush now. I'm not going anywhere in a hurry." The back gate latch clicked. "Here's your dad now." She gave Nick one of her looks. "Not a word, you. This is my job. Take Simon into the front room." She stepped into the kitchen and pulled the door closed.

Nick ordered my silence by putting a forefinger to his lips. He pressed his ear against the door, frowning with concentration as he tried to eavesdrop. I squeezed away into the opposite corner by the coalhole. I'd never hear Gran's mischievous threat about Jimmy again.

Nick tiptoed over to me. "I can't hear a single word."

Through the misty veil of the net curtain, we watched Dad pace to the outside lavatory. Nick cupped his hands around my left ear.

"Come on, let's go and listen. I bet you anything in the world that he's crying."

The thought of my strong, dependable father crying in the toilet was an image that I couldn't bear to visualise, and when Nick tugged me towards the kitchen, I twisted free from his grasp seconds before he pulled the door open. The meagre daylight from the small window glowed on the kettle sitting atop the cooker, highlighting the crater in its red metallic surface from when Steve had clouted Tim over the head with it years earlier.

Mam turned from the sink and, with her hand sparkling with washing-up liquid bubbles, grabbed the sleeve of Nick's school jumper, stretching the thin navy-blue wool as he tried to wriggle free. "And where do you think you're off to?"

"The loo."

"Your dad's in."

"I know. I don't need to *go*. I just want to see if I can hear him crying."

Mam's hand whizzed across the top of his head in more of a karate chop than a slap, and she shoved his shoulder. "Get back in there now, and let's have no more of your nastiness." Her push propelled him towards the living room. "Go on, get in." With damp fingers, she swept back a snake of hair that had wriggled from her slide. "I really do wonder about you at times, Nicholas."

Nick barged past me, and as I followed into the back room, I counted his heavy footfall upon the stairs. My bare knees slotted into the indents left by his on the saggy cushion in Mam's chair. I rested my arms across the back and pressed my chin into the prickly weave of my cardigan sleeves. As soon as Dad emerged from the toilet, I scuttled into the front room. Replicating my earlier kneeling position on the heavy armchair beneath the window, I shrouded my head with the lace curtain, and with tearful eyes, I observed the empty street. I'd always enjoyed Gran's reminiscing about her friends, but they were echoes of a world I had no access to, and one not relevant to mine. I was safe from death because Mam and Dad were alive and younger than Gran, who'd been practically ancient. When I was much younger, I'd cried when she told Mam that I wanted looking at just because I asked her if she remembered the dinosaurs. I gripped the white cotton antimacassar between my fingertips, shivering as I recalled Mam's question to Nick a few moments earlier: "Will you cry when I'm gone?"

I'd stared at the empty street, unaware of how soon the shadow of bereavement would completely envelop our lives again when breast cancer claimed my beloved Mam's life.

And now, on this last evening of the seventies, I stood in front of my bedroom window with a bunch of flowery curtains grasped in each hand. I stared at my seventeen-year-old face reflected on the cold pane.

Without any upstairs heating, the temperature was a chilly reminder of the frosted ornamentation sparkling on the inside of the windows at our old house. I drew my cloth-filled fists together and shut out the dark night and New Year's Eve for good. I'd go to bed and wake up tomorrow when it was over and done with.

There was a tapping on my bedroom door. "Are you coming down to the Sycamore, Son?"

Brimming with self-pity, I was unsure how I wanted the final scene of the unfortunate pantomime that was this decade to play out. "Two secs, Dad." I jabbed the silver pause button of the cassette player, halting my homemade compilation of singles from the past few years.

He poked his head around the door and immediately his eyes flitted to the album displaying black and white photos of Mam that lay open on my bed.

"I dunno, Dad. I think I'll stay in."

His sigh wasn't the exasperated huffing that Tim frequently made at the slightest inconvenience, but one heavy with resignation.

"I'm not telling you what to do, Son, but I don't think it's a good idea to sit in the house on your own on New Year's Eve. Tom and Betty are having a do after the midnight chimes from London come on the wireless, and Little Nancy has promised to play the piano." He ruffled my hair just as he did when I was so much younger. "Tom's even booked that man who dresses up as a woman to come in and do his act, so it will no doubt turn into a bit of a jolly-up."

"What man who dresses up as a woman?"

"Angela Britvic."

"Not Angela Vandella?"

"No, Son. She does the striptease."

I laughed at the daft names of the two drag artistes who Tim trekked to see in the Radford pubs. "Oh, I don't know what to do, Dad. I feel in such a muddle sometimes. It's like there's too much inside my head."

"I understand, Son. As a family, we've had awful things to contend with, and you more than most. What happened was so wrong."

He reached down and lightly traced a forefinger around Mam's face. It was my favourite, a black and white close-up he'd diligently hand-tinted into colour.

"After your mother died I feared that you'd never be...well again. You used to sit on your swing in the back yard, but you didn't swing. You loved swinging, which was why I built you one. But you sat there, staring at your feet and singing the words from that song in the hit parade. Over, and over, and over again."

This was the first time I'd heard any of this, and I wasn't sure if I wanted to hear more. "Was it 'Hot Love'?" I couldn't resist picking at the scab to see what was underneath.

"No, it wasn't T. Rex. It was the one that Tim was always whistling. You remember. That Scottish woman with the dreadful voice."

"What Scottish woman with the dreadful voice? Which song?"

He raised his head and looked at the ceiling, making the back of his neck ripple into a sausage of flesh against the constriction of his white shirt collar. "Where's your mother gone, where's your mother gone?"

He paused. My watch had never ticked so loudly.

"I woke up this morning and my mother was gone, far far away."

This was not the moment to allow my pedantic nature to take charge and correct his misquoting of the lyrics.

"Sometimes you'd be there for half an hour or more. Not swinging, just sitting, looking down, and singing those same, awful words. I didn't know what to do. I felt so helpless. I knew that you were grieving, but there was nobody that I could confide in. I was terrified that some do-gooder would take you away and put you into an institution."

Sickly disorientation sucked me into the quicksand of lost memories. The saggy softness of my bed was replaced by the rigid seat of my swing. Beneath my plimsoled feet, ants streamed in regimented lines through the diagonal indents in the blue bricks of the path. The crows on the factory roof cawed raucously, and a boy somewhere sang parts of a song from the charts with mournful monotony. Peppery bile stung the back of my throat. I shook my head, refusing to aid the distressing recall.

"Sorry, Son. I didn't mean to upset you."

"Honestly, Dad, I'm okay. It's you that I'm worried about."

"Don't worry about me, Son. I'm your father. I'm all right. I have to be." He cleared his throat. "So are you coming down with me?"

I acknowledged the signal that the subject was closed. "Okey-dokes, I'll just get changed."

Once the door was closed, I contemplated his unburdening with horror. The novelty song hit called "Chirpy Chirpy Cheep Cheep" had topped the charts six months after Mam died. The ripples of my bereavement extended far past that devastating Sunday morning in January when he told us that she was dead, and they continued to spread throughout my life.

Reeling from Dad's unnerving recollection, I needed to return to firmer ground and evoke something that I had been in control of, not flashbacks to the traumatised behaviour of my junior years. I jabbed the pause button on the cassette player which released the end of Tom Robinson's "Glad To Be Gay," and my rocking mental boat was immediately steadied. The song had become my personal anthem, and so empowered by it, I'd proclaimed my homosexuality at work when I was sixteen. My clumsy tape edit segued the applause at the end of the song into the growling bass beginning of "Something Better Change" by The Stranglers.

"Yeah, something *had* better change," I grumbled at the American gay magazine *Blueboy* that I'd been reading that afternoon. The liberating magic contained within its pages was bittersweet. I was uplifted by the world portrayed within, yet simultaneously depressed because I longed to be able to wear a *Ready For The 80s* T-shirt like the one that hugged the taut pectorals of the man in a mail order advert. The hated excess flesh on my chest made this an unattainable desire. There was no way I could wear such an amazing item of clothing, and I shrugged out of the protective armour of the baggy earth-brown cardigan Mam had knitted for Dad before I was born. He'd always worn it when he rolled about under the car doing repairs, and I'd tugged on it to get his attention when I was young. He'd lightheartedly chided me, "Watch out, Son, it'll be a foot longer if you keep doing that, and I'll be wearing it as a frock."

In recent years, the cardigan had become convenient camouflage for my unsightly chest, yet if I sniffed the chunky stitches hard enough, I could still detect the Gun Gum exhaust filler that he'd used. My fingertips rubbed against something prickly in the depths of one of the pockets, and my investigation showed a fine line of seeds. During which of our countless countryside jaunts had Dad collected them? When Mam was alive? Or was it after she died? Inevitably, my mind wandered along sombre paths of reminiscence that always led back to Mam, just as if I was sitting on her lap as Dad drove us along the winding country lanes in his vintage black Alvis Firefly.

Dozens of printed eyes stared down from my gallery of posters

Chucking Putty at the Queen

that documented a decade of my musical obsessions. Unsurprisingly, Marc Bolan numbered the most, beginning with the free poster from his *Electric Warrior* LP, which had been my main Christmas present in 1971. Submerging myself in the deep ocean of his songs had temporarily diverted me from the pain of Mam's death that dominated my existence since the beginning of that year.

Other faces represented a portion of the crossroads where my musical and sartorial tastes lay: Eno, the flamboyant synthesiser player from Roxy Music, Freddie Mercury, and from the pages of *Titbits*, pictures of the jewellery-bedecked celebrity pianist, Liberace, and the exotic wrestler, Adrian Street. Their glamour rubbed up against the guttersnipe grimaces of ripped and torn punk rockers The Sex Pistols, The Clash, and Generation X.

In my mid-teen days that seemed a million years ago, I'd pinned a poster of American television cops Starsky and Hutch close to my pillow. I chuckled, remembering how as soon as I'd returned from the paper shop, I'd folded the glossy sheet vertically in half so that only Starsky showed, wrapped in his own baggy cardigan, legs encased in denim jeans faded to a soft hue of periwinkle as he stared at me with his swarthy, come hither look. I cringed to recall how just before I turned the light off, I'd dreamily whisper, "Goodnight, Starsk" and lie back, hoping that my dreams would contain a romantic visitation from him. This celebrity crush in the middle of the seventies guaranteed my watching of the energetic cop show with devoted fervour, as the video tape in my head recorded his every movement and each of his drawled sentences.

But now, all of it must go. I promised myself that I'd dedicate the first day of 1980 to wiping my slate clean and to converting my bedroom into a more mature haven to represent what I was determined would be the new me. I didn't want to be anyone else, just a happier version of myself.

I shrugged into the heavy, oversized 1940s black serge suit that I'd bought for a fiver from one of the charity shops in town. When I first wore it, Tim stared at me as if I were naked, then guffawed, almost choking on a mouthful of cheese Quavers, and the force of his hilarity sent fragments of the puffed orange snack onto my jacket.

"What you got on?" He laughed again and proffered the yellow packet, its silver lining shining through the gaping mouth of the glossy plastic. "D'ya wanna Quaver?"

183

"No, ta. I've got enough on my jacket already."

He laughed again. "It looks like you nicked it off one of the old tramps down the park."

I didn't care, and I revelled in his reaction as my attire was my current mode of expressing my difference to the rest of society. After pinning a one-inch *Public Image Limited* badge to the left lapel, I flicked my bedroom light off and descended the stairs to where Dad waited for me in the hallway, helpfully holding my walking sticks in readiness. When I stepped out from our house for the last time in 1979, it was imperative that when the calendar turned, I would achieve a positive change in my life. As the T-shirt slogan in the magazine proclaimed, I was ready for the eighties.

21

SOMETHING BETTER CHANGE

As the final minutes of the 1970s ticked by, Dad and I squeezed into a corner at the end of the bar of the Sycamore Inn. Both of us agreed that we were relieved to see the back of the challenging decade. Above the expectant, tipsy hubbub in the overcrowded room, the piped music still bore a selection of Yuletide songs, and although I groaned at the beginning of Slade's perennial hit, "Merry Christmas Everybody," I had to heed its lyrics and look to the future.

The strings of fairy lights hanging behind the bar were no longer cheery, but tawdry melancholy blobs of colour, as were the sagging stretched strands of twisted crêpe ribbons radiating from a tissue paper bell in the centre of the ceiling. The opposing ends of these ornamental lengths were tethered to the walls beneath glittery bunches of plastic holly or cardboard placards bearing seasonal wishes in a gold Germanic typeface. Depressingly adhering to tradition, they'd remain pinned to the burgundy flock wallpaper for another week until the official end of the festive season. How I yearned to rip the garlands and streamers down, to throw open the doors and let the cold, fresh air sweep everything away. Out with the old and in with the new.

Snake hiss shushes subdued the cheerful chatter. Dozens of expectant eyes checked the Home Ales clock above the bar.

Brian the binman yelled, "Fifteen seconds, get ready. Here we go!" and the communal countdown began.

When the first chime from Big Ben resounded from the portable radio behind the bar, Tom the landlord matched it with a dozen deafening peals of the big brass bell usually reserved for calling last orders. With the sound of a hundred champagne bottles being opened, the smoky space above our heads became a galaxy of multicoloured paper trails rocketing from party poppers. Always the joker, and therefore a source of irritation for many regulars, Scouse Barry clutched a can of Silly String in each hand and ejected the aerosol-propelled contents over the celebratory crowd, covering heads and shoulders with tangles of neon spaghetti. Having sat in anticipation of midnight with her wrinkled, aged fingers poised above the chipped ivory keys of the ancient upright piano, Little Nancy bashed out the opening chords of "Auld Lang Syne." Her vigorous playing made the empty beer glasses on top of the piano tinkle in accompaniment, whilst Dad and I formally shook hands and wished each other happy new year. Of course, nobody remembered the following verses, and mumbled approximations of the sentimental words were replaced with cheers and claps when Little Nancy segued into "Roll Out The Barrel," instigating the start of a small conga line that clumsily shuffled around the tables and chairs.

My silly grin at the jolliness was wiped away when I turned around and saw Dad hunched into the corner with his back to me, his head bowed low, and his shoulders shaking. Oh no, he was having a stroke or a heart attack. In my mind, the fairy lights were replaced with the blue flashing ones on top of an ambulance as it raced away from the pub to take him to the hospital emergency admissions. My childhood fear of his death was sickeningly overpowering as I reached out to him. But before my hand got to his shoulder, he spun around. Two lights flashed at the base of his neck, and his eyes had a devilish glint that I hadn't seen for years. He was wearing the illuminated bowtie that Mam had bought me from the Sign of Four trick shop after we'd been to the dentist for my check-up. Unbeknownst to her, I'd smuggled it into school the next day. Our headmistress had quickly confiscated my sartorial novelty after I'd activated it during assembly. Now Dad was randomly pressing the connectors to the battery which I surmised was in his jacket pocket, making the thin green cotton bow flash erratically. I hadn't seen it for ages and thought that Tim had chucked it out in one of his over-zealous Sunday morning tidy-ups. As I laughed, a scrawny arm blemished with bronzed kidney spots and a wrist adorned with jangling jewellery thrust past my head towards Dad.

"Happy new year, Sid! Giz a kiss, me duck."

The squawky parrot voice from the past burst my balloon of memories. It was Reenee, the garrulous, effusive friend of Aunty Lu and Mam. She wriggled between us and pecked Dad on the cheek, then nudged me.

"I know you're the baby of the family and you're all grown up now, but you're not too bleddy big to have one an' all."

It was hard not to gag on the invisible cloud of asphyxiating perfume as she tiptoed to reach my cheek.

She gave Dad a daft, inebriated smile. "He's the dead spit of Betty, isn't he?"

The landlady drifted behind the bar bearing a plate of sausage rolls secured beneath stretched cling film that reflected the overhead lights in white zigzags. "Hey there, is somebody taking my name in vain?"

"No, duck, not you. I'm talking about his late and much beloved mam. They say that the Lord takes the good when they're young," Reenee sounded as if she was reading from the deaths' column in the *Evening Post*.

"Somebody shift them empties," Tom requested of nobody.

I added them to the collection crammed precariously atop the piano until it resembled the glassware section in Jessops, the posh department store in the Victoria Centre. I was just in time as a surge of bodies pressed us against the velour-padded bar. The crush coincided with the arrival of the free sandwiches, carried regally high on aluminium serving trays by Jo, the perpetually scowling pensioner barmaid. Dad called her "the faithful retainer," whilst Tim less charitably nicknamed her "the old misery" and reckoned that she looked like a bullfrog wearing bifocals. She'd made it obvious during the past few weeks that she disagreed with the pub being granted an extension until one a.m. Yet despite her getting paid double time, and Tom forking out of his own pocket for a taxi to take her home, she continued to vociferously warn that allowing people to booze so late would end in trouble.

Just before chucking out time the previous night, she'd clutched the gold crucifix hanging from a thin chain around her wrinkled, leathery neck. "All this carrying on. It's not right. It's ungodly." Her raspy voice had taken on a sombre tone. She closed her eyes as if experiencing great pain. "'Then the Lord rained on Sodom and Gomorrah sulphur and fire from the Lord out of heaven.'" She crossed herself and opened her eyes. "You mark my words; it'll end in tears."

When more plates were borne aloft and then lowered onto the bar, Reenee nudged me, her eyes wide. "Look at them boggers! Pickled eggs *and* gherkins an' all. What a bleddy nosh-up."

She lunged to reach the plates and was submerged in a wave of swaying, hungry drinkers. Clad in a frilled black and red blouse, with each raised hand bearing a sandwich and with a stick of celery gripped between her lipstick-smeared false teeth, she resembled a St. Ann's version of a flamenco dancer biting a rose and playing castanets. With considerable difficulty, she handed me the celery.

"Ode onto that for a minute, duck." With scraggy, chicken-claw fingers, she peeled the slices of white bread apart and wrinkled her nose. "They're a bit stingy with the potted beef, but it don't matter. I heard Tom say they're bringing out some dripping sandwiches in a minute."

I only realised the high level of her intoxication when she shook her head, tears twinkling between her over-mascaraed eyelashes.

"Your mam used to make a lovely dripping sandwich. I used to tell her, 'Betty, you make the best dripping sandwich this side of St. Ann's Well Road.' You know, there wasn't no one what could touch your mam's dripping sandwiches." She smiled wistfully. "She didn't tell everybody this, but she used to put pepper in 'em. 'That's my secret, Reenee,' she'd say. 'A little shake of pepper, and Bob's your uncle.'"

She narrowed her sparkling eyes, snatched the celery from me, and nodded to the end of the bar where several people were loading their paper plates with mini sausage rolls, sandwiches, and triangles of pork pie. Stored hamster-like for safe keeping, pickled onions distended the cheeks of several male revellers as they shoved their way through the crowd towards the seating.

Reenee harrumphed. "They're not even from round here, that lot. I know them. They live down near the Wessy."

The Westminster Abbey pub was about a quarter of a mile away. Reenee was affronted by these interlopers who demonstrated their disregard for the unseen boundaries delineated by loyalty to boozers. I didn't mention that she'd come five miles by two bus services from Broxtowe, where she'd been relocated after the demolition of the old way.

Her eyes grew large and round as she pointed rudely across the room at a laughing, obviously drunk, pale-faced woman with a dyed black bouffant, waving a cigarette around as if she was conducting an orchestra.

"And *her*, that's Sheila Hobson's eldest, and *she* lives right at the top of Donkey Hill, so don't you tell me this is her local. Someone once told her that she looked like Elizabeth Taylor, and she's been acting like she bleddy is ever since." She burped. "Pardon me, I'm sure. And I'll tell you summat else: *she* had no right to wear white on her wedding day."

This was the kind of gossip that I loved to hear when Mam took me round to Aunty Lu's and I joyfully discovered that Reenee was there. The queen of judgement tutted and glared across the room.

"They're only here for the free grub. Talk about owt for nowt. They'd best not take all the bleddy gherkins, or I'll have summat to say, new year or no new year."

A woman who celebrated her expansive girth and insisted that people call her Fat Pat shoved towards us. "Oh, give over, Reenee, and pass us some of them cheese and pickle before they're all gone." She elbowed past Dad to reach the bar. "Oh, sorry, Sid. I didn't mean to spill your pint."

Dad pressed himself further against the side of the piano. To my delight, Little Nancy thumped out, "My Old Man Said Follow the Van." It was one of my favourites. Mam used to have me in fits of the giggles when she'd burst into a spate of cockney dancing in the front room at the old house, lifting her apron and swirling it above her knees.

Dad placed his empty pint glass onto the bar, extracted a five-pound note from his wallet, and twitched it between his fingers before laying it on the bar. "Do the honours, please, Son, and also get a port and lemon for Little Nancy. I'm going for a piddle."

As I watched him swallowed by the celebratory melee, the sediment of my memory was disturbed, and a panic from nine years earlier covered me in a gritty cloud of flashback.

Dad and I were in the supermarket doing the Saturday shop and as usual, I was piloting the trolley. He consulted the list I'd written in various coloured felt pens the previous evening.

"Righty-ho, Son, we're cracking on. Next up is coley. I'll go to the fish section, you wait here. I'll be just a tic."

He threaded through the busy shoppers, turned the corner and was gone. I tightened my grip on the smooth plastic of the trolley handle until it creaked. It was just like shortly after Mam died and he'd popped out to the shop next-door-but-one for a loaf. By the time he'd returned, I was a gibbering wreck, convinced he'd been run down by a car and killed, making me an orphan. Under the glaring supermarket lights, that same terror tightened my throat. I sucked air through my nostrils and blew it from my mouth as the black hand of the overhead clock swept the seconds away. My ears drummed. This time he really wasn't coming back. I knew it for sure because a couple of weeks earlier I'd overheard him tell Tim that a bloke in the pub had advised him, "You should put that youngest lad of yours in a children's home and get on with your own life." I shoved the trolley until I reached the corner of the unit and stopped at a crossroads where avenues of highly polished lino stretched. I whirled around, anxiously scanning the heads and backs and faces, but none of them were my dad. Where had he gone? Who could I ask for help? My fingers became vicious hooks of anxiety digging into my soft, sweaty palms as I slid right back to my first day at nursery…

I didn't realise that Mam was going to leave me there. I thought she'd be with me all day, doing all the lovely things with me that she'd promised that children enjoyed there: painting, playing in the sand pit, and listening to "miss" reading us stories.

Inside the gate, Mam kissed me and stoked my hair. "Have a lovely time. I'll be back later."

Her statement shocked me more than when Steve had deliberately burst the big balloon of a Black lady's head with three coloured feathers sticking out of the top that she and Dad had bought me at Goose Fair. Because I'd adored it so much, each year they bought me a similar balloon and each year, Steve spitefully popped it with the hot tip of his cigarette.

"Where are you going?"

"Home, I've got a steak and kidney pie to make for dinner and a pile of ironing taller than you."

I stared as she stepped onto the path at the side of the park. The teacher closed the heavy iron gate, slid the bolt across, and turned a big brass key in the lock. I was a prisoner.

Mam blew me a kiss and sauntered up the path as if she hadn't a care in the world.

"Mam, come back. I don't want to be here." I scuttled alongside her, separated by the spiked black barrier and when I could go no further, I reached out between the railings, clutching frantically at thin air. "Mam, come back. Please don't leave me." Tears burned my eyes as I stamped my feet and yelled, watching as she turned a corner and was gone. Hearing giggling, I spun around. The other children stood in a crescent behind me, pointing at the hot wetness dribbling down the inside of my

Chucking Putty at the Queen

bare legs.

And so, beneath the supermarket's bright lights, I squeezed my thighs together, hoping it would stop the urgent pain in my bladder, dreading a repeat of that day at the nursery. I jumped out of my skin when a hand rested on my shoulder.

"What are you doing up here, Son? I asked you to wait by the margarine." Dad placed a plastic-covered polystyrene tray of white fish and a stubby golden jar of mustard on top of the groceries. "Are you okay? What's the matter?"

"I wondered where you'd gone. I thought you'd run away."

"Run away? I'm not going to do that, Son. I only went to get some Colman's. You know how Tim likes mustard with his fish."

I desperately needed to hug him but instead, I tugged my parka from where it lay over the trolley, wriggled into it, and pulled it tightly closed. Unlike my very public tears, the result of my relief that had soaked the crotch of my green corduroy jeans must remain hidden once more. "I was scared that you'd gone forever."

He ruffled my hair, pulled his handkerchief out, and dabbed at my cheeks. "It's okay, Son. I'm not going anywhere other than to get some cream crackers. You wait here."

Gripping my walking sticks as hard as I had the shopping trolley handle, I watched him disappear through the New Year merriment into the pub passageway. The celebratory cacophony irritated me into drinking my pint too fast, as if the deep gulps would hasten Dad back more quickly. My vision was set on the door. Of course he hadn't had a heart attack in the gents and fallen dead. Don't be stupid, of course there wasn't a fight in the passageway during which he'd accidentally been on the receiving end of a misplaced punch and lay lifeless on the dirty floor tiles littered with fag ends and splashes from spilled pints. I gritted my teeth, hating myself for succumbing to that same fear that had cursed me since Mam's death. I couldn't keep on like this, allowing my sanity to be compromised by the emotional toxicity of my earlier years, but when Dad finally reappeared, squeezing through the drinkers gathered in the doorway, dread slipped from my tensed shoulders like a heavy blanket of snow from rooftops during a rapid thaw.

He grinned at me, but before I could offer to buy him a drink, I saw a lanky, boss-eyed woman called Blossom shove people out of her way as she zoomed towards us like a laser-guided missile. Because of her sticking-out ears, flared nostrils, and dental problems, Tim had nicknamed her Plug, like the Bash Street Kids character in *Beano*.

"Happy new year, Mester Smalley!" Her drunken attempts to place a tissue paper party hat on Dad's head only resulted in it slipping from his bald pate. "Ode up," she spluttered from between her four protruding front teeth. "Gizza minute."

My eyes almost fell from my head when she removed a small grey nub of chewing gum from her mouth, stretched it until it split in half, and pressed the two bits to the sides of his scalp. She then attached the flimsy pink and yellow crown.

"It int going nowhere now, duck." She kissed his cheek. "Happy new year!"

Dad remained unruffled. He'd never be intentionally rude to anyone and so gave her a rather forced smile. "And a happy new year to you, Plu–Blossom."

Her goofy grin quickly changed to a look of alarm as her shoulders uncontrollably bucked. "Urgh, I'm gonna spew."

When she clamped a bony hand across her mouth, displaying the dark blue tattooed 'hate' which complemented the 'love' on her other fingers, Dad stepped as far back as he could and reached forward to gently push her away from him. "A most ladylike statement. I suggest that you go outside for some fresh air."

As she elbowed through the bodies towards the door into the car park, he pulled the decorative crown from his head, folded it neatly until it was a small square and slipped it into his jacket pocket. Then he lifted a paper napkin from the bar and twitched the chewing gum blobs from his head. "Blossom." He scrunched the napkin into a tight ball and placed it into the ashtray next to the brown stub of his cigar. "Such a pretty name for such an ugly girl."

My explosive guffaw shook the crêpe paper holly dangling just above me. As my mirth diminished, a familiar squawk grabbed our attention.

Dad looked around. "Oh, Christ, Son. It goes from bad to worse. Here's Reenee back on the warpath."

Mam's old friend could hardly stand as she forced herself between us and tried to throw her arms around our shoulders. Her condition was what Tim would describe as "steaming." With me being taller than Dad,

Chucking Putty at the Queen

she had to clutch at my suit jacket to steady herself. It was my pride and joy, and it would piss me off if her talons caused any damage.

Either through tears or the temperature of the overheated pub, her heavily applied mascara looked as if ink bombs had been chucked at her face. She sniffed morosely, and her bottom lip trembled. I guessed that the gin I heard Aunty Lu tell Mam that Reenee was a "real bogger for" had already taken its emotional toll.

She shook her head. "Betty would of loved it, wunt she?"

Her clumsy attempt to put her arm through mine caused my lager to slop from the glass. Irritation spiked through me. "Would have."

"Eh?"

"Would have, not would of."

"Yer what?"

"You said that my mam would *of* loved it. It's would *have* loved it, not would *of* loved it."

She stared as if I'd just announced that Mam wasn't really dead, and we were just waiting for her to come in and join us for a singsong.

"Int he just like yo, Sid? All proper and correct and polite. Betty would of..." The muscles in her scrawny chicken neck seemed to have lost their strength. Her head half fell backwards, and her eyes rolled.

Dad's hand shot up to support the back of her head. "Steady as you go, Reenee."

She gulped, and her watery eyes made me wonder if she was about to burst into tears.

"I was just sayin' Betty would *have* been dead proud to see him all grown up. She would *have*, Sid, wouldn't she? She would *have*."

"Yes, Reenee, she would."

She gripped her talons into my shoulder more forcibly. "But she can't. She can't, can she?"

Thankfully, a yell from the doorway prevented her snivelling transforming into a full-blown waterfall of gin-soaked misery. "Taxi for Reenee! Taxi for Reenee!"

"Oh, gawd, that's for me, int it? I'll have to go. Now, Sid, don't try to persuade me to stop. Not even for poor Betty's sake. Our Hilda and Maud are expecting me early tomorrer for a walk round the Arboretum." She clicked open her handbag and scowled. "Where's me bleddy earrings? I took 'em off before we did the hokey cokey in the carpark 'cos I couldn't be doing with losing 'em. They're too precious."

I nodded to the sparkling plastic jewels dangling on each side of her neck. "You're wearing them."

A scraggy claw flew to each ear. "So I am. I must've put 'em back on after I'd picked Doris up after she fell over." She hiccupped, then leaned towards me and narrowed her eyes as if she were about to divulge a great secret. "She just can't hold her drink, that one." After another hiccup, she lightly tapped her earrings. "Do you like 'em?"

"They're very pretty."

"Ta, I won 'em on Hook-a-Duck at the fair yonks ago."

"Taxi for Reenee!" This time, the man's tone was sharp with impatience.

"Oh, bleddy hell, I'd best go." She pecked both of us on our cheeks, sniffed a few times, and mumbled, "Poor Betty," before she weaved through the jammed crowd and was gone.

Dad closed his eyes and pinched the flesh at the bridge of his nose as he always did when he was weary. "I know that she means well, but I could have done without that tonight, Son. Are you all right?"

"Yeah, I'm all right, but she was a bit much. All that going on about Mam."

Dad stuck out his bottom lip and blew upwards through his moustache. "I know, Son. I don't mean to be harsh or unkind, but right now, we're in the 1980s. We have to move on. I sincerely hope that the next ten years will be kinder to you than the last ten were. You've been through too much already."

"*Me*? What about *you*?"

"I'm fine. Now, let's have one for the road."

When he turned to order a couple more pints, I stared at his head as if the shiny baldness were a crystal ball which would show me my future. Whatever lay ahead, it *had* to be less miserable for me, and somehow I must make it so. Squashed amongst the revellers still proffering either genuine good wishes or booze-inspired temporary sincerity, I was too overwhelmed to figure out how I'd make the upcoming years a success. When Dad handed me a drink and grinned, I made my New Year's resolution that in this new decade, as my record by The Stranglers dictated, something better change.

22

HAPPY HOUSE

The glowing crimson numbers on my bedside digital clock silently morphed to the first seven a.m. of the 1980s. After breakfast, I returned to my bedroom and revisited the cassette I'd played the evening before. "Something Better Change" picked up where I'd left it, a raucous reminder of my New Year's resolution. Within an hour, I'd cleared the walls of my posters and stored them in my wardrobe.

Since the previous summer, I'd attended physiotherapy at the General Hospital for two hours, five days a week to hopefully alleviate the pain caused by the unique and complicated constrictions of my crippling disability. Gruelling regimes were invented by the department head, Mr Galbraith, who frequently devoted his Saturday mornings to aid me. Even though the facility had closed from December 21st for two weeks, the devoted physiotherapist still undertook the thirty-minute drive from his rural Derbyshire home and opened up the gymnasium to ensure minimal disruption to my exercise regime.

"No rest for the wicked, laddie," he'd say and grin. "Worse things happen at sea."

As he'd served in the Royal Navy, I thought that if anyone should know that, it would be him. However, with the New Year's celebrations following a weekend, I'd been afforded a brief respite before resuming attendance. My usual self-reward after each exhausting session was to slowly head to Selectadisc, where I'd leisurely flip through the racks of second-hand LPs in a quest for kooky and uncompromising music. Another favourite destination was Central Library from where I was able to loan six books and six LPs at any one time for no cost. The sale of blank cassettes must surely have boomed once I embarked on a mission to create my own eclectic and illegally copied musical miscellany. My thirst for new audio experiences was unquenchable, and I rapidly developed a catalogue of classical pieces and a collection of jazz titles that were often so annoyingly discordant that, as I cringed at the shrieking trumpets,

I reassured myself of how arty and urbane I'd become. And when Tim banged on his bedroom wall, yelling condemnation that they were "a sodding racket" preventing his Saturday afternoon kip, I knew that I'd attained an enviably ethereal level of cultural refinement.

I cherished those hours spent within the book-lined canyons which were a direct consequence of the prosaic school education I'd received. I was determined to develop cultural enlightenment, and as I basked in the warmth of my self-styled sophistication, I loaned volumes by Balzac, Gore Vidal, E.M. Forster, W. Somerset Maugham, and myriad other inspirational wordsmiths that were my intellectual superiors. I reclined on my bed reading slender publications of Verlaine, Rimbaud, and Baudelaire, rejoicing in my relaxed literary investigations and secure in the knowledge that, unlike in the school library, when I returned these books, I'd no longer have to keep one eye on the door for fear that my foes would discover me and beat me up again.

Tucked into a shadowy corner of the top floor was a shelf whose plum-coloured strip of Dymo tape categorised the line of hardback books as Interior Design. I lugged a plastic bag containing an inspiring trio of heavy tomes homewards, the elasticity of the handles stretching with each of my faltering steps, but thankfully not snapping. I gawped at the sumptuous rooms on the glossy pages. Inspiration painted my imagination, and I soon set about planning an alternative world that, although contained within my bedroom walls, would be unrestricted by my inventiveness: a sanctuary to characterise my distinction from other human beings. Once more I assured myself that I didn't want to be someone else but just a happier version of me. Until I solved the problem of how to eschew the self-doubts about my physical appearance and summon the courage to actually do something about meeting other gay men, I would barricade myself from orthodoxy with books, music, and the varieties of luxuriant foliage that enhanced many of the rooms within the library loans. That would be just the mental tonic that I needed.

Therefore, in April 1980, the objective of one particular post-physio wander was to visit what Tim called "that posh plant shop up Derby Road." Weary and aching from the Herculean exercises of my activity in the gym, I left the General Hospital behind and moseyed along the Ropewalk, admiring its sturdy Georgian and Victorian buildings. My previous stays in hospital had imbibed me with a sense of institutionalisation which continued with the daily physio regime that dominated my life. Despite the connotations of ill health, I easily succumbed to the melancholic genius loci that attracted me to this part of my home town as I connected with my own medical history. I cautiously navigated the paving slabs, occasionally tapping their uneven levels with the black rubber ferrules of my walking sticks as a blind man would with the metal tip of his white cane. I paused before the architecturally pleasing frontages, many homing the private practices of surgeons and consultants. My psyche was imbued with the sombre sense of belonging to this area as again, I yielded to an emotional disquietude that I perversely didn't want to lose. Even the harrowing memory of visiting my terminally ill mam and her not recognising me couldn't diminish the morbid magnetism of these streets. Although she was dead, she'd once resided here, and I was certain that the dark red Victorian bricks of the foreboding hospital linked her to my soul. Our old house was long demolished, and I believed that being surrounded by the same sturdy buildings where Mam was once a patient strengthened my spiritual bond to her—one which I was terrified would become irretrievably broken with the passing of time.

Exhausted, I finally reached the plant shop. Once through the door, I was enshrouded by enormous, luxuriously leafed palms and a noticeable elevation in temperature and humidity. I carefully traversed a meandering course through the sultry, dark green interior and peered around. Above me, the succulent zig-zag fronds of giant Boston ferns hung in the black-painted ceiling space. Within the misty gloom, I could have been Henry Morton Stanley during his quest through the foreboding African jungle to find the missing nineteenth century explorer Dr Livingstone. I hugged myself. This was just what I wanted, and my mind's eye pictured me reclining on my bed surrounded by greenery. But upon reading the price written in violet inky swirls onto a butterfly-shaped tag, I gasped as if I'd finally discovered the missing adventurer. In 1980, £5.99 was an incredible sum for one plant, and I'd need at least two of the green monsters if my bedroom transformation was to be as successful as I'd planned. I contemplated my quandary. I could buy an LP and a couple of singles for the price of one of these plants, and following weeks of waiting, my priority purchase that day was the debut album, *Strange Boutique*, by The Monochrome Set.

I jumped when a lanky man with cropped blond hair and an oversized black Zapata moustache appeared, the lilies and vines which decorating his Hawaiian shirt aiding his camouflage within the sweltering man-made jungle. He approached, hissing mist from an ornate galvanized plant sprayer onto a captivating display of exquisite tiger orchids. Their lichen-blemished terracotta pots stood upon the curly twirls of a wrought iron étagère which I immediately added to my mental list of must-haves. I could just see it standing on my windowsill, and passers-by would pause and point at its elaborate wonder, contemplating which urbane person owned such an elegant object. My fantasy was disrupted by a slug of sweat sliding down the back of my neck just as Kate Bush's appropriately titled song "In the Warm Room" filtered through the foliage from an unseen source. Mr Moustache was advancing, and I needed to make a decision before my impulsive temperament nudged me into purchasing plants that I couldn't afford. And how would I get them home? My intrinsic vinyl addiction won over nature, and I chose the LP that I'd ached so long to be released. I'd have to postpone the transformation of my St. Ann's bedroom into a sophisticated San Francisco pad. I navigated my way through the rainforest and, with the tinkling of the shop bell diminishing with each of my footsteps, I headed down to Selectadisc.

After Dad announced that he was going to retire five years earlier than he was due to, he took the occasional Friday off work to use up his holiday entitlement. On those days, he'd visit a street market in a suburb north of the city to buy meat from the mobile butcher who set up his van there. After stocking up with chops, sausages, a weekend joint, and a pound of chitterlings if the butcher had them, he'd meet up with his friends Ken and Evelyn for a lunchtime pint and a cheese and pickle cob in the Greyhound.

I'd repeatedly hauled the heavy coffee table books back to the library to renew them, impressed and stimulated by the swanky abodes. One Friday, when I stumbled into the house and plonked the colourful bag on the table after another of these tiring visits, Dad asked me why I just didn't call the library on our newly installed telephone to extend my loan.

"I didn't think of that." I imagined a pair of donkey ears sprouting from my head as in the cartoons on the television. Dad slowly turned the pages, pointing out the interiors he admired most, commenting on where I'd slipped a torn strip of paper to mark rooms crammed with jungly foliage.

"Some of these places remind me of my old colleague Syd and his pal

Chucking Putty at the Queen

Bill's place. Do you remember it?"

There was no way I'd forget the afternoon some years ago when Dad took me to the two men's incredibly furnished bungalow. As a thank you for Syd designing the groovy birthday invitation for my ninth birthday party, I'd drawn a picture of him and Bill standing by the coconut shy at the works' sports day. I thrust the sheet of paper towards Bill.

He chuckled and patted his stomach as he handed it to Syd. "Looking at this, I think that I could do with losing a bit of weight."

My eyes just about fell from my head when they ushered us into the living room. The walls were covered with chocolate-coloured cork tiles, and the glow from polished aluminium lamps low to the ground projected shadows of enormous palms with slender fingers that stroked the buttermilk ceiling. I gawped at a towering grid of polished wooden boxes filled with books and LPs, but my delight turned to horror when I looked around and saw a well-groomed hound reclining on one of the sofas, its coat shining like pleats of cream silk. It raised its head and regarded me with regal disdain. I was afraid of dogs and when I took a step backwards, Syd was at my side, having obviously noticed my fright.

"Don't worry. This is Marlena. She's the queen of the house."

"Well, one of them," Bill mumbled.

The dog yawned, exposing brilliant white teeth, then stared at me with shiny, shoe-button eyes. I moved closer to Dad and put my arm around his waist. I tried to be brave even though I was terrified it would jump up and bite me. Despite the accelerated thudding in my chest, I feigned nonchalance. "Dad, what breed is it?"

"A hairy whippet."

Bill guffawed and slapped his beefy thigh, which attested to his weekend pastime as a rugby forward prop. "Oh Sid, you stole that from Julian and Sandy."

Dad had never mentioned these friends before. I looked up at him. "Who are Julian and Sandy?"

"You remember how your mother used to have the wireless on when she was doing Sunday dinner? There was a show called *Round the Horne*."

I shook my head. If a radio programme didn't have pop music on then it passed me by. "No, I don't remember."

"Julian and Sandy were a couple of out of work actors."

199

"Chorus boys," Bill chipped in. Syd shook his head and frowned at him.

Dad cleared his throat. "You know Kenneth Williams in the *Carry On* films, Son? Well, he played Sandy."

"And Hugh Paddick played Julian," said Bill.

I wasn't really paying attention because I needed to keep my eye on the sofa. Despite her dainty name, the dog looked as dangerous as a shark to me. She slid from the emerald corduroy and stretched with long front legs extended, her back stretched into an inverted arc, and her rear end in the air. When she stood erect, she was just about up to my chest. I took another step backwards, and Syd chuckled.

"Marlena's an Afghan Hound. She won't bite. You can stroke her if you like."

Instead, I slid around Dad until he was a barrier between me and the large, elegant dog.

Syd clicked his tongue. "Come on, girl, down the garden." He stepped over to a plate glass French door and slid it open, banishing the reflections of the room and revealing a wide, paved desert surrounded by spiked ornamental grasses and small bamboos erupting from squat turquoise pots. When Marlena swept past me, I daringly reached out and laid my fingertips above her spine, my light touch rippling the smooth surface of her silken coat that flowed like reeds in a slow-moving stream. Despite my impulsive act of bravery, I still breathed a sigh of relief when Syd slid the door closed behind her and walked back over to Dad and Bill.

The soles of my shoes sank into the softness of the burgundy shag pile carpet as I approached a slender platinum record deck and a space-age amplifier that stood on a shelf seemingly growing from the wall. I looked under and around it but could see no brackets or other form of support. This really was an incredible home. My addiction to records, their labels, and artwork was already well-established, and I was overjoyed when I recognised the sleeve for Dexter Gordon's *Go*. Dad loved jazz and owned this LP on the legendary Blue Note imprint, and I often asked him to play my favourite track on it, "I Guess I'll Hang My Tears Out To Dry." A poignant vision stoked my memory when I remembered how, on one Sunday morning, Dad succumbed to my pestering and put the disc onto the small record player in the front room. We sat side by side on the settee as I read the credits on the back of the sleeve, even though I'd done that so often they were as familiar to me as my face in the small mirror above the kitchen sink when I brushed my teeth.

Mam came in with a clean net curtain for the window. "Well, what a surprise. You're listening to that song again."

Dad chuckled. "Simon's request, of course."

Mam leaned over Dad, and her lips brushed the top of my head. "You're our sentimental son, all right." Then she kissed Dad's bald pate. "I wonder where he gets it from."

Our own home would soon be demolished and even without Mam there, I still loved it to bits, but I would have adored to live in this amazing bungalow. I could just see myself drowning in the emerald corduroy sea, happily trapped between the oversized icebergs of white cushions as my T. Rex single played on the fabulous record player. On the wall, slim silver frames restrained aggressive daubs and vibrant splodges of multicoloured oil paint, and beneath them, lacquered shelving the colour of ripe cherries bore a collection of bizarre sculptures. I stared at one and when Syd laid his hand on my shoulder, I jumped out of my skin as if he'd let the dog back in, and it had nipped me.

"This one's called 'Venus & Adonis.' It's inspired by Greek mythology."

Thrilled that I wasn't being treated like a child, I put my head on one side, nodded knowingly, and scratched my chin just as I thought an art lover should, pretending that I understood, even though it just looked like a bashed-up lump of concrete with two bits of bent copper pipe sticking out of it.

Bill appeared, rattling ice cubes in a glass which he raised to Dad. "Would you like a drink? We're having gin."

"I'd better not; I'm driving."

"What about an espresso then?"

Syd laughed. "Honestly, Bill, you can't wait to show off your new Gaggia."

Dad gave a thumbs-up. "That'll do the job. I think that the last time I had one was in Italy."

Bill winked at me. "How about you, sir? An orange juice or something similar?"

"I'd like what it is that my dad's having, please."

The kitchen doorway framed me as I watched Bill operate the steaming, hissing, shiny silver machine. The enveloping aroma of freshly ground coffee beans even seemed to smell deliciously dark brown and reminded me of when Penny and Marge took me to the Kardomah on King Street in town. I couldn't believe that these two men had their own machine.

When we were leaving later, I poked my head around a partly open door, one of only two in the hall. The walls inside were panelled with something that resembled huge slices of charcoal, and on a dark grey carpet stood a vast, low bed covered with an unwrinkled, intensely indigo bedspread that stretched out like a waveless ocean. At each side, elegantly angular black side tables were topped with chrome lights in the shape of flying saucers. I'd never dreamed that such a fabulous, mind-blowing home existed.

Dad, Syd, and Bill were still talking about camera exposure speeds or something. Mam would have called me, "a nosey crow," but I pushed the other door open anyway. The room was an office complete with a telex machine, electric typewriter, filing cabinets, and a vast board with various memos pinned to it. The room seemed to contain most of the telephony equipment that Dad photographed in his job. The walls were covered with what looked like hessian. I wiped my fingers against my jumper just in case they were mucky before I gently stroked the rough surface.

"Are you all right?"

I pulled my fingertips from the hessian as if it were alive with electricity. So deep was I in my admiration of the unusual décor, I was unaware of Bill standing in the doorway. "Yes, thank you. That's a weird settee." I pointed to a beige mattress folded over, with slats of pale wood behind it.

"It's not a settee, it's a futon."

"A what?"

"Futon. It's Japanese and folds out into a... Hang on, I'll show you." Like a magic trick, he unfurled the mattress. "They're very practical and space-saving. If we have someone to stay, then this is the easy solution. We can have an office and somewhere for a guest to kip, rather than have another bedroom that's hardly used."

A cough alerted me to Dad's presence.

He raised his eyebrows. "Before you ask, Son, no, we can't have one."

Syd squeezed in and pinned my picture to the notice board. "There you go, Simon. Pride of place."

My cheeks burned whilst Dad looked at his watch. "Come on, Son, we mustn't outstay our welcome."

The gravel beneath the car tyres scrunched pleasingly as Dad manoeuvred his Rover down the drive.

"Dad, why, in that office room, if there's a fyootwun—"

"Futon."

"Futon. If there's a futon, why is there only one proper bedroom with that massive bed in it?"

He stopped where the gravel met tarmac, flicked the indicator and looked left up the lane, then turned the steering wheel clockwise as we set off home. "Because it's only Syd and Bill who live there, Son."

With those memories of the fantastic bungalow stirred like fallen leaves in the wind, I closed the cover of one of the gorgeous library books and smiled at Dad. "Yeah, there should deffo be a photo of their place in here. I remember those palms they had, and the futon." I reached for another of the books. "I've got a great idea. I could dismantle my bed and just have the mattress on the floor."

"Not a good idea with your bad leg, Son. How are you going to get up and down from it? You have enough trouble as it is."

He did have a point. As I contemplated ways around this oversight, Dad tapped the cover of *California Homes*.

"I'll tell you what, Son, you must come with me to the market one Friday when I go to meet Ken and Evelyn. There's a chap there selling house plants. I'm sure you'll find something to suit."

After physiotherapy the next week, Dad met me outside the hospital, and we drove across town. By this time, he'd downsized his motor, regrettably having sold his Rover 100 and replacing it with a black Morris Minor. I'd joked that I couldn't imagine Dad owning a car of any other colour. With another four miles added to the odometer, relief coursed through my muscles when I awkwardly extracted myself from the front passenger seat. Sensation tingled as it returned to my numbed limbs when I stretched. "Good-oh. It's not busy at all."

The soles of my shoes half stuck to the splattered mosaic of discarded chewing gum blighting the paving slabs when I stepped towards the market. Grubby blue and white striped plastic canopies protected the wooden stalls, adding a continental gaiety despite the discarded drinks cans and tumbleweed balls of scrunched newspaper blown by a stiff breeze.

Dad held his hand out, palm upwards. "Bugger it: rain. I've left my umbrella at home."

I had no time for his weather update. "Wow, Dad, look at that lot." I pointed with one of my sticks towards the angled shadows from a modern church where a vendor stood apart from the others. Above a hand-painted sign, Ted's Plants, the planks of his stall looked as if it would snap beneath the weight of multiple pots bursting with greenery.

"Hang on a tic, Son. Just watch these slabs; they're very uneven. You wait here. I'll go to the meat wagon, and then we'll go over to the plants together."

But patience was a stranger to me, and when Dad joined the crowd of shoppers eager to buy discounted meat, I hobbled over towards the plants with a pair of enormous Boston ferns in my sights.

The stallholder nodded. "Mornin', duck."

I guessed that the big, dishevelled man visible behind the foliage was the eponymous stallholder. I greeted him as if we were old friends. "Ayup, Ted. How much are the ferns, please?"

"Int there a price on 'em? There should be." He leaned forward and began to rummage with thick, dirty fingers between the fronds until he retrieved a piece of torn cardboard printed with the ornate red K of Kellogg's. He looked at it, turned it around and shoved it towards me defiantly as if I'd accused him of hiding it. "I told you it was here. £1.99 each, or two for three quid."

This unkempt bloke and the tatty piece of an old cornflakes box scrawled with the price were the antithesis of the trendy-looking man in the shop in town and his lilac-inked butterfly shaped tags. I looked around, scanning the shoppers. Where *was* Dad? The paving slabs dropped away as the sickening surge of childhood insecurity overwhelmed me. I was back in the supermarket, watching him disappear around the corner of the shelves. The crowd in this small marketplace blurred and swayed. I crimped my eyelids together, trying to repel the bitter sick surge of worry that he'd deserted me and cleared off for good. *Stop it, stop it, stop it.* Fear and nausea collided, and as my grip tightened on my walking stick handles, I knew I would never be free from the curse of insecurity, even though at the beginning of the new decade I'd vowed to myself that I'd no longer allow myself to be tortured so. I was a grown man, no longer a child!

"You all right, mate? You look a bit queer, like."

I opened my eyes. The marketplace no longer rolled and pitched, and I laughed my relief. If only the stallholder knew the truth. I wanted to say, "I'm more than a *bit* queer," but instead, I fingered the sweaty wad of pound notes lining my trousers pocket. Finally, I could make real my bedroom dream. But before I could extract my money, a short, dumpy woman in a transparent rain mac shoved past me, the smoke that drifted up from the cigarette clamped between her lips trapping like a grey veil in her plastic rain bonnet. She tugged at the ferns until the tip of a frond snapped off. How dare she? I'd already visualised them hanging in my bedroom with fine unbroken trails from joss sticks weaving through them.

Ted scowled at her and protectively encircled the plants with his arms, pulling them towards him as if he was preventing infant twins from stepping into a busy road. "Do you bleddy mind?"

The woman shrugged. "Sorry, duck, I thought they was artificial."

"Well, you thought wrong, didn't you?"

The woman dropped the remnant of her cigarette to the dirty paving and rearranged her rain bonnet. "Yer too bleddy pricey any road. Only a mug would pay that."

Watching her shuffle away, my impatience got the better of me, and I blocked the front of the stall by placing both of my walking sticks wide. No other interloper was going to get those plants because I wanted them. No, I didn't want them, I *needed* them, and after thrusting three pounds to Ted, they were mine. Again I looked around for Dad, chiding myself not to be so stupid. Of course he hadn't run off. My impulse purchase overrode the fact that having to use two walking sticks prevented me from carrying this ready-made jungle. Thankfully, Dad was on his way over to me. He clutched large plastic bags full of glistening meat, the transparent corners glowing with gathered blood as if he were a props man heading for the set of *The Texas Chainsaw Massacre*.

Supplementary plant paraphernalia placed around the stall included macramé hangers dotted along their knotted lengths with dark wooden beads. The reality of making my bedroom how I wanted it to be was within my affordability, and the now-smiling Ted was soon slipping my five-pound note into the mouth of the worn brown leather money bag tied around his substantial waist.

Once we were back home, Dad didn't have chance to have a cup of tea as I insisted that he drill into the plasterboard ceiling either side of my bedroom window. Sturdy hooks were installed, and the macramé attached to those, into which I carefully titivated the riotous ferny fronds until they looked just so.

"Very stylish, Son." Dad wound the grey flex of his drill into loose circles around its handle. "If you've done, I'm going to have a cuppa and a sit down before you can dream up another project for me."

I lit a gardenia-scented joss stick and slipped it into the hole of the crushed seashell-embellished wooden holder I'd bought for the purpose, remembering how Tim had scoffed when he'd seen the wrapper that it came in.

"Handmade from Himalayan cypress? Is it bollocks. More like knocked up out of an old orange box from down the back of Sneinton Market." He tossed the packet onto my bed. "You'll believe owt, you will. It's just bleddy hippy rubbish, so don't you start pratting about with drugs. Things like this are just the start of all that."

I chuckled at the memory, watching a narrow strand of incense smoke rise from the glowing ruby tip until it fanned out into wispy grey mare's tails through the lush foliage of my new ferns, just as I'd hoped it would when I stood on at the market stall. Reclining on my bed, I smiled with contented, superior suaveness. My room was beginning to look just how I imagined the pad of a gay man in San Francisco would look.

Over the next few days, my imagination blossomed. I went to the Reject Shop in town and bought a five-foot wide bamboo blind for the window. To inject more atmosphere, I clamped a pair of aluminium industrial photographic studio lights to my bed head. Dad used to have them in his tiny photographic dark room at the old house, but they'd remained stuffed in the top of the wardrobe in the back bedroom ever since we'd moved here. I replaced the high-power bulbs with those of a lower wattage and, after considerable meticulous luminary experimentation, I angled the beams to highlight the ferns from beneath, creating gargantuan, fuzzy charcoal spiders that crawled across the ceiling and down the walls, reminding me of Syd and Bill's amazing home. I rapidly rendered the overhead light redundant; it was too invasive, too harsh, and just far too mundane for someone as tasteful and chi-chi as me.

From the shadowed depths of the airing cupboard, I extracted the black and gold curtain that used to be at the bottom of the stairs in the old

Chucking Putty at the Queen

house and stapled it to the plasterboard wall. Further delving amongst the towels and sheets produced a frizzy blanket covered with mis-matched squares and oblongs in varying shades of green and yellow. I had no idea where it had come from, but it was just the job, and I stapled that to the wall too. I stepped back to admire my handiwork, pleased with this macho modern look which I was sure would be all the rage in the Castro. This was fab. I'd promised myself that something better change, and it had. Oh, yes, the eighties were definitely going to be my decade.

My enthusiastic creativity was unstoppable, and I saw potential in even the most mundane objects. In the back yard stood four cement breeze blocks left over from one of Tim's projects. I struggled up to my bedroom with them, and when Tim got home from work, I asked if he could get me a couple of scaffold boards.

"What do *you* want with scaff boards?"

"To make bookshelves for my bedroom."

"With scaff boards? Are you bleddy barmy? What do you want to prat about with them for? I've got some lovely lengths of mahogany at work; I'll make you a proper bookcase. Call it an early birthday present." Tim was proud of his capabilities as a joiner and was as passionate about wood as I was of collecting records. However, it would inevitably take the best part of nine months before I saw the finished product.

"No, ta. I need something *now*. I'm creating a West Coast utilitarian vibe." I sighed, as if explaining basic addition to a simple child. "So it *has* to be rough and industrial."

"What the fuck are you on about, West Coast whatever it was? You're bleddy wappy, you are." He shoved a hand down the back of his jeans and scratched vigorously. "Rough and industrial. Have you told Dad about this?"

"'Course I have," I lied. "He thinks it's great. Aw, go on, Tim, get me some. I know what I want."

He shook his head and continued scratching. "I'll tell you what you want: you want bleddy looking at, that's what you want." He delved further inside his jeans and grimaced. "I reckon I've got a splinter in me arse." He extracted his hand and examined an object clasped between his forefinger and thumb. "Huh, it's only a bit of dried-on Cascamite. I dunno how that's got there." He flicked the hardened spot of wood glue across my room. "Have it your own way, but I'm telling you, you'll never get full-length scaff boards down the hall, round the corner, and up the stairs. Not without cutting 'em in half. Yeah, that's what I'll do, I'll cut 'em in half up at work on the band saw when I'm on overtime next weekend."

"Cheers."

"But I'm not doin' it for nowt."

"I knew there'd be a catch. How much?"

"You can go up me allotment next week and trim the privet hedges."

"But there's miles of them."

"That's the deal. You do me hedges, and I'll get you your scaff boards."

True to his word, late on the following Saturday morning the earth shook as one of the firm's lorries belted up the road at the back of us as if in a scene from one of Tim's favourite films, *The Hell Drivers*. But unlike Stanley Baker and Patrick McGoohan, who raced their dumper trucks to see who could deposit the largest load of construction rubble in the fastest time, this was a competition against the clock to see how quickly Tim and his mate Terry could unload and manoeuvre the truncated timber upstairs, and then clear off to the boozer.

With my unconventional bookcase completed, I congratulated myself on my supremely minimalist artistic statement and beamed at the shiny spines of my homosexual bookish bounty bought from Mushroom Bookshop–the cherished volumes by Andrew Holleran, John Rechy, James Baldwin, Christopher Isherwood, and Larry Kramer–which I proudly displayed on the rough timber.

My shadowed fern canopy was soon augmented with more macramé holders supporting cascading lengths of grape ivies, tradescantia, and spider plants. The cumulative effect soon prompted Dad to comment that my room was a cross between the public library and the hot house at Kew Gardens, and that he'd soon need a machete to get in.

Yet my dark unhappiness flourished beneath this abundant Amazonian fertility. Beyond the perimeter of the bedroom, my private jungle succumbed to the concrete reality of the awaiting outside world. As I sat reading *Gay News* with my unlit pink triangle candle on my bedside table, I vowed not to stay hidden here but venture further afield and seek my as yet undiscovered tribe, just as Dr Livingstone had quested into the jungle.

Illuminated by the soft glow from a string of white fairy lights that I'd persuaded Dad to let me use just until next Christmas, I lay back against my pillows. Although their covers were from Brentford Nylons, my imagination readily converted the harsh fabric into hand-stitched Madras silk. I periodically sipped from a wine glass filled with pineappleade and sighed contentedly at how avant-garde and unconventional I'd become. However, the commonplace soft drink was not sufficiently cosmopolitan for the new, cultured me, and to exemplify my elegance, I bought hand-wrapped individual sachets of jasmine tea from a health food shop in Hockley. At that time, the thoroughfare wasn't the trendy area it evolved into in the following century. Instead, the shops beneath the tall Victorian buildings comprised of everyday stores including butchers, haberdashers, a pram shop, a supermarket, cobblers, optician, and a fascinating surgical appliance emporium. All rubbed shoulders with what Dad distrustfully branded as "fly-by-night catch merchants selling hippy tat."

My refinement gurgled down the drain when I opened the lid of the tin tea caddy to find it devoid of the misty white squares of jasmine-perfumed tea leaves. I bet Tim had carried out his threat to take them to work "just for the craic" and remembered him elaborating that he couldn't wait to see the faces of the lads up the yard when he mashed a pot of jasmine tea. "They'll think I'm a right poof."

Exhausted after my physical endeavours at the hospital, I really didn't want to traipse all the way back into town, and remembering their slogan, "It's all at the Co-Op," I ambled down to the shopping precinct. Upon my request for the exotic beverage, one of the assistants, Marilyn, scratched her scalp, and repeatedly clicked her tongue as if to demonstrate the effort of thinking.

"But jasmine's a plant, int it? Me nanar had one down the bottom of her back yard outside her bog when I was little because she reckoned it covered up the smell." She shook her head. "But I don't think you can make tea with it, duck. Let me go and ask the manager."

She returned with John, a man of Mediterranean appearance with ill-fitting dentures and eyes that resembled the liquorice and aniseed flavoured Pontefract Tea Cake sweets that Gran had fervently loved. He placed his hands on his hips whilst giving me an up-and-down look worthy of my favourite camp entertainer, Larry Grayson. I wouldn't have been surprised to see him run a finger along the shelving and indignantly comment, "Ooh, just look at the muck on here." Instead, he pouted and tapped a rapid rhythm with one black slip-on shoe on the shiny lino floor tiles.

"Well, you're *quite* the adventurous one, aren't you? *Jasmine tea*—I've never heard the like." He paused and raised his eyebrows. "*Most* people round here drink PG Tips or Co-Op's own." His sing-song voice gurgled as if he were battling to keep his false teeth from falling out of his mouth.

I raised my own eyebrows and shook my head. "Well, I'm not most people round here."

He flapped a pulpy hand. "Ooh, there's no need to get all *huffy* about it, I'm sure. I was just *saying*, that's all."

"It's okay, really. It doesn't matter if you haven't got any. I'll go to the health food shop in Hockley."

He gave an excited squeal as if I'd just told him he'd won a million pounds on the football pools. "Ooh, the *health food shop*. In *Hockley* of all places! Get *you*!" He ran a hand over his thinning hair and sighed. "You know, Marilyn, young men these days... They're beyond me." He lightly pressed a forefinger to my sternum. "And you know this one here, when he was little, well you'll *never* guess what he used to do."

I groaned because I knew what was coming next: he'd go on about when I was younger and used a blue felt pen to insert a full stop between the T and R on every block of TREX cooking fat stacked on the refrigerated shelves so that it looked like T.REX. I'd remained undetected for weeks until one afternoon when, bent over with my face cooled by the artificial temperature, I only had another six blocks left to alter.

"Gotcha!"

Sweaty fingers and a thumb handcuffed my wrist. My blue felt pen dropped onto the white blocks as I was jerked upright. "Ow, gerroff. You're hurting."

It was John. He reached down and grabbed my pen. "If I let go, do you promise not to run off?"

I giggled. "What, in *these* heels?" With my free hand, I tugged at my purple bell bottoms to reveal the women's boots that I wore at every available opportunity.

He released my wrist. "Well, I must say I'm surprised to find that it's *you* who's been doing it. I've been wondering *forever* who was vandalising my cooking fat, and all the time it was *you*."

I bobbed a curtsy, then twirled, certain that the cerise sequins emblazing T. REX across the shoulders of my net curtain cape would

Chucking Putty at the Queen

sparkle like neon fuchsias beneath the harsh lights. "Well, who did you think it would be?"

"You cheeky bogger. This is vandalism. I should call the police." He scratched his stubbly jowls. "But I don't like to get involved with them, so I'll let you off with a private warning." He wagged a forefinger. "Don't do it again."

"May I have my pen back, please?" I held my hand out.

He unclipped the lid from the end, sheathed the nib, and slipped it into the top breast pocket of his overall. "No, you bleddy can't. I'm confiscating it forever. Now be on your way, or I really will ring the police."

I huffed and tossed my head. The fronds of my multicoloured crêpe-paper wig rustled as I flounced towards the doors. "Betcha won't."

I stared over his shoulders at the changed landscape beyond the plate glass windows. The weak saplings that had been planted on the once-new precinct were now sturdy young trees, the women's boots no longer fitted me, and my glittery raiment was faded and pushed in a box beneath my bed. Thankfully, before the grinning manager could resurrect the memory of my felt pen activities for Marilyn's entertainment, I was saved by the bell ringing at the tills.

"John, the dividend stamps machine's got all jammed up again."

"Hang on, Sylvia, dear, I'm on my way." He smiled at me and gulped as if he'd swallowed the invisible sweet in his mouth. "Nice as this is, I can't stand here chatting to you about the old times. *Some of us* have got work to do."

I followed him as he swished towards the agitated Sylvia.

"Thanks for your help anyway." The metal door frame grated on the tiles when I shoved it open.

"Oi, Simon, bring me a jasmine tea bag back from the health shop for my afternoon cuppa, won't you?"

I paused in the doorway. "How do you know my name?"

Deftly rolling a blue paper ribbon of dividend stamps, he giggled coquettishly and arched his thick black eyebrows. "Oh, come on. *Everyone* round here knows *your* name."

211

23

HERE COMES A SATURDAY

REGARDLESS OF THE ELATION I'd gained from my interior design adventures, I remained in a state of frustrated, lonely stagnation. Apathy festered, contaminating me with deep depression about the futility of my existence. I was going nowhere fast. What was the point in celebrating my difference? As a consequence of such weltschmertz, I eschewed my homemade post-punk gear. The energetic graphics and provocative sloganeering with which I'd adorned the numerous shirts now seemed pointless.

On bin day, I pulled them from the metal hangers in my wardrobe and with arms laden like a contestant in a grab all you can in sixty seconds competition, hurried downstairs and hobbled to the back of the rumbling wagon. "Hang on, mate. I've got these." I tossed them into the stinking metallic mouth and watched the crushing jaws close on not only the vibrantly decorated cotton but also on my confidence. If only I could so effortlessly discard the debilitating paranoia that continued to poison me like an untreated infection. Shadows moved within shadows. Voices mocked me although there was nobody around. I searched for footprints that had disturbed the smoothness of the front lawn, and pigeons cooing on the rooftop became the threatening murmurs of my adversaries.

Beneath the weight of this psychological malaise, I refused to be noticeable. I flattened my mess of hair and donated my oversized black 1940s suit to the charity shop from where I'd bought it. I became mundane and pedestrian, dressing in clothes more suitable for someone fifty years older. My sense of self had eroded like wind-whipped sand dunes, with my spirit bleached the same beige as the baggy clothes I used to disguise the despised flabbiness of my chest. And when I donned a chunky knit, caramel-coloured cardigan adorned with chocolate brown lapels and two-inch-wide circular wooden buttons, I realised that my surrender to conformity was complete. I'd turned into the man who advertised sensible clothing for seniors in the back of a Sunday paper.

I succumbed to an evening routine of going to the pub with Dad, where we sat with his pals Ken and Albert around a circular table with a Formica top the colour of overripe damsons. In our quartet, I was the only clean-shaven one, as all three ex-servicemen wore handlebar moustaches, and Albert augmented his facial hirsuteness by sporting impressive lambchop sideburns.

    I sometimes thought that an onlooker may have considered my being in the company of much older men as something unusual or perhaps piteous. But to me, it was neither. Their established masculinity attracted me, and I relished the myriad conversational topics of this trio of seasoned home brewers, bakers, and gardeners. I knew the best soil in which to grow sweet peas for maximum floral yield, the assorted complexities of fermenting oak leaf wine, and I'd been educated in which yeast was preferable to bake the perfect cottage loaf. These lighthearted opinions sat cheek by jowl with more profound considerations on politics and social issues, although they strictly abided to their rule of never discussing religion and football, the two subjects that Dad maintained were "guaranteed to create a falling out." I listened and learned, remembering Dad's advice that if you have nothing sensible to say, then say nothing, and when I occasionally chipped in with my opinions, I hoped that they didn't regard me as a silly seventeen-year-old. Yet I remained unfulfilled as I revelled in the cosy, manly companionship of sagacious debate and of being a junior member in this intimate club in which Dad and Ken puffed cigars and Albert sucked at his pipe, all three expelling columns of fragrantly woody smoke that hovered above us in churning graphite clouds worthy of John Constable's atmospheric brushwork.

    Each night, as a lone moth drawn irresistibly to a flame, I returned home to once more flutter through my gay magazines. The faces of the models had become as familiar to me as those in our family photo albums, and I knew the narrative of the lascivious stories by heart. I devoured enticing reports of a world alien to mine, one in which I could join a vibrant community of friends with whom I'd visit nightclubs, restaurants, and discos. And as I clicked off my bedside light, I dared to dream that within such a Utopian new life, I might even find love.

    But until the manifestation of that currently unreachable event, my only respite from mediocrity occurred in the vaults bar of the Chase pub at eight o'clock on Saturday nights. The jukebox was unplugged, and the dazzling neon tubes overhead were extinguished and replaced by four

Chucking Putty at the Queen

flashing-coloured bulbs on the front of Disco Jim's twin turntable mobile rig. Draped over the dartboard next to the untuned upright piano, the electric anaconda of his six-foot rope light pulsed golden twinkles that transformed the dirty miasma of cigarette smoke into a council estate bar room version of the northern lights. Every weekend, the entertainment began when the countdown introduction of Dan Hartman's hit "Instant Replay" launched two-and-a-half hours of excruciatingly loud music from present and past top twenties.

But the flickering, shining, ear-splitting escape wasn't the Trocadero Transfer disco in San Francisco or the legendary Studio 54 in New York, those bacchanalian arenas where gay DJs spun wonderfully exhilarating twelve-inch singles. This was just a ramshackle mobile disco in the local pub, with a collection of seven-inch records ferried to the premises in wooden Babycham boxes. There were no shirtless men gyrating as they sniffed bottles of amyl nitrite, their sweaty torsos smeared with reflected spangles from dozens of spinning mirror balls. Here, the patrons attempted shouted conversations above the ear-splitting volume of the Nolan Sisters, Dr Hook, and The Police. Nevertheless, I relied on the temporary escapism it provided, and the vastly diluted glimpse of a scintillating nightclub future that I desperately hoped to be a part of one day.

One Saturday night at chucking out time, giddy after I'd recklessly matched Tim pint-for-pint, I stumbled down the steps from the pub and landed face down on the concrete slabs of the shopping precinct. "I'm not pissed." I manoeuvered into a sitting position and examined my hands. "It was just me sticks gave way." I blew on my throbbing palms.

Tim hauled me to my feet, retrieved my walking sticks, and checked that I wasn't seriously injured.

"You okay?"

"Just about."

"I'm off up the chippy for me favourite. Are you coming?"

"No, I'm going home. That shook me up a bit."

Tim strode away on his mission to buy half a deep-fried chicken, a portion of chips, and a couple of pickled eggs, all covered with curry sauce. It was a dead cert that in the morning he'd complain, "My guts are off. I dunno why," and attribute his gastric discomfort to a bad pint, which unfailingly was the fault of a negligent pub landlord who hadn't cleaned the beer pipes out properly. My grub-loving brother maintained that this ad-hoc supper combination was not only "bleddy lovely" but essential sustenance after downing eight pints of bitter. I just wanted to get home and ensconce myself within my imaginary San Francisco apartment. I'd cosy up in bed beneath my palms and ferns and immerse myself in the pages of Andrew Holleran's *Dancer from the Dance* until my drunkenness made his lines of prose sway on the page like telephone wires on a windy day.

As I staggered homeward bound, my two walking sticks seemed to have developed independent lives, determined to ignore my forward command and preferring to move sideways or backwards instead. Each time I blinked to rectify the double image of the wobbling line of parked cars, the cloudless night sky became populated with blue, red, yellow, and green UFOs that the flashing disco lights had burned onto my retinas. I weaved unsteadily past the back of the shops where the smell of boiling fat polluted the air as it spewed in grey clouds from the metal chimney above the chippy. Splayed creamy fingers of illumination reached out to me from the streetlights on the precinct, highlighting the square paving slabs that were cracked into quarters from the weight of delivery lorries, forming miniature, jagged mountain ranges.

My dormant paranoia erupted like a beery belch. My progress was being watched from behind the half-open wooden gates of the chippy. Through the irregular clatter of an extractor fan, my ears sucked in the urgent whispered alert, "Here he is." My schoolyard foes, now young adults, were ready to ambush me. There was no protection in the temporary vision-robbing blackness back here. Although Tim was only twenty yards away, he may as well have been in the Old Market Square, oblivious to my peril as he waited within the bright lights, no doubt relishing the greasy smells of his favourite post-pub eatery. The buses were no longer running, and all was silent apart from the nerve-jarring fan. Emboldened by a surge of lager-fuelled confidence, I refused to endure a repeat of those attacks at school. I lurched towards the gates where the neglected paint peeled in autumn leaves of crisp brown gloss. Even if my tormentors fulfilled their promises to kill me, I'd take on those bastards whose unforgiving regime of bullying had made my life hell.

"Come on then. You don't scare me anymore." I raised one of my walking sticks and thwacked the gate. The impact of wood on wood

Chucking Putty at the Queen

resounded like a spy film gunshot but prepared as I was for confrontation, I still jumped out of my skin when a ginger cat leaped past with something white and floppy dangling from its mouth. Otherwise, the area that stank of rotten fish and stagnant water was lifeless. Though I hadn't achieved any retribution, I was proud of my display of retaliation. I continued my unsteady walk home with my chest puffed out as if my unremarkable cardigan were a military tunic adorned with medals for bravery.

The next morning, I sat at the table in my usual place facing the large picture window, squinting against the sunlight dazzling from the cellulose sheets that Dad had made the lean-to greenhouse from. I closed my left eyelid to block Tim making light work of his breakfast. When Dad placed a similarly magnificent fry-up in front of me, I thought I'd faint.

Tim grinned as he energetically cut a well-cooked sausage. He leaned forward, a brown smear of Daddies sauce on his unshaven chin. "What's up with you?"

"I feel rough."

"I can see that. Your eyes look like piss holes in the snow."

"Cheers." I blew slowly through my pursed lips, hoping that it would alleviate my nausea. "How much did I drink last night?"

Tim laid his knife precisely on the edge of his plate as if it were an expensive new chisel and clapped me on the back. "I had eight pints, and you kept up with me."

His admiration was so strong that anybody would've thought I'd won the Nobel Peace Prize. *Eight pints.* For over a year, the same thing had happened each weekend, and yet again, I thought of the records that money could have bought instead of being wasted on beer. My queasy mind and empty stomach collided, and I pushed my tarmac tongue around my sandpit mouth as an angle grinder shot sparks across my vision.

Hoping to halt the uncontrollable roundabout in my head, I massaged the clammy flesh of my forehead. "I feel dog rough. I might go back to bed." My moist palms cushioned my hot face, which I imagined melting like an almost-spent candle, my features slowly distorting and dribbling down the inside of my arms. "I don't half feel off. Perhaps I had one of those bad pints you're always on about."

"Well, there's nowt up wi' me." He stuffed a large slice of juicy blue-grey mushroom into his mouth.

Dad had bought them from the market the day before and upon his arrival home, he'd triumphantly announced, "Blueys with breakfast tomorrow."

Then, the thought of this breakfast delicacy filled me with delightful expectation but now, I would rather have eaten sand as I watched Tim slide another glistening, slug-like slice into his mouth.

"You wanna know summat? If you can't take your ale like a man, you shouldn't drink it."

His mushroom-muffled judgment was the last thing I needed. I peered at him from between my fingers. "Come off it. You're twenty-seven. I'm seventeen. You've had loads of practice."

"We've all gotta start somewhere. You wanna get some of that grub down your neck. That'll settle your guts. And, ayup, if you don't want them sausages, I'll have 'em for my snap tomorrow."

Even though eating the fried breakfast was the last thing I wanted to do, there was no way I'd let Tim have my sausages to add to his Monday elevenses at work. After several deep breaths, I half-heartedly chewed, wincing at each fingernails-down-a-blackboard scrape of Tim's knife against his plate. I hoped that eating breakfast and drinking a couple of cups of strong, sweet tea would curtail the lump hammers impacting on the inside of my skull. I closed my eyes and exhaled, hoping to repel the nausea that had surged when egg yolk swirled slowly into the juice of my plum tomatoes and blushed the bronzed slice of fried bread. My hangover compounded the wretched, negative reality of my stifling life, and I once more lamented my lack of gumption to change my situation and to get out and meet other gay men.

Tim burped and tapped the edge of my plate with his knife. "Tell you summat, you about chewed that John's tabs off last night."

"John?" Sweat bloomed on my forehead. "What John?"

"That big bloke with the 'tash like Groucho Marx."

Until that moment, when my heart thrust the blood through my veins with sickening urgency, I didn't know it was possible for my temperature to rise and drop simultaneously. I frowned as if I were trying hard to remember but knew full well who Tim was talking about. Oh, shit. What had I said? My breakfast rebelled and threatened to reappear as the replay of the night beneath the flashing lights fast-forwarded.

John was an anomaly amongst the weekend parade of suits, ties, jumpers, and cardigans. He looked as if he'd stepped from the American gay magazine *Blueboy* that resided in my bedside cabinet. He perfectly fitted the description I'd read of the Castro Street Clones, the burgeoning subset of gay male culture who wore short back and sides haircuts and adorned their top lips with moustaches. They favoured the macho lumberjack garb of checked flannel shirts, faded jeans with keys hanging from a belt loop, and sturdy work boots. We were only a few months out of the seventies, and a substantial proportion of the male population still had what my young nephew called "big hair." But, similar to the men in my magazines, John's was cut short, and a thick black moustache covered his top lip, its darkness blending with his jowls and chin that were permanently dirtied with stubble. Although I covertly studied him, the disconcerting thing was that he stared at me. *He stared a lot.* Despite the thick golden band that encircled the third finger of his left hand, I never saw him accompanied by a woman. Whenever I'd seen him on the street from afar, he was always alone. Occasionally, a white miniature poodle pranced daintily at his workboot-shod feet as he strode purposefully to wherever he was going. He looked so masculine that I would have expected him to own a Doberman pinscher or an Alsatian. Within the crowded pub, he appeared solitary and barely engaged with fellow drinkers. If he sat at a table with other men, it wasn't as one of their mates but rather, he was just taking advantage of a vacant stool.

As weeks passed, I began a less cautious appraisal of him. Every time I did so, I was met by his coal black eyes, framed by thin-rimmed spectacles. Increasingly emboldened by the pints of lager that I'd necked to soothe my own Saturday night fever, I'd begun to recklessly stare back at the beefy man who stood out from the crowd just as I had in my flamboyant, homemade glam gear when I was younger. As with my sartorial appearance back then, nobody else looked the same.

I fell back to earth with a bump when Tim tapped the end of his knife on the table.

"So what were you gassing on about? I didn't know you knew him."

"I don't."

"Well, you had your heads together, and you were going on about summat."

"It was nowt much. I really can't remember. Disco Jim had his volume turned up dead loud as usual." My stomach churned, and a fresh wave of clamminess made me want to vomit. Oh, god, this was terrible. Slanting rays of reflected sunshine highlighted the frizzly top of the tea cosy, converting the cropped pile of threads into a multitude of hairy caterpillars. If only I could recall what I'd said to him. How we'd even got talking was lost in the sludge of alcohol-addled memories.

Tim raised his empty plate and licked away the greasy residue of the fry-up, smacked his lips, and burped. "Bleddy lovely, that was, Dad. Ta." He shoved his chair back and stood up.

When he clapped me on the back, I thought my eyeballs would fall out and join the scarlet tomatoes on my plate.

"And I'll tell you summat for nowt. If you're that hungover, you wanna come down the pub with me for a Sunday livener. A few dinnertime pints will sort you out."

"Ugh, don't. I'll never drink again."

Tim wiped away the dribble of brown sauce still on his chin and leaned towards me, frowning. "I got to admit, you do look bleddy rough. If you're not coming for a few pints, you want to get some of that orange juice in the fridge down yer neck."

My fork thudded on the tablecloth. Orange juice. *Oh no*. I closed my eyelids and fell into a black hole of recent memory…

As usual, I'd joined Tim in the bar and although he was no great conversationalist, I couldn't shake the sense of abandonment when he went to join his mates gathered around a table in the corner. A raucous wedding party arrived, laughing and light-heartedly complaining about the rain. Across the room, the plate glass windows were a mosaic of dribbling jewels created by the headlights, indicators, and brake lights of vehicles passing by outside, complementing the flashing colours indoors. My heart juddered when I recognised a familiar figure at the back of the party. Clad in his usual attire, it was obvious that he wasn't a member of the jolly matrimonial crew.

The influx swelled the revellers in the bar and before I knew it, John was at my side. His elbow jostled my arm.

He nodded. "Sorry, mate."

I looked into the dark eyes that were closer than they'd ever been and gripped my glass so tightly I expected it to shatter. "You're all right. I haven't got enough left to spill."

"Eh?"

I leaned my head in closer. "I said I haven't got enough left to spill." His hair smelled of the delicious dampness of fresh rain.

His chuckle was deep and rich. "That gets me out of buying you a pint then."

A man in a hideous pin-striped suit shoved past him towards the bar, and now we stood shoulder to shoulder. If only I could stop my legs from quivering.

He nudged me. "Dunno where this lot's come from. They seem pissed up already."

"Yeah."

"You're Tim's brother Simon, aren't you?"

He knew my name. But then again, most people in this room knew I was Tim's brother, so why should his statement make my legs tremble so violently? "Yeah, I'm the baby of the family."

His grin revealed a flash of even, white teeth beneath his luxuriant moustache. "You're not that much of a baby. I'm John."

"Ayup, John." *What do I say now?* I watched the pin-stripe suited man weave through the crowd until he reached the beer crate podium where he handed Disco Jim a spirits' glass then yelled something in his ear.

Trapped within the crowd, there was no let up in the pressure of John's upper arm against mine.

Disco Jim tapped his microphone. "One-two, one-two. Even though they'll be in their Welsh honeymoon suite already, this is one for the bride and groom from the best man, Wayne."

The abrupt change in music couldn't have been harsher. The opening refrain of the ghastly novelty song, "Day Trip To Bangor" was received by cheers and whoops from the wedding party.

"Oh, not this. I can't stand it."

I only just heard John. This was my chance to forge a bond by agreeing how crap the song was and also to hint at my homosexuality. Even though my head was spinning and the level of the room see-sawed, I congratulated myself for my flash of inspiration. "I can't stand it an' all. I've just bought the single by Orange Juice. It's called 'Blueboy.'" I raised my eyebrows and nudged him, anticipating his eager acknowledgement of this significant code word, waiting for him to confess that he bought the same gay magazine as me.

"You what?"

He moved his head closer to mine. Vibrant colours from the three-hundred-watt reflector bulbs played over his unshaven features and converted his thick moustache into thousands of stained-glass shards. I leaned in as close as I dared. Surrounded by the flashing electric disco lights of the twentieth century, his musky aftershave, redolent of pine and damp earth, suggested a location more natural and organic than the brash bar room. The drunken scriptwriter in my head rapidly wrote our life together. In a widescreen romance, we sauntered hand-in-hand through mist-shrouded coppices as the russet rays of an autumn sunset glowed between the ridged, reddish-brown trunks of sky-scraping fir trees.

He stopped beneath the secretive canopy of dark green undulating in a gentle Pacific Northwest breeze and turned to face me. "I can't hear you."

Flashing disco lights replaced the fingers of shimmering evening sunlight. The two glasses of Dad's potent home brewed bitter I'd had before leaving the house reacted with the lager swilling inside me in reckless, alcohol-inspired audacity. I winked. "It's called 'Blueboy.'" I nudged him. "You know, *Blueboy*, like the American magazine for men." I searched behind the prism-reflecting lenses for a signal, but he only shrugged.

"Never heard of 'em." He shook his head, then raised his glass and drained the remaining deep brown ale, his Adam's apple bobbing in his thick, bristly neck with each gulp. "I can't be doing with this crowd."

My back was against the wall as he placed his left hand on my right shoulder and stretched across me to place his empty glass on the shelf above the darkened jukebox.

"I'm off then. Me missus will be on at me that I've been out too long. See you, mate."

The sickening hollowness in my midriff couldn't have been more devastating even if he'd ripped out my heart and drop-kicked it across the pub car park. "Uh, yeah. Cheers."

He pushed through the crush of bodies to the door. In the corridor he paused and looked back through the glass panel. From the stories in the pages of *Blueboy*, I knew what should happen next. I'd follow him outside, and we'd go to his place. But that scenario couldn't play out with his wife waiting at home. To quash my devastating sense of loss, I imagined her standing on the doorstep looking at her watch as he sheepishly approached, a rolling pin-wielding toothless harridan whose greasy hair framed her warty face. My unfounded jealousy raged. She was probably boss-eyed as well. That handsome, masculine man deserved better, and that was me. I was clueless, completely naïve, and head-swimmingly drunk.

Tim laid his knife and fork on his empty plate. "So what were you on with? You looked very pally-pally."

"I can't remember. Summat and nowt, I suppose."

He carried his plate towards the kitchen. "Well, if you're not coming for a pint, I'll get meself ready."

More boozing was the last thing I wanted as hangover hammers continued their attempt to destroy my cranium. I sipped my tea. This was definitely the morning after the night before. I suppressed the acidic ocean in my stomach rearing up. The path of my life journey was heading in a desperate, dangerous route, and I had to do something to alter its course and find friends like me. Otherwise, I'd take a step in the wrong direction and get queer-bashed by a married man who dressed like the models in my gay magazines.

24

DOWN IN THE SUBWAY

"You don't want to go giving the glad eye to married blokes in the pub; you'll get yourself duffed up. I keep telling you: you need to get down town and meet other puffs."

Jacqui was right. I drained the last tepid inch of PG Tips and put my mug into the bowl filled with steaming, lemon-scented soap suds. "It's not that easy, though, is it?"

"Why not?"

"'Cos it's not."

"Why?"

Instead of answering, I opened the back door. "See you Saturday."

"Hold up, don't get all huffy and go flouncing off."

"I'm *not* getting all huffy and flouncing off."

"Yes, you are."

Frustrated by having no solution to my lonely predicament, I hovered in the doorway as if my friend would magic one up.

"So, are you going down the pub tonight?"

"Oh, I dunno."

"Well, if you do, promise me you won't go giving the glad eye to married blokes."

"There's no need to tell me a second time. I'm not *that* daft."

Jacqui finished her own tea and shook her head. "I'm not so sure."

As each of my slow steps took me closer to home, I pondered my situation. Adventuring into town to explore the gay scene wasn't as cut and dried as she assumed. She knew how hung up I was about my reliance on a raised orthopaedic shoe and having to use sticks to walk but regardless of our close friendship, I wasn't ready to confide about the flabby flesh on my chest that also prevented me from achieving my goal.

When I entered our living room, Tim was sitting at the table.

"Ayup, look what I found!"

"Oh, not *that* thing!"

It was a novelty circular jigsaw that was a present from Uncle Harry and his wife, Marjorie, on the first Christmas after Mam died. Dad was insulted that they'd posted it to his workplace instead of bringing it to the house.

"Your Aunty Marjorie is an out-and-out snob, Son. The worst kind of suburban social climber. She looks down on St. Ann's, even though she's from the same background as us."

Tim shook the box. "You gonna help me do it?"

"No, I'm not."

I had no patience with jigsaws, let alone stupid circular ones, and turned to go upstairs.

Tim shook the box. "Hold up. Don't go. I'll check that it's all here. If there's any bits lost, you can help me find them." He slid the box open. "One. Two. Three..."

As if he were a hypnotist counting someone into a trance, I drifted off, recalling an incident on a crisp Sunday morning in January 1973 which had really set the brotherly cat amongst the pigeons...

Dad and I were in the kitchen, and after I'd badgered him to let me help, he relented and suggested that I peel parsnips in preparation for roasting them in beef dripping.

"We'll do them slow and low, Son. Slow and low."

He allowed me to use the sharpest knife, although not without a degree of foreboding.

"Concentrate on the job in hand, and remember that it's a knife, not a microphone, so please don't use it to sing T. Rex songs into. I don't want to be fishing slices of your fingers from amongst the parsnip peelings."

I'd already peeled several when through the back gate slats there was a flash of turquoise.

"Dad, look at that car!"

We stared up the yard as it swooped down the parking area and pulled up next to Dad's Rover 90. My rakish Uncle Harry alighted from the driver's seat and swaggered to the gate, clicked the latch, and let it swing wide. I lay the knife on the draining board, pulled the back door open, and skipped up the path onto the pavement. "Uncle Harry! Wow, what kind is it?"

He nonchalantly shrugged his shoulders, pulled the collar of his sheepskin coat up, and took a drag on the tiny stub of a cigarette. Then he tipped the rim of his trilby hat so that it was almost on the back of his head. "A 1957 Cadillac Coupe de Ville."

I moved my fingertips towards the bonnet. "What a fabulous colour."

"Don't touch. It's a special American paint job and cost me a fortune."

I breathed my reverence as if it were an incantation. "A 1957 Cadillac Coupe de Ville with an American paint job." For a split second, I tremored with traitorous regret for loving the exotic name and jaw-dropping hue that were far more glamorous than the black Rover 90, but nevertheless, I pirouetted, clapping my hands. "Oh wow, oh wow, oh wow. It's a real live, two-finned Caddy just like in 'Chariot Choogle.'"

"What language is *that*?"

"It's a T. Rex song from *The Slider* and Marc Bolan sings about a two-finned Caddy, short for Cadillac. And one of the two tracks on the B-side of 'Telegram Sam' is called Cadillac although Marc spells it with just one L." The flats at the top of the parking space became unfocused and wobbled slightly, so I took a deep breath. "And now here's a Cadillac right in front of my very own eyes."

Dad came to my side and rested his hand on my shoulder.

"Hello, Harry. You look like a second-hand car salesman."

I was still contemplating how the glamorous vehicle shone with streamlined angular ostentation next to the bulky, regal solidity of Dad's car when I noticed two spectral figures in the back seat. I crouched to have a better look, wondering if the unmoving heads and shoulders were showroom dummies. Dad had mentioned in the past that Uncle Harry did a lot of "buying and selling of tat and anything that he can make a few bob from."

Dad bent down next to me for a couple of seconds then resumed his upright position. He frowned. "Who's that in the back? You've not picked up a couple of tarts again, have you?"

When Uncle Harry narrowed his eyes, I realised why Dad reckoned that he was shifty.

"No need to be snidey, Sid. That was an innocent misunderstanding, and you know it. Don't keep dragging it up. It's Marjorie and her mother."

"What are they doing sitting out here in the car? Aren't you coming in for a cup of tea?"

Uncle Harry looked at his feet and kicked at an empty Player's No. 6 cigarette packet with the toe of his fawn suede shoe. "No, Sid, I won't this time. We were just passing through the area, so I thought I'd show you my car."

"Just passing through?"

The severity of the chill in Dad's voice could have created more icicles to join those already hanging from the roof tiles of the nearby houses.

"Yes. there's a burst water pipe, and we were diverted down Sycamore Road, so I thought, you know, as we were practically passing the door—"

"You thought you'd come and show off."

"Don't be like that, Sid."

"I'm not being like anything. But surely a quick cuppa won't hurt. It's such a long time since Simon saw you."

"Yeah, I've got my new T. Rex album, so I can play you 'Chariot Choogle,' and you can hear all about the two-finned Caddy."

Uncle Harry ignored me and avoided looking at Dad. He shot a glance at the glamorous car. "I'd best not, Sid. It's not me; it's Marjorie and her mother."

"What is?"

Uncle Harry took a deep breath. "They won't come in because it's a council house."

Dad stared at him as if he'd suddenly grown another head. "They won't come in because it's a council house? But Marjorie's mother was born in Radford. What's *she* got to be uppity about?"

"She's not uppity, Sid. You know that win on the pools let us buy a house, and Marjorie says we mix with a better class of people now we're not council." Uncle Harry flattened the cigarette packet beneath his shoe, then nudged it to the edge of the grey kerbstone until it fell into the litter-filled gutter. "She loves it. She holds coffee mornings and is doing flower arranging at the church now, and she's even been invited to join the Residents' Association." He flashed Dad a sideways glance. "And I've been accepted by the golf club." He gave a palm-upwards gesture to the Cadillac. "So what do you reckon to my new beauty then, Sid?"

I slipped my cold, dry hand into the warmth of Dad's, and he gripped my fingers until I thought they'd snap like old twigs.

"It's certainly snazzy, Harry, although many people would regard it as vulgar. Mother used to say that money can't buy love nor good taste. Now, if you'll excuse me, I have to continue preparing dinner for the lads. As you know, I'm on my own since Betty died, and I can't afford the time

Chucking Putty at the Queen

to stand around chatting. Give my regards to Marjorie and her mother." He churned his mouth and twisted the tips of his handlebar moustache. "I hope they're comfortable in the back seat of your new beauty, and I apologise for mistaking them for a pair of tarts. Enjoy the drive home to your better class of people in Edwalton."

He released my hand and, after a smart about-turn, he strode down the path and through the back door. Uncle Harry pinched his cigarette between thumb and forefinger, sucked hard at it until his cheeks hollowed, then flicked the nub away to where it rested on the tarmac like a red sequin against black velvet. Without looking at me, he slid into his spectacular car.

"Can you believe it? My own brother said that I look like a second-hand car dealer."

After aggressively reversing to the top of the car parking area, he did a nifty manoeuvre, and the Cadillac shot off down the road in a blur of kingfisher colours.

In the kitchen, Dad handed me the knife. "Right, Son. Let's get back to peeling parsnips."

"It's a very flash car, Dad, isn't it?"

"Yes, Son. Your Uncle Harry's always been a bit of a spiv."

I pulled the bag of unpeeled parsnips towards me. "How many more shall I do?"

"A half dozen? A dozen? What do you think, Son? How many have you got there already?"

"Hang on, Dad, I'll have a count up. One, two, three, four..."

"Four ninety-eight, four ninety-nine, five hundred...five hundred *and one*?"

I opened my eyes. "You've counted wrong."

"I haven't then."

"You must have. It's a five-hundred-piece jigsaw."

"It don't matter." Tim reunited the two halves of the box, rattled the pieces inside, then farted. "Cor, my guts are off again. I think I'll lay off the ale during the week."

I clamped a hand over my lower face and took several steps backwards. "You need to do summat. That stinks like bad drains."

He grinned and enthusiastically shook the box. "I'll have some Alka Seltzers in a bit when I have another go at this. Are you gonna give me a hand with it?"

The fiendish puzzle had been a nightmare the first time and ended up being swept back into its box unfinished. I grimaced at the memory of how annoying it was. "You *are* joking, aren't you?"

"Suit yerself. Yeah, a few nights in'll sort me out. I'll have that pot of whelks from the fridge, and there's that big packet of peanuts, and that new jar of piccalilli an' all. I'll ask Dad for a few bottles of that Geordie Bitter he brewed. I'm all set for a good night in."

"Thought you were laying off the ale?"

"Home brew don't count. It int the same as going down the boozer, and I'll save meself a few bob." He tapped the lid of the box. "And I'll get this jigsaw done an' all."

I thought about my own jigsaw existence. I had all the straight edges connected, but the middle remained a confusing jumble of pieces. As much as I would have liked the handsome, swarthy John from the pub to be a significant part of my life, he belonged to a different, already-completed puzzle and would never fit into the imagined picture of my future gay happiness.

My disconsolate loneliness continued to delude me that I'd meet my true love in an unorthodox way. It would be *me* who finally discovered Quentin Crisp's fabled, elusive *Great Dark Man*. I couldn't wait to be in the arms of the masculine, hirsute-faced dreamboat who would not give two hoots about my bad leg and flabby chest. In my overactive fantasy, a bird's-eye view showed me at a Belfast sink, joyously worshipping at the altar of domestic drudgery as I handwashed his dirty socks and filthy overalls after his week of hard graft under the lorries that he fixed for a living.

My certainty of this belief intensified after I read a two-part story in *HIM* magazine which centred around a young man who was fixated on a butch older bloke whom he'd seen several times in the same location. He'd hung about until they met and, in a perfect fairytale ending, they set up home and lived happily ever after. Each night in bed with the already well-thumbed pages crumpled in my gripping fingers, I religiously revisited the tale, taking strength just as a devout person would gain solace from the Bible. After closing the magazine and clicking off my side light, I snuggled down and wrapped myself in the narrative. Just as I'd wished for Christmas Day to arrive when I was much younger, I impatiently yearned

Chucking Putty at the Queen

for this fictional romance to become reality.

Then, an unexpected light bulb moment arose when I was reading the adverts in the back of the newspaper, thus providing me with a way in which I could hopefully assimilate myself with others like me. The film *Cruising* was playing at the Odeon cinema. It had already gained a degree of notoriety for its blatant depiction of the gay leather scene in New York City and simultaneously attained instant infamy with a large faction of the gay community who complained that it exploited homosexual men by portraying us as abnormal, sadistic sex freaks who were intent on murdering each other. Filming in New York was interrupted by multitudes of gay men blowing whistles, playing loud music from portable stereo tape decks, and yelling through loudhailers. Upon its commercial release, placard-toting crowds picketed outside cinemas. If there were to be demonstrations here, I could engage in some exploitation of my own by using it as a chance to meet other homosexuals without having to lay myself open to judgemental scrutiny in a pub or club. I could wear my pink triangle badge to confirm my sexuality. I was bound to meet someone, surely, even just to talk to. What a great idea. I'd have a quick bath and then head down town.

I stepped from the tub. Condensation draped the bathroom mirror like a dirty lace curtain. I wiped it away with a face flannel and instantly wished that I hadn't as I stared at the reflection of my atrophied leg and the busty flesh on my chest. Not for the first time, I damned the family doctor's misdiagnosis of my leg injury and his unwavering insistence that I was suffering from rheumatoid arthritis in my knee. It was laughable that he believed my pain and ungainly gait would be remedied by Dad rubbing embrocation fluid into my right knee every night. If only he'd immediately sent me for an X-ray, then the dislocation of my hip would have been exposed sooner, and I wouldn't be in this ugly, crippled state now. The psychological ramifications from the endless litany of taunts made by local kids about my bad leg, and the still-raw memories of being attacked at school reinforced my opinion that my walking with a pronounced limp, needing to use walking sticks, and having to wear a raised orthopaedic shoe made me a lesser man than others. And here I stood, kidding myself that I was going to town with the hope of connecting with other gay men and perhaps meeting that apocryphal great, dark man. The droplets on my skin cooled along with my enthusiasm, and I rebuked myself for allowing this ridiculous self-delusion. I hated my appearance, so why would anyone else like me? The steam in the small, muggy room quickly re-shrouded the mirror and once more hid my shameful secret. I pushed open the window, allowing the steam to churn out through the same gap that I'd eavesdropped on Dad talking to the police after I'd chucked putty at the queen only three years ago. I had been so cocksure of myself then. Where was that spirit now? Behind me, with the gurgling last breath of a drowning man, the final inches of dirty bath water drained away and took my temporary wave of confidence with it.

Weeks passed and, secure in my bedroom surrounded by plants, books, and music, I frequently felt that I was living a monastic existence on a remote tropical isle, only needing to venture out when my spiritual supplies needed replenishing. Mushroom Bookshop was one of my sanctuaries. I'd begun visiting occasionally after school, although I never bought anything. I'd earmarked the money that Dad gave me at the start of every week to pay for five days of school dinners for the more crucial kind of purchase: thrilling punk rock singles.

The bookshop was a calm haven that provided respite from an increasingly alien world. Its huge plate glass windows were the perfect environment for a small collection of Swiss cheese plants which reached up with dark green open hands through the delicate lazy haze of joss stick smoke, and on bright days, the rough wooden floorboards shone with minuscule, twinkling prisms from stained glass sun catchers suspended inside the windows by lengths of thin thread.

Tim collared me one Tuesday when he came home from work. He chucked his haversack into the cupboard under the stairs and then headed to the fridge as he always did, even though it was less than an hour until the evening meal. I turned to go upstairs when he grabbed my shoulder.

"Ayup, I want a word with you."

"About what?"

"You know Snotgobbler, dontcha?"

Tim's scruffy, unsavoury associate had a sinus condition which led to his apt nickname. "Yeah. Why?"

"I had a pint with him in the Corner Pin last night, and he said he saw you goin' into that hippy bookshop in Hockley the other day."

"So?"

"So you want to keep out of there, that's all."

"Why?"

"'Cos it's full of bleddy druggies and weirdos wearing baggy hairy jumpers, and they sell joss sticks and all crap like that." Tim's eyes widened as he grabbed my forearm. "Snotgobbler told me that one of the women even had all coloured beads woven in her hair." As if this outrage wasn't enough to dissuade me from future attendance, he looked over each shoulder with the exaggerated caution of a movie spy. "Me and Black Ernie went past it the other Sunday morning when we were having a mooch round town waiting for the Milton's Head to open. Do you know what was in the window?"

"Well, as it's a bookshop, I'm guessing books?"

"Don't be a smart arse. No. You won't guess."

"Well, tell me then."

"There was a bleddy *cat* sitting inside the window." He rotated the cube of cheese he'd selected towards his mouth, then paused before he took a bite. "*Inside the window.* And that was when the shop was *shut.*"

"I don't think that a cat sitting in a shop window is a crime, Tim."

"Well, it isn't right, is it? Not when the shop's shut."

"When should it be there then?"

"That don't matter. It shouldn't've been there when it was shut. I'm just telling yer for your own good. Keep outta there and away from them weirdos."

"And their baggy jumpers."

"Don't you cheek your elders. Just keep away."

Tim's misguided warning didn't stop me going. Sometimes I wish it had, as it was there that an incident occurred which exemplified my ineptitude at forcing the hand of chance to change my life.

On an autumn afternoon cloaked with the doleful premature darkness of midwinter, rain sloshed in turbulent torrents from the overwhelmed Victorian gutters high above Heathcoat Street and splashed up from the pavement as if millions of diamonds were being hurled from the rooftops. The soaked slabs glowed with the pools of amber that spilled from shop windows, stretching towards each other but not sufficiently to form a single lagoon of light. Within the shelter of Mushroom's doorway, I hooked my walking sticks over one arm and removed my spectacles to wipe away the raindrops that crystallised my world. The door was yanked open from the inside, and I was almost bowled over by someone leaving. One of my walking sticks clattered to the ground. I stepped back onto the wet street, my one free hand shielding my newly dried lenses from the downpour. In front of me, surprised dark eyes widened beneath dense, black brows on a square-jawed unshaven face.

"Oh, sorry, mate. Didn't see you." My unintentional assailant bent down, picked up my stick, and handed it to me surprisingly gently for such a bruiser, then stood to one side, gesturing to the still open door. "After you."

Beneath the protection of the shop doorway, I stared after the viciously shorn bull clad in a black leather jacket and army camouflage trousers. When he was on the opposite pavement, he turned and looked over his broad shoulders through the steely lines of rain, then continued on his way, his heavy boots splashing puddles into platinum coronas. At the end of the street, he looked back at me, then disappeared around the corner of the building. The anxious sensation of loss made me glance at the ground, wondering if I'd dropped something. Then I recognised the mental disquiet as that which I'd suffered in my younger years when Dad went out of my sight, no matter how momentarily. But why should that fear of being deserted devastate me now? This bloke had nothing to do with me and, unlike Dad on that day in the store, this stranger wasn't coming back.

A fortnight later, the shop bell pinged. It had sounded several times during this visit, but something told me to look to the door. The eyes that had stared at me in my dreams now stared in the awake world. The bruiser left the shop and crossed the road, where he leaned against the wall next to the barber shop and shoved his hands deep in the pockets of his camo trousers. Familiar fear transmitted a jerky Morse code of painful warning down my bad leg. I was going to get queer-bashed. These fascist thugs were fearless, and there'd be no protection for me once outside this haven that represented what his ilk despised. Never far from my mind, the gut-twisting memory of the vicious attacks on me at school overrode my common sense, and I looked around, hoping to see a back door through which I could escape. I thought that I was safe here. Clearly, I wasn't.

"We're closing in five minutes."

I flinched as if the words were a clenched fist thrust at me and almost dropped the copy of EM Forster's *Maurice* that I'd been pretending to

read, having stared at the same page for so long, the lines of words were black prison bars ingrained on my retinas. "Oh, sorry. I'll take this, I think."
"Good choice. It's a classic."
Tim's warning about the inhabitants of the shop sprung into my mind like an I told you so jack-in-the-box when she tugged at her sloppy purple, orange, and green jumper, but I couldn't laugh. Maybe if I hadn't been so stupid, then I would have heeded him and ceased my visits here.
I'd be safe.
But the danger didn't come from the pale-faced woman in front of me, smiling as she toyed with one of the coloured wooden beads threaded onto her white dreadlocks. It came from a few yards over the road. She pushed in the book spines that protruded from the shelves and resumed her position behind the counter. I unsteadily moved towards her, laid the paperback on the wooden top, and proffered a five-pound note.
She frowned at my shaking hand, then looked up. "Are you all right?"
"Yes, thanks, I... Um..." My mind raced back to school. If my two best friends were unable to prevent me from being beaten up, then I doubted that this lady could offer any protection. What could I tell her? Would she think I was mad if I told her that a thug was waiting across the road to pulverise me? I checked over her shoulder to see what he was up to. The barber was closing up his shop, and the bruiser was gone. Or was he? Maybe he'd crossed over and was lurking in a doorway on this side of the road, waiting to jump me as I left. I leaned further against the counter and scanned the reflections of this side of the street in the windows opposite. There was nobody there.
"Are you sure that you're all right? You're very pale."
"I'm okay, thanks. It's just that my bad leg's hurting."
The street outside was deserted. I set off for home, pretending to shelter in doorways from the rain but really checking that I wasn't being followed. Though even if I was being followed, what could I do? A lone, straggly length of coloured lights glowed with pathetic loneliness in the window of a shop selling hand-knitted baby clothing. I cut down Convent Street at the back of the Palais, where orange Dayglo posters announced the dancehall's upcoming events. This was the quiet thoroughfare which became notable to me when I was sitting in the outside toilet at the old house. The latch of the back gate clicked, and I heard Steve and Tim talking. They stopped, unaware of my presence on the other side of the

door. I bit into my fist when Steve bragged to Tim that he'd beaten a bloke up and "left him for dead on that little street at the back of the Palais." Within a few seconds, I heard them greeting Mam in the kitchen, and it was safe for me to carefully open the toilet door, hoping that the creaky hinges wouldn't alert Steve to my presence. As soon as I stepped into the living room, Steve grabbed me and sat me on his knee.

"Where you been, dagger arse?"

"In the loo."

Tim's head shot up, and he glanced at Steve. "I'm goin' upstairs."

Steve jigged me up and down on his knees and tickled me to make me laugh. I made myself as floppy as possible, and he tugged and tossed me about like a galleon on a tempestuous sea.

Mam called through from the kitchen. "Give over, Steve, he's only just had his tea. I don't want the carpet covered with it."

I let my arms go lifeless, and Steve grabbed my wrists, briefly using my own hands to slap my face.

"What do you keep hitting yourself for?"

I twisted free and slid my hands down to the pockets of his cardigan. "What have you got today?" It was a daft game we'd play, and usually I'd extract a handkerchief, a packet of twenty Player's fags, and a box of matches. But this time my fingers connected with something hard. I pulled out four shiny metal circles joined together and fixed to a bar. I turned it around beneath the glow of the overhead light.

"What's this?"

"Stretch your fingers out."

"No, you'll twist them backwards and try to break them."

"I won't. Not this time, I promise."

"You promised before."

"Giz your fingers and stop being so yitney."

Yitney was local slang for cowardly, but I thought that not offering Steve my fingers was merely sensible.

"Come on, dagger arse. Open them up, and I'll show you what it's for."

With my hand shaking, I splayed my fingers out. Steve attempted to slip the thick metal rings over them just as Mam shot in from the kitchen, her eyes glaring.

"Stephen! What do you think you're playing at? Put that away. You'd better not let your father see it."

Steve laughed as he slid the knuckleduster from my fingers and returned it to his pocket.

It seemed a lifetime ago. Mam was dead, and Steve was in jail. I continued along Convent Street and shivered, not only from the rain dribbling down my neck but also at the thought that my soft young fingers had once connected with the cold metal that Steve had used in his vicious attack on another man.

Rainwater gurgled along the gutters and swirled in shallow pools above the blocked drains. Although Christmas was over a month away, the desolate street already carried a murky, pre-festive sadness, and I viewed the upcoming, inescapable celebrations with foreboding. Even though I'd be surrounded by family members, I already anticipated the aching loneliness that exemplified the rut in which I was well and truly stuck. I'd drink too much lager in the pub and gaze with increasing recklessness at the butch men obviously uncomfortable in their recently unwrapped sweaters or matching shirt and ties. I'd yearn to be with one of them as one half of a romantic Christmas twosome. And of course, later on, after necking some of Dad's delicious but potent homemade wine, I'd grow even more maudlin and torture myself with memories of Christmases when Mam was alive.

That evening, I sat once again with a cup of tea in Jacqui's kitchen. I peered over to the square Tupperware container half-filled with biscuits. "Haven't you got any pink wafers?"

"No. You had them all last time."

"Giz a coconut ring then."

"Get it yourself. I'm not here to serve you biscuits all night." She nudged the container towards me. "You know what the problem is, don't you?"

I selected two of the circular biscuits and held them up to my eyes like spectacles. "What, that men don't make passes at girls who wear glasses?"

"You big wally. No, you won't get anywhere like this, and you shouldn't be trying to pick blokes up in the street."

"It wasn't the street, it was a bookshop, and I wasn't trying to pick him up." I tapped the top of the wooden mug tree standing on the worktop. "This is new."

"Two quid from the Reject Shop, but don't go fiddling about with it. I know you; you'll snap it. And stop trying to change the subject."

We stared at each other in awkward silence. "So, come on, clever clogs. What's the answer?"

"I've told you before: you'd be better off finding this bar that's mentioned in your paper."

She was right, of course. Even though I'd visited Mushroom frequently in the hopes of seeing the bruiser, I never clapped eyes on him again. Weary of my ridiculous fantasies and lack of courage, I was determined that now was the time to be in contact with other gay men, and I knew just where I'd find them. I'd deal with the problem of my chest somehow, but now I just needed to make contact.

The most direct way for me to access my gay salvation was via a gloomy subway beneath the abominable Maid Marian Way. The Hearty Good Fellow was an unremarkable pub on the corner of a cheerless parade of shops that lined the upper stretch of the ugly, two-lane asphalt thoroughfare that slashed through the town, effectively divorcing that part of the city centre from the more bustling, well-populated rest. Despite the preposterously romantic name, it easily acquired the damning accolade as the "Ugliest Road in Europe."

Falling victim to frequent vandalism, the tunnel's neon lighting panels in its ceiling seldom worked and travelling beneath the muted rumble of the overhead traffic amplified a creeping sense of unease. Passing strangers emanated invisible anxiety and tended to be instinctively sucked towards the grimy walls. To walk in the middle of the passageway was confrontational. Should you see more than one person at the distant opposite end, it provoked a disconcerting sensation of being trapped within the traumatic scene from *A Clockwork Orange* in which Alex and his Droogs savagely brutalize a vulnerable drunk.

I'd begun a supplementary evening regime of physio, which necessitated me using the subway. The twice daily exercises knackered me and left me uncertain as to their efficacy. But I trusted Mr Galbraith and did what I was told. The subway was challenging enough in the daytime but as dusk faded into secretive nightfall, it became shrouded with foreboding. When the shops closed, other than Nottingham Playhouse several hundred yards away, there was nothing to attract citizens to that part of town. If you were alone and encountered another male, you never allowed your eyes to connect as you approached. That would be completely foolhardy. You drew a breath and pressed on

Chucking Putty at the Queen

with the muscles in your back taut and your vision adhered to the floor or sideways to the advertising posters. The inanely grinning faces that recommended washing powder, cat food, toothpaste, and chocolate bars were frequently disfigured and amended with swirls of misogynistic, racist, and anti-gay graffiti. The scrawled short, sharp slogans appeared to be in the same hand, making me wonder if there was an embittered, friendless man sitting alone in a darkened room devising them, then sneaking out in the early hours armed with a thick marker pen and a head full of hate. When you arrived at the other end of the subway, you realised that the throbbing in your ears was not solely from the traffic thundering above, but also because you'd been holding your breath like a novice swimmer attempting to complete an underwater length for the first time.

On an uncharacteristically chilly July morning, the sombre grey sky diffused the sun into a dismal orb as I left home and trudged to catch the bus into town for my daytime physio session. At the terminus, I took a detour to Selectadisc to buy *Crocodiles*, the first album by Echo & the Bunnymen that was released that day. A fleeting tremor of mutiny almost persuaded me to nick off from my two hours of painful physical procedures and return home to play it. Just this once wouldn't hurt. But guilt weighed as heavily as the four-pound sandbags that would soon be attached to my right ankle in the gym. It was imperative to adhere to the workouts which were intended to ease my disability, even though a deep-seated awareness told me that engaging in the exhausting exercises was futile. I remained just as crippled as when I first embarked on my regime a year earlier in July 1979. Instead, I chose to reward myself by savouring the anticipation that was already building, knowing that during the strenuous session, it would increase in strength as I weakened with fatigue.

Unsurprisingly, the buoyant good feeling generated by my new LP evaporated when I descended into the mouth of the gloomy subway where a microscopic newsagent's kiosk was indented into the wall a few yards from the entrance. Taped to a display case holding a mosaic of cigarette packets, a notice written in a poor imitation of medieval lettering advised, *Abandon Hope All Ye Who Enter Here*.

I paused to buy a magazine and some mints, such virginally innocuous purchases considering that my peripheral vision was besieged by the glossy covers of pornographic periodicals. The tiny teeth of small metal bulldog clips gripped the magazines to vertical lengths of parcel string, and in the disruptive breeze that twisted through the opening to the outside world, the lurid pages fluttered like adults-only Tibetan prayer flags. I fiddled in my jeans pocket for a five-pound note whilst trying to make it obvious that I wasn't looking at the titles that my brother Tim had sandwiched between his mattresses.

As if complementing the typeface of the notice, the emaciated newsagent resembled a medieval soldier peering with docile hostility from behind battlements of high-stacked daily papers. He probably assumed that I was yet another lustful young bloke whose perturbed discomfort made it difficult to ask for the magazines full of female flesh. If that was what he was thinking, he couldn't be more wrong. Standing before the neon-lit, retina-burning rabbit hutch, the daylight splurged at each end of the dark tunnel to remind people that there was the salvation of a vitamin D dose within several dozen strides. "Good morning!"

"Yeah? What's so good about it? You're not stuck here all day."

Heat flushed my cheeks at this unexpected misery. "*NME* and some extra strong mints, please."

He placed my order in the gap between the battlements. "Just them then?"

"Yes, ta."

"You don't want owt else?" He winked, nodding at the magazines, and with orange tipped fingers, sideswept a grey band of greasy hair over his shiny pate. "Nowt to be embarrassed about, lad."

I decided to make a stand against his impertinence and assumption that I was straight. "And if you've got one, I'll have a *Gay News* as well."

"Oh, I see. The Hearty's not open yet, if that's where you're headed."

His snide remark didn't warrant an answer. I gathered my change and continued to the hospital.

Spanning the next few days, his sarcastic remark smouldered, making me resolute to visit the gay bar in the Hearty Good Fellow. Even though I was continually pulled down by the unhappiness generated by my physical appearance, I could just go in and have a look. I didn't have to stop long, just go and see what it was all about, and maybe connect with another gay man who'd understand my dilemma. I wasn't so naïve as to expect that I'd instantly find what the *Gay News* classified adverts called an LTR, a long term relationship.

A picture parade featuring the photos from my magazines flipped through my head with each ascending step from the subway, and I emerged grunting and panting onto the pavement as if I was a soldier reaching the end of an assault course. Across the bottom of Mount Street stood the pub. My private battle was over, and here I was, winning for once. In a reckless moment, excitement overrode my worries about my injured leg and flabby chest as I stood before the portal. One of the two doors was ajar, and its hinges gave a tortuous, horror film groan when I pushed it open. With a drumming in my chest, I crossed the threshold. In the gloom, an illuminated cigarette machine glowed spectrally at the bottom of a set of steps leading up to the bar and on my right, another set descended into blackness, the entrance barred by an aluminium barrel and an A-frame board with a notice: *Private Party. No Admission.* Sucking air into my lungs, partially in preparation for climbing the stairs and partly for bravery, I trod on the first step, desperate to escape my mental isolation and to join my gay comrades. At the top, in the seconds before shoving open the door and entering a gay bar for the first time, I was gripped by the toe-clenching sensation of being perched at the edge of a towering diving board. I'd come so far on my journey, and hauling myself up the psychological steps to reach where I now stood had been prolonged and lonely. I was determined to meet others like me. Washed with a wave of optimism, I didn't just want to tentatively dip my toe into the pool but to gloriously divebomb into the depths and emerge, splashing joyously. I shoved the door open and was immersed in the familiar pub odour of stale beer, cigarettes, and deep fat frying. The bar top needed revarnishing and at the end, a tall woman moved a cloth slowly around an ashtray. With her titanic bleached bouffant, dazzling diamanté earrings and an impressive cleavage barely restrained by a leopard skin print blouse a la Bet Lynch from *Coronation Street*, closer inspection was required to tell if she was a real woman or a man in drag.

When she blinked her eyes, her splendid, undoubtedly false eyelashes seemed ready to disobey the adhesive that secured them to her lids. "Yes, duck?"

The deep, husky tone evoked Tim's words of wisdom on the subject: "You can always tell if it's a tranny because they have big hands and an Adam's apple."

The barmaid's mitts were suspiciously on the large side, but my scrutiny of the front of her neck was foiled by a wide purple velvet choker studded with what looked like shards of pink coral. I would have killed for such an item in 1972 and for several delirious seconds, I indulged in a giddy vision of my brothers' disapproval as I sat at the dinner table wearing it.

She drummed her talons on the bar, dragging me into the present. "Yes, duck?"

"Sorry. A pint of lager, please."

"Owt else?" She nodded sideways at the menu board. "The cobs are today's."

One glance at the pummelled, wrinkled crusts imprisoned beneath the transparent plastic dome made me question her statement. Instead, I focused my attention on the assorted nibbles hanging from cardboard displays. "Some scratchings, please."

"Just you watch your teeth on 'em." She tossed a packet onto the bar. "We had some Yank tourists in last week. They'd been up the castle." She placed the pint on the bar and leaned forwards. "They asked for *three haffsa ya best Nadd-ing-ham bidda and some traditional English bar snaaax.*"

A gurgling chuckle accompanied her memory as I smiled politely at her risible impersonation.

With a blood red fingernail, she tapped the white cellophane. "I said to him, 'Here's a bag of tramp's toenails.'" She giggled. "You can't get much more traditional than them, can you?"

"Did he like them?"

"He stuffed his gob full then spat them into the ashtray. 'They're too hard,' he says. 'I've broken a tooth.'" She bellowed with laughter. "Honest to God, he said he was going to sue us. I told him not to be so bleddy sucky and didn't he know what scratchings are? I mean, like I told him, they're scratchings not bleddy marshmellers, aren't they?" She slid the bag towards me. "Just them then?"

"Yes, ta."

She pushed the amber-filled glass further towards me. "Here you are then, duck. One pint, nice and cold."

The first large gulp extinguished the heat of my nerves as I surveyed my first gay bar. The smoky room was anything but gay in both senses of the word. It was just like any other boozer that I'd been in with Tim and Nick. Before I'd entered the pub, I'd had to sidestep an inverted V-shaped notice board that advertised *Pub Grub,* and here behind the

Chucking Putty at the Queen

barmaid, white letters impaled into a black plastic noticeboard displayed the menu. As my eyes travelled down the unadventurous list, it was obvious that they'd either lost or run out of some of the plastic letters. The E in sausage cob was a pound sign, the L in saveloys was an upside-down number seven, and beefburger had become *be fburger*. The frame of the synthetic board rested upon a heated glass case containing several sweaty-looking sausage rolls and a trio of extraordinarily orange pies bathed in the atomic glow.

An elderly couple sat side by side as if posing for a remake of Grant Wood's famous 1930 painting, *American Gothic*. Two pairs of eyes stared at me with sullen resentment as if I'd gate-crashed a poorly attended funeral wake. It seemed disrespectful to disrupt the graveyard quiet. Uncomfortable and embarrassed, I looked over to where a man leaned over the sarcophagus of a dark blue jukebox. His deflated stance made me wonder if he couldn't make up his mind which song to select or whether to give up on life altogether and jump out of the window. Eventually his coins clattered into the machine. "Do Nothing" by The Specials blasted from the inbuilt speakers. I took another draught of my lager and contemplated Terry Hall as he mournfully asked how could he be anybody else? I couldn't be anyone else, and I certainly didn't *want* to be anybody else. I still wanted to be me, but I didn't want to be alone. I wanted gay friends. The further lyric about living a life without meaning struck home, but at least I'd made my first move towards living a gay existence.

The record changed, and The Specials were replaced by the familiar intro of The Beatles' "Eleanor Rigby," magnifying the deep melancholy of the lifeless room where cigarette smoke hung in the unmoving mist worthy of a moonless cemetery in a creepy film, and when Paul McCartney sang of all the lonely people, I knew I should call time on this futile exploration. I was getting nowhere fast. Had *Gay News* got it wrong? Something was amiss with this morbid scenario, and I didn't have the courage nor the motivation to ask if it was the gay bar. I drained my pint and before the bottom of the glass touched the patchily varnished wood, the barmaid reached out for it.

"Same again?"

"No, ta. I'm off."

Depression and self-pity dropped on me as I descended the stairs into the small foyer and was submerged into the ghostly illumination from the cigarette machine. I perched on a metal beer barrel next to the warning, *Private Party. No Admission*. Yeah, that was about right. Should I find whatever I was looking for, it would no doubt turn out to be a private party with no admission for me. From my resting point in the cool, shadowed entrance area, I gazed through the half-open door that framed the passing pedestrian parade of everyday life. The dazzling summer sun defined the moment in stark shadows and bleached brightness. If only my life was so easily delineated, but it remained fuzzy-edged. Like when Dad rotated the knob on his Rolleiflex camera, I'd tried to bring my life into a sharp focus but had failed. I hauled myself up and set about the return journey home. Forget my gay liberation. The quest to find my tribe was over. With the resignation of the vanquished, I'd go to the local pub with Tim that evening where I'd drink too much lager and eye up men from behind the bars of my self-imposed prison.

BOOK TWO

After

25

IN THROUGH THE OUT DOOR

JANUARY 1982. SIGNIFICANT NUMBERS from my life fluttered through my mind like the discarded pages of a desk calendar blown by the wind. It was eleven years since Mam died, four years since I came out at work, and two years since I'd vowed that the 1980s would see my emancipation from a monochromatic existence. After a lacklustre beginning to the decade, my disenchantment had reached an unbearable level. It seemed to be my destiny to evolve into a late-teens version of the pensioners in the pub: old before my time. Finally, frustration at my lassitude erupted in unexpected self-empowerment. Determined to avoid such a miserable, beige-coloured fate, I vowed to pilot my life towards brighter horizons. Following a consultation with a surgeon who'd agreed to remove the pappy flesh on my chest that for so long had prohibited my happiness, I still found that my psychological disturbance was not so easily remedied, and I remained resigned that I could do nothing to resolve the problem of my bad leg. I stagnated in a mentally unmoving backwater of heterosexual family and friends, and as much as I loved them—or most of them—the imagined voices of my own tribe called to me with increasing volume from afar. Discouraged by my earlier fruitless attempt to discover those gay kinfolk, the positivity now engendered by my newly flat chest dictated that I must double my efforts. I needed to embrace the fulfilling acceptance that would validate me after such an exhausting wait.

I was three months away from turning twenty when I replaced the receiver of our telephone in the hallway and wiped my sweaty palm on my trousers. The bloke at Nottingham Gay Switchboard had just informed me that their small, informal social gatherings each Monday and Thursday would be a gentle way to ease me from my isolation. Twenty-four hours later, I marched up a narrow passage leading from Mansfield Road, jabbed the button next to the only door, and waited.

Footsteps drummed on stairs, getting louder. My quickened breathing made me light-headed, and I cast a final glance to where the entrance to the street framed what I knew was already my old life. When I heard the door being opened behind me, I turned to face my future.

A fresh-faced man wearing a rugby shirt smiled at me. Threadbare, periwinkle blue jeans covered his legs, and grubby Slazenger trainers encased his feet. With his chestnut hair in a classic short back and sides he epitomised sporty, good health. I recorded all this visual info within a couple of seconds, which was so easy for me as I'd spent my life surreptitiously absorbing details of how men looked, measuring every inch of stretched denim; and my binocular eyes zooming in on a glimpse of chest hair between the buttons of a white shirt. In the world I'd left behind, I knew not to be caught looking, but surely here I should be free from such caution.

"Hi. Can I help you?"

"My name's Simon, and I live up the road, and I phoned last night and spoke to a bloke. I can't remember his name even if he told me. I think he just said, "Gay Switchboard," and I told him that I need to meet other gay men because I feel really isolated, and it's great going out with my straight mates who know I'm gay and don't care, but anyway, he told me about the meetings here and suggested that I come down, so I have done because I'm really lonely."

He smiled and stepped aside. "Come in. Don't worry. You're home now."

I lurched against the door frame, my vision swimming. "I've waited such a long time for this."

He laid a hand on my shoulder as I wiped my tears away. "Hey, it's all right. You've made the first move towards your new gay life."

I followed him up three flights of stairs, each step loaded with increasing triumph.

"I'm Carl, by the way," he called over his shoulder when we turned a switchback to the next level.

Unable to compete with such athletic energy, I leaned against the wall as Carl waited at the top, the palm of one hand flat against a closed door like a fireman testing for contained heat.

"Are you ready?"

Only several steps separated me from my complete liberation. My face prickled by the time I'd joined him. "I just need a couple of seconds. This is the best thing that's happened to me." Whatever was on the other

Chucking Putty at the Queen

side of the door would change my life forever. This was it. "Okay, I'm ready."

Carl pushed the door open, unleashing a fragrant warm wave of coffee and cigarette smoke. "Hey, everyone. This is Simon."

Within a pocket-sized room, its walls papered with a tattered patchwork of notices for CND, Amnesty International, Prisoners' Aid, and numerous telephone advice lines, several men sat around a low G-Plan table, its timeworn, laminated wooden circumference scarred with scorched fingerprints from where cigarettes had been balanced and allowed to burn down. Mugs of tea and coffee surrounded a white plastic ashtray bearing the Cinzano logo and on a chipped-edge earthenware plate laden with biscuits, a handful of chocolate fingers pointed to malted milks, fig rolls, and rectangular pink wafers. They were the ones that Mam liked best when we had a biscuit selection box at Christmas.

All except one of the assembled men greeted me as if I was a long-established friend. A man sporting a huge yard-brush moustache was reading the latest *Gay News*, and I wanted to leap in and comment that I had that current issue to show that I was one of them.

But I remained silent. I was new and didn't know the etiquette. I jumped when a slim man placed a hand on my arm. His sad, watery blue eyes gave the impression that he carried the weight of the world on his shoulders and was ready to burst into tears.

"I'm Bill. What's the weather like up there? How tall are you?"

"Six feet five."

"And what have you done to your leg? Why do you use a stick?"

"I dislocated my hip when I was fifteen, and it went undiagnosed. Then it all buggered up, and I've been like this ever since."

"Oh, you poor thing. Have a pew and take the weight off."

The armchair creaked worryingly when I inelegantly lowered myself onto it, almost knocking the coffee table over when I stuck my bad leg beneath it, converting the contents of the mugs into miniature stormy brown oceans. "The eagle has landed." Embarrassment of my disability provoked my uncomfortable quip as I looked around at the men with mild disappointment. I'd half-hoped that this inaugural meeting would resemble a gathering of the Village People fan club. But there was no leatherman, construction worker, cowboy, native American, US cop, or soldier. They were men who ranged from their twenties up to their fifties, all unremarkably attired apart from the one absent in the chorus of welcomes, who could have been an extra from the 1971 comedy film, *Carry On at Your Convenience*. I could hear Mam telling me that it was rude to stare, but it was a challenge not to gawp at his rust-coloured corduroy 1960s overcoat, the collar topped with a light tangerine fake fur trim, and its front decorated with bronzed buttons the size of small saucers. It was splayed open wide enough to display a blue satin shirt with a cream Peter Pan collar, which I bet even had balloon sleeves. I would have killed for it when I was ten. His white jeans were tucked into tan Cuban-heeled, pointy-toed cowboy boots bearing purple leather cut out letters spelling *New York*. The thought that he may be going to a fancy-dress party flashed uncharitably in my mind.

Guarding the empty fireplace, three bars of an electric fire radiated in vivid scarlet and cast a ferocious glow onto the stubbly face of a burly, stern-looking man in his late forties resting against the low window ledge. My attraction to him was instant. He was very much my type, with dark shadowed jowls that indicated he needed to shave twice or perhaps three times a day. He was dressed in a suit of deep charcoal, which was offset by a white shirt and dark blue tie, and I absurdly thought that he didn't *look* very gay. I thrilled to imagine that he could have been a plain-clothed copper, or involved with the government, or even a high-ranking military officer. But no medals adorned his suit jacket. Instead, a small black badge with green capital letters CHE discreetly studded the left lapel, and once more I resisted the urge to assert myself by stating that I owned a similar badge that I'd bought from Mushroom Bookshop, and that I knew what the Campaign for Homosexual Equality was. In an earth-quakingly gruff voice, he was in agitated conversation with a thickly moustached, lanky man awkwardly crammed into a chair nearby, his tight jeans-encased legs jutting angularly in the confined area.

He poked a finger onto his leg to illustrate his point. "After all, it's a matter of basic human rights."

As if he'd noticed me looking at his badge, or to perhaps ensure it was safely pinned to his lapel, the burly man rubbed a thick thumb over its shiny surface.

"Yes, we have to fight back against these fucking fascists."

From beneath dark hairy caterpillars, his eyes locked with mine briefly, then away as he continued his debate with the other man. When the doorbell rang, Carl jumped up from a tatty armchair that looked as if it had been gnawed by a dog, and bounded towards the doorway, almost knocking over a squat table lamp whose gingham shade bore an oval scorch mark where the bulb must have touched it.

He yanked the door open. "I've got it."

"Well, keep it to yourself. We don't want to catch it."

The corny response came from the *Carry On* man. Of course, none of us in that room in January 1982 could ever imagine how devastatingly prescient his wisecrack was to prove. He dragged on his diminishing cigarette, then exhaled so hard that the smoke jetted across the room as if leaving the engine of a fighter plane.

"Jesus fucking Christ. She never stops, that one. Is she still doing tons of speed? Shovelling that shit down her neck will kill her one day if I don't do it first. All that dashing about and jumping around. She gets on my fucking tits."

Dad had a firm belief that you could enter a room full of one hundred people and take an instant fancy to someone or, similarly, an immediate dislike. This was one of those latter moments. Within seconds of my arrival, spiky instinct told me that he was trouble.

"Now, now, Vernon. Don't be nasty." The lustrous black curtain of moustache adorning the upper lip of the man sitting opposite him didn't move with his admonishment.

Vernon leaned forward with his cold eyes gleaming. "Don't you *dare* tell me off, Peter. You're not bossing teenagers around in your classroom now, you know."

He ground his cigarette onto the ashtray, then snatched a golden packet of Benson & Hedges and a gilded cylindrical lighter from the tabletop. As he reclined with one leg crossed over the other, bobbing his foot, he moved the packet to his mouth and extracted a fresh cigarette by gripping the end with his lips, thin and tight beneath his clipped moustache. The lighter sparked with repeated flicks of his thumb until a flame flickered and held. As he touched the steady yellow crocus to the cigarette tip, he looked over to me from beneath his sandy fringe. I hadn't seen such a hostile look since school. As the smoke rose in a quivering grey line, he glared at me if he'd just fired a six-shooter at my head and missed. With his thin lips tightly pursed as if trying to hold words in, my established relationship with paranoia warned me that something was up, and that he was biding his time.

He jerked the cigarette to his mouth and sucked strongly, before throwing his head right back and launching a colossal spout of smoke upwards where it joined the hovering nicotine storm clouds.

The man in the chair by the window had finished his conversation with the burly man. He unfurled himself from the chair and leaned over the table with his hand extended. "Hi, and welcome. I'm Greg." He jerked his head to the burly man. "And he's Jim. Have you come far?"

I turned my back on Vernon and shook Greg's hand. "No, I live less than a mile away."

"A local lad then." Greg's eyes smiled but I couldn't see his mouth beneath the bushy moustache.

"*Lad*."

Ignoring the voice of common sense in my mind telling me not to, I turned around and looked at Vernon who blew a line of smoke towards me. Throwing caution to the wind I coughed and flapped my hands. "Oh, what a smell of sulphur." When the others laughed at the *Wizard of Oz* reference, I knew I'd hit the right spot. Vernon leaned towards Peter and muttered something before returning his stare to me and projecting a laugh rather too loud and too forced, immediately ushering me back to the chilling snickering and whispers in the school corridors that preceded me getting beaten up. But now I was resolute that I would not be intimidated, not when I'd only just realised my dream. Too many of my formative years were soiled by hiding away, of jumping at my own shadow, of watching fearfully from behind my bedroom curtains, terrified of my enemies. And here, during my liberation, those same sensations threatened to ruin this momentous milestone. No, I wouldn't be discouraged or thwarted by some prat who looked like he was one of some tacky novelty combo who had entered the *Eurovision Song Contest* in 1975.

Peter nudged Vernon. "Oh, don't be such a bitch. You never say anything good about anyone."

Vernon continued to glare at me with cold eyes. "Come off it, Peter. You think it, and I say it. Since when did you turn into fucking Snow White? I mean, just look at her. She's like little Dorothy from Kansas just landed in Oz. She's only been here five minutes, and she's already going gooey over Greg." He dragged on his cigarette and blew the smoke towards me once more. "Some virgins have no self-restraint. She's obviously

Chucking Putty at the Queen

desperate for it."

Bloody hell, I'd only been with these men for a few minutes and one of them openly hated me. Vernon slightly wobbled his head, which made me wonder if he had what Aunty Lu used to call "a condition."

Since childhood, I've had the ability of being able to stare for at least a minute without blinking. Now it was time to utilise my uncanny skill, and I stared back. After several seconds, Vernon dropped his gaze and again whispered to the uncomfortable-looking Peter, who shook his head.

"Oh, don't start."

Vernon reclined, his foot still agitating, and his eyes thin slices of blatant dislike. "Are you all right over there, Dorothy... Dottie... Dot."

When I ignored him, he leaned forward to transfer his cigarette to the ashtray, then clapped his hands.

"Now listen, everyone. Shut up gabbing and pay attention to me. I've had a great idea." Once he had everyone's concentration, he pointed at me, the clear varnish glistening like ice on his fingernail. "I've decided that from now on, this one here is to be called Dot." He paused and surveyed the assembled men. "Short for Dorothy of course, because she's from Kansas, and she's never had a man before. She's here looking for a husband but she's not fucking having mine, so she can keep her goddamn eyes and hands to herself."

I'd never heard anyone say goddamn in real life and assumed that the hideous New York boots had something to do with it. He relaxed back onto the chair, beaming with blissful satisfaction as if he was a mother who had just learned that her only child, previously thought to be a simpleton, was now going to university to study advanced thermonuclear dynamics. Despite his evident dislike of me, I was nevertheless taken aback at the unexpected diatribe unleashed in the intimacy of the smoky room. This was my big debut, and this camp idiot was having a go at me for nothing. I'd hoped to find friends but had already made an enemy. It was school all over again. I'd been a fool to hold such grand expectations of my emancipation, of finally turning my back on past hatred. I placed my hands on the chair arms and began to push myself upright. "I think it's best that I go."

"You stay there." Jim half-rose from the windowsill. "And *you*..." He focused his dark glare on Vernon. "You pack it in. You should remember how you were when you first came out. You were like the Virgin Mary, so give over. The lad's only just come here. You need to remember how hard it can be."

"*Lad? Lad?* That's the second time in five minutes I've heard that word. A lad only in your twisted fantasies, Jim." He jabbed his cigarette towards me and scrunched his nose and mouth as if I were emitting a foul odour. "She's got to be thirty at least, and as to all of this *'only just come here'* business, well, she can *only just* fuck off back to whatever local slum she's limped out from."

"Steady on." Jim's half-closed lids converted his dark eyes to black lines.

"I don't want her here. What's the matter, Jim? Have you already marked Dot as your next virgin to conquer?"

I was in the firing line and had no idea what I'd done wrong.

Vernon flashed me the most insincerely sweet smile. "How old *are* you, Dot, dear? Does your mother know you're out this late? No wonder Jim's impressed; you look so young! *Do* share your secret. Is it Pond's Hand Cream or Oil of Ulay? Maybe it's chip fat because you're such a *local lad*, and I'm sure you *lads* must eat loads of chips."

A page turned in a book at the back of my mind, showing an image of a crumbling brick wall, the torn poster pasted upon it bearing the legend, "Those who cannot remember the past are condemned to repeat it." I couldn't forget nor escape my own subjugated past, and right now, I acknowledged the childhood weaknesses which had caused me to be the victim of bullying for far too long. Tonight was to be my dazzling diamond dream come true, and it had already turned as black as the night behind the small window. Eyes watched me as intently as if I were a participant in a chess tournament. I had to do something, so I did my best to replicate Vernon's smarmy smile. "I'm nineteen and judging by looks, I'll always be fifteen years younger than you, *dear*." I glowed inside when my weak rejoinder produced a ripple of laughter from the compact cluster of men.

"Oh, Dot, you've got a fan already. It's obvious that you're the next on Jim's list of rent conquests." He smirked. "You see, Dot, dear, you being a virgin from Kansas and all of that, you won't know that Jim here has all the good-looking *lads* to live at his house as lodgers, especially those who have run away from home when their mummy and daddy don't want them anymore because they found out they're queer."

I couldn't have been more shocked if he'd thrown the contents of his mug into my face. How could a gay man use the word that those outside this small office fired as part of their verbal weaponry against us? It was an unforgettable component of the chanting at the school gates as I fearfully approached the waiting mob, "Here he is. Here's the queer," before they set upon me, punching me until I fell to the ground, where they continued their assault with their feet.

Vernon fixed his eyes on the burly man sitting on the window ledge. "And if they can't afford the rent, there's another way to pay, isn't there, Jim?"

Who knew how I'd been the cause of this nastiness, but one thing was certain: having come this far, I wasn't going back. Jim glowered as if he would get up and throw Vernon through the window down three storeys onto the iced pavements below.

Oh, how I wished that he would.

"Pack it in." Greg's deep voice tersely interjected from beneath the chestnut canopy of his lustrous moustache. "God, you can be a nasty bitch at times, you really can. I don't know why I bother with you. You have to pour your vitriol on everyone, don't you? What a great welcome. What fabulous gay support you've provided to someone who's where you were not so long ago." White teeth gleamed beneath the curtain of moustache. "Sod this for a lark. I'm going to the pub. Are you coming?"

26

BURNING WITH OPTIMISM'S FLAMES

ONCE MORE I WALKED through the subway beneath the dual carriageway. Although velvety darkness plugged each end, the usually broken lighting blazed surprisingly, making the tiles shine with the brilliance of a cleaning product advert, and at the join of floor and walls, soapy bubbles congealed where a maintenance crew must have swilled away the quintessential combination of vomit and urine. Perhaps the council had decided to improve the dark and dangerous underpass in honour of my journey, one that I'd made countless times before when attending hospital appointments, and one more memorable on my ill-fated quest to find the gay bar.

However, the difference on this freezing night was that after such a long and lonesome wait, I was in the company of other gay men. Flanked by Bill and Peter, we followed Greg, who forged ahead with determined strides as if he was the standard bearer of a righteous army marching me towards my salvation. If only my depressed and lost younger self could have looked into a crystal ball to see me as I fearlessly embraced this liberating adventure. My cheeks ached so much from my ecstatic grin that I visualised it going not only from ear to ear but also right around the top of my head.

"Oi, you fucking queers!"

The verbal violence rebounded from the gleaming walls, and we whirled around as if in well-practised choreography. But instead of the mob of vicious thugs I'd expected to see, it was only Carl, who panted as he laid his palms on his knees.

"Your faces! I knew that'd get your attention. Haven't you heard me shouting? I've been trying to catch up since outside Yates's." He grimaced as he rotated his left foot, then raised the leg of his jeans to reveal the binding of creamy bandage visible between blue denim and black sock. "This bloody ankle injury isn't as healed as I thought it was." It was several hundred yards from the popular pub, so it was no wonder that he was coughing as he caught his breath. He grinned. "I know you're eager to get there, Simon, but it's not a race."

We continued on past the closed newsagent's stall, now protected from nocturnal burglary by a grey metal shutter, and when we arrived at the end of the tunnel, a power surge in my electrified imagination transformed the grim steps leading up to the street into the illuminated stairway on *The Larry Grayson Show*. Although I wore dark jeans and Tim's chunky knit fisherman's jumper in the colour of a midnight ocean, I fantasised that I was resplendent in an Arctic white suit just like that of my favourite camp entertainer. But instead of descending as Lal did with nimble gaiety towards the certainty of a rapturous audience, I strenuously ascended towards the unknown, wondering what kind of audience awaited me. This time was so different to my earlier exploration. The bronze rail aided my climb, although I imagined clasping a neon tube of blazing pink. At street level, I waited for my heart rate to settle and half closed my eyes, pretending that the everyday cars zooming past us were elegant, polished limousines. My fervid expectation was stimulated to such an intensity that I half expected to see Gay Bar in flickering letters over the doorway like those backstreet dives in the TV series, *The Streets of San Francisco*. My baptism had so far not only invigorated me but had also metamorphosized a drab January Nottingham evening into one of breathtaking American glamour.

The pavement ran in an iced trail beneath the concrete canopy for the length of the block, right past Brentford Nylons where Dad had bought me a continental quilt for my seventeenth birthday. How many hours had I'd laid swathed beneath its luxurious warmth, fantasising about meeting other homosexuals. And finally, here I was, one of this band of merry men on Maid Marian Way.

Greg beckoned me from the pub doorway. "Come on, new boy, it's celebration time. I'll buy you a pint."

When he turned towards the pub entrance, a wave of gauche, absurd ebullience overtook me. Ignoring common sense, I confided in Vernon with giddy exhilaration. "This is a dream come true. I can't believe it's happening." I didn't care that I sounded like an over-excited boy who was hopping from foot to foot in his pyjamas in front of a beautifully wrapped mountain of presents on Christmas Day morning. "And Greg's buying me a drink on my first visit to a gay pub." Too late, I realised my error in allowing euphoria to make me drop my guard in front of this new adversary. Vernon grabbed the sleeve of my jumper and pulled me away from the others towards a grey concrete rubbish bin.

The tiniest gleam showed through his slitted eyelids. "Now you listen, Dorothy, and you listen good. I don't know if you're just plain fucking stupid, or if you're trying to piss me off, but let's get one thing straight from the start. This sure ain't no Emerald City, and what's more, Greg and me are together. He's my affaire. Get it? Me and Greg. Greg and me. We're an item. A couple. A twosome. And do you want to know something else? If we could get married in this crummy, godforsaken town then we would."

The breath that powered my derisive guffaw churned in white clouds around his face, much as his cigarette smoke had choked me earlier. "'Crummy, godforsaken town?' Which episode of *Peyton Place* did you get that from?"

Vernon dragged forcefully on his cigarette, making his cheeks concave so much that I thought his face would implode. The last few millimetres of the white shaft diminished to a scarlet glow that matched the hot fury in his cold eyes.

"He's only being nice to you because he feels sorry for you having that gammy leg, but you don't fool me by playing Little Miss Innocent. You should've heard yourself earlier." He placed a forefinger against his chin, raised his eyes to the dark sky, and mimicked the syrupy voice of Marilyn Monroe when she sang, 'Happy Birthday' to President Kennedy. "Oh Gweg, what's the gay scene like? Oh Gweg, I'm a virgin. Oh Gweg, I've never wevver even been kissed before."

"Get lost. I never said that."

Vernon shivered and tugged the collar of his awful coat up high until he resembled a frilled lizard. "I'll tell you what it's like, Dorothy. It's tough, and it's hard out there in the meat market, and it's about the survival of the fittest. You limping around is really going to hold you back, so why don't you give up now and piss off back to Kansas before you embarrass yourself even more? Nobody wants to fuck a cripple, and trailing around after Greg like a lost puppy won't get you anywhere. Just you remember that he's mine, so keep your hands off him. Comprende?"

He thrust his hands into the large white patch pockets sewn onto his coat with thick red stitches, making the taut material resemble over-filled strawberry jam sandwiches. With a snort, he swished towards the pub doorway where our small entourage stood with breath rising in impatient locomotive clouds. How I hoped he'd slip in those stupid boots and break his neck.

Greg waved at me. "Simon, are you coming or what? Time for your celebration, and I'm buying you a pint. Is lager okay?"

Vernon barged through the men as he headed through the entrance. "Get out of my fucking way."

Bill stepped over to me, his eyes watering in the frigid wind that had chilled the tip of his nose into a red rosebud. "I don't exactly know what that bitch said to you, but I can guess it was the famous 'hands off' speech. We've all had it at some point."

I slipped off my spectacles and rubbed my eyes that stung from a combination of the bitter wind and impending tears. "I dunno. Perhaps this was a bad idea. I've had enough shit in my life already. I don't need more enemies."

Bill sighed. "It's easy for me to say, but just ignore him and try to stay out of his way."

"But I was so looking forward to this moment, and that wanker's ruined it."

"Listen to the voice of experience, dear. It's only ruined if you let it be so. This is your fabulous time, and it'll only happen once. I for one won't let it be spoiled for you. Ignore her, dear. She's just a spiteful queen who has vitriol in her veins instead of blood." He squeezed my arm and winked. "Come on, time for your grand entrance. Oh, how I envy you."

"I suppose if he's called me Dorothy, then he must be the wicked witch."

"Which witch, dear? Remember there were two: one from the west and one from the east."

"The Wicked Witch of the East Midlands."

Bill clapped his red woollen gloved hands together and chuckled. "See? You're learning already. I can tell there's more to you than meets the eye."

"Thanks."

"Now let's go in. I'm gagging for a drink and if Greg's in the chair, then I want a crème de menthe, dahlink."

I hesitated as he stepped into the pub. Irrational uncertainty froze my mind on this bone-chilling night. It seemed that my delicate champagne flute filled with fizzing expectation had turned into a grubby pint bottle of curdled milk. Twenty-four hours earlier, I'd danced a jig of delight at finally ending my isolation, when the heat of my excitement was so intense that I thought my mind would melt. Now I already had an enemy and my going into the gay bar could easily replicate the hell of my school days. Who else would there be to carry the same instantaneous hatred of me that Vernon made no effort to conceal?

For the second time this evening, I convinced myself that I had to go home. I should've done it earlier. I'd already endured too much aggro, and I didn't need any more from the likes of Vernon. That morning in my bedroom, when I'd drawn back the curtains and viewed the snow-covered, regimented rooftops beneath the cloudless, bleached denim sky, I wholly believed that it was the dawning of a new era.

But what would Jacqui say if I told her that I'd chickened out? It wasn't an option to turn tail and flee back to a life where my socialising was restricted to estate boozers and the circuit of pubs in town. I couldn't give up now when I'd travelled so far along the yellow brick road to reach my very own Oz.

27

GOING UNDERGROUND

AND HERE I WAS again, entering the Hearty Good Fellow, preparing to triumphantly climb the stairs to the gay bar. Vernon had assumed role of Akela in our compact troop and shoved his way to the front where, to my utter confusion, instead of ascending the stairs as I had on my fruitless exploration eighteen months earlier, he did a swishy about-turn and squeezed past the A-frame noticeboard which still bore the same warning: *Private Party. No Admission.*

I grasped Carl's arm. "Where's he going? The sign..."

"Oh, don't worry about that; it's there to keep the straights out."

So that was why my earlier reccy had proved unrewarding. The set of stairs were interrupted by a small landing, and from there, they descended further into the pub's bowels that glowed scarlet from a naked bulb. Already I was comparing this current situation to my younger years of sitting on Mam's lap as we read my favourite book, *The Inquisitive Elf*. But tonight, I was no scarlet-clad waif in pointed turquoise footwear stealing down a twisty stairwell towards a witch's subterranean lair beneath an ancient tree. Tonight, I was a trembling, six-foot-five, broad-shouldered, nineteen-year-old man wearing his brother's wood glue-speckled fisherman's jumper and undertaking the last stage of a journey to a new life with other homosexuals. A few more steps, and the ennui of my existence would end.

Our progress was abruptly thwarted by a fuss at the bottom of the stairs, where Greg was being scolded by Vernon. With his thin lips moving against the short dark curls surrounding Greg's ear, he looked up the stairs, momentarily spooking me. The bloodbath glow of the overhead bulb accentuated his demonic glare, and I didn't have to be super intelligent to know that I was the subject of his remonstrations.

This impromptu drama created a claustrophobic backlog of my companions, who shuffled as if we were stuck on a broken escalator. To think that a few feet above us at street level, the straight world continued:

passengers waited at the bus stop with chilled impatience, and traffic navigated clockwise around the grassy island bearing the huge placards advertising Barbara Windsor as *Aladdin* in the Theatre Royal pantomime. Those everyday people were unaware that I'd rubbed my own dull lamp until it gleamed, and the gay genie had finally been released.

The performance at the bottom of the stairs ended when Vernon lightly slapped Greg on the side of the head, then called up the stairs, "All right ladies, it's showtime."

This was it. No mix up of being in the wrong place at the wrong time. To the left, a bashed slatted wooden door bore a faux bronze sign marked *Gentlemen* in Victorian script, but there was no similar plaque which designated *Ladies*. In front, a similar one with a matching adhesive sign cautioned it was for *Staff Only*, and on the right, a slightly larger pair were topped with reinforced glass that rippled with indistinct shapes and colours. The dulled thud of a four on the floor beat synced with my pounding pulse as I smirked knowingly at a notice that reiterated the warning at the top of the stairs. Being a member of an exclusive club, I now knew that it didn't apply to me.

Vernon was obviously intent on making an entrance, but his ta-da moment was thwarted when he pushed his shiny-nailed hand against the door, and it encountered resistance. He shoved forcefully. There was a yelp, and he whooshed through.

"Well, you shouldn't fucking stand there, should you? Stupid old queen."

The rest of us shuffled in chain gang style. I didn't want to look up until the very last second, so I focused on a bronzed strip separating the concrete floor and a purple and dark green carpet. For the second time that evening, I stood before a life-changing threshold. Once I crossed it, nothing would ever be the same again. This was it. I stepped forward and looked up.

In front of me was a darkened, smoky room some thirty feet in length, its low ceiling covered with shining chrome clouds of crumpled cooking foil which reflected multi-coloured starbursts from myriad fairy lights attached to them. With incredible, disconcerting appropriateness, Linda Clifford's 1978 frenetic disco version of "If My Friends Could See Me Now" fanfared my arrival. A few single men sat on leatherette seating that hugged the wall in a reversed, elongated C shape, whilst others

Chucking Putty at the Queen

congregated on stools clustered around circular tables topped with swirly burgundy and orange Formica. The length of the wall was covered with a montage of film and pop stars, beefcakes, and pretty boys. It was easy to see that as the gallery was updated, new pictures were stuck randomly over the older ones, leaving perhaps an eye, a smile, or part of a trademark haircut showing. I grinned to see the poster of American telly cops *Starsky & Hutch* which I'd had on my bedroom wall. I could never have foreseen me looking at it in a gay bar.

On my left, the compact bar was an oasis of low luminosity from the beer pump displays, and the chunky ochre pottery lamp which sat atop it wouldn't have looked out of place in *Man About The House*, one of my favourite 1970s sitcoms. From beneath its oatmeal hessian shade, an ellipse of amber spilled onto the purple countertop where several shallow pools of beer reflected the pretty psychedelia of more hanging lines of fairy lights. I adored how their colours floated in the silver foil firmament, hazily diffused by a milky way of cigarette smoke that remained unmoving despite the effort of the nicotine-tarnished Xpelair extractor fan high on the wall.

I knew that my eyes were like saucers and that my mouth hung open gormlessly as I continued to survey my new world and the pictorial parade of pin-ups which so fascinated me. Rubbing shoulders were celebrity footballers Georgie Best, a bubble-permed Kevin Keegan, and local legend Ian Storey-Moore, and all were pinned next to Rock Hudson, who grinned a Hollywood studio smile at Doris Day. Gleefully, my younger years were represented by a large poster of Marc Bolan, one of the many of him from the *Jackie* magazines that had adorned my bedroom walls. The Sweet pouted with unconvincing coyness like four brickies wrapped in Bacofoil, whereas the American contingent of perfect white teeth was represented by the Osmonds and David Cassidy. I was instantly seduced by this tacky underground Utopia, but my elation deflated when one man nudged his companion, nodded at me, and then whispered something to him. That old enemy of mine, paranoia, effortlessly reared its destructive head, and I gripped my walking stick so tightly it wouldn't have surprised me if it splintered into small fragments. When Bill touched my arm, I jumped as if he'd stabbed me.

"It's your first time. Congratulations." The sparkling multicoloured galaxy reflected on his spectacle lenses. "Are you all right?"

"Um, sure. It's fab." I lowered my voice. "But why are they all looking at me?"

"Because it's feeding time at the zoo, dear." His hot breath caressed my ear as he purred lasciviously. "The animals are hungry, and you're the fresh meat."

I recalled Vernon's remark about the meat market as Greg handed me a pint of lager.

"Congratulations! Happy coming out."

His resounding bass salutation caused a couple of nearby men to smile and nod, and when they raised their drinks to me, I knew that I was in my new home. But just as I lifted my own glass to them in return, a jostle at my right elbow slopped the frothy-topped lager over my fingers.

"Oops, sorry. I'm so clumsy." Vernon smirked. "Accidents will happen."

If I'd been more reactively masculine like our Tim, then Vernon would've been picking his teeth up from the sticky carpet. But I wasn't like my tough brother and inwardly cheered when Vernon waved at someone then pushed away from us through the crowd.

Bill smiled at me again. "He's so tiresome. Remember, just ignore him and try to stay out of his way."

Including the duo behind the bar, I counted thirty-six men and, as at my meeting at Gay Switchboard earlier, they were unremarkable. There were no ostensibly stereotyped characters there: no studs and chains, no cowboy chaps, no hard hats. Just ordinary blokes like I'd seen in dozens of pubs, except that they were all homosexual.

The euphoric celebration of "If My Friends Could See Me Now" ended, and in the hush that followed, my overworked intuition warned that eyes were upon me. The jukebox clicked, and the next record began. Disbelief washed over me along with the lilting waves of Dusty Springfield's "Son of a Preacher Man," which Penny and Marge bought for me when I was six. I'd adored it so much and entertained Mam by mimicking Dusty's flamboyant hand gestures that I remembered from *Top of the Pops*. And at this very moment in this underground room, the song was a talismanic assurance that I'd made the right decision in telephoning Gay Switchboard...although I wasn't about to perform my Dusty routine here.

My height enabled continued scrutiny of the walls as I returned to our group and dipped in and out of the conversation whilst attempting to eavesdrop on what other men were saying, hoping to glean further gay education. I looked around and caught a bloke staring at me. I studiously examined the gallery, hoping that the glow from the red light bulb through the window would mask my burning cheeks. I'd never known there were so many gay icons. Next to a huge poster for *Cabaret,* with its ornately stylised vaudeville lettering, a denim-clad *Six Million Dollar Man* was taped next to a black and white Burt Reynolds flaunting his hirsute chest. *Butch Cassidy & the Sundance Kid* squinted in the desert sunshine, Shirley Bassey pouted with sparkling attitude, Marlene Dietrich simply stared, and surly Marlon Brando idled against his motorcycle in the iconic leather jacket pose from *The Wild One.* Inevitably there was Judy Garland, arms flung wide as she stood frozen forever in a stark spot-lit finale, and representing one of Tim's favourite westerns, *She Wore a Yellow Ribbon,* John Wayne gazed from dead fisheyes with a thick moustache adorning his top lip.

Beneath the electric spectrum glowing on this subterranean community, I stood intoxicated, a willing addict after only one fix of this new drug. Dusty's husky tones hushed and faded before being rudely replaced by the syn-drum blast of a rollicking disco song I'd never heard before. It was an immediate, urgent hit with me; one of those tunes that after one hearing, I sweated with a feverish, anxious determination to learn what it was. Whenever I entered a new pub, my priority was to check out the jukebox and, bearing in mind Vernon's spiteful opinion about how my limp would affect my chances of meeting someone, I self-consciously moderated my gait and slowly meandered through the forest of men towards the source of the exhilarating music. As I leaned over the glowing silver and pink plastic chest to peer at the paper slips displaying the songs, someone squeezed my backside. Oh god, I'd just had my bum pinched in a gay bar. I didn't know the etiquette surrounding such an action, so I didn't look around to discover the culprit and continued to investigate the musical selection. The machine contained a catalogue of camp: Dusty Springfield, Shirley Bassey, Judy Garland, both unrelated Lees (Peggy and Brenda), and Helen Shapiro. More personal favourites, Bobbie Gentry's "Ode to Billie Joe" and The Kinks' "Lola" slipped in between a healthy selection of Tamla Motown, classic sixties and seventies pop, and a sunshine splash of chart reggae. Hoping for a repeat of the buttock pinch, I bent further forwards and peered through the Perspex panel to read the handwritten wafer of paper next to selection E2: "Love and Desire" by Arpeggio. I promised myself that the next day I'd visit Rob's Record Mart, the second-hand vinyl emporium. He was sure to have a copy amongst his disarray of deleted discs that was so beloved by rare vinyl collectors.

Before I could slide a ten pence piece from my pocket to play it again, the mechanism clicked as the aluminium arm delivered the next selection. As soon as the introduction to Charley Pride's "Crystal Chandeliers" crackled from the speakers, my sunny disco elation parachuted back into a dark landscape of relentlessly frustrated and depressing nights in the local pub with Tim, evenings filled with sweaty beefburgers covered with cremated onions, plastic bags of cockles and whelks from the travelling seafood seller's wicker basket, and worst of all, my easy surrender to Tim's question, "You having another one?" after he'd drained his seventh pint. Hearing this tristesse ballad was evocative for all the wrong reasons and exemplified the poison of the lonesome lifestyle that I'd self-empoweringly eschewed this very evening. I shuddered as I recalled the many inebriated Bank Holiday weekend dinnertime sessions when, at closing time, my forlorn existence stretched through the afternoon with the unbroken loneliness of a desert.

When I returned to the island of our group knotted in the middle of the room, a short man who was the double of the comedian Ronnie Corbett winked at me, and I hoped that he wasn't the phantom bum-pincher. Drunk on a potent cocktail of twinkling colours, loud music, and the camaraderie of other gay men in this glittering grotto, I just had to share my gay bar baptism and grabbed Bill's arm.

"I just had my bum pinched when I bent over the jukebox."

"I'm surprised it took someone so long, dear."

Cautiously finding my feet in this new environment as if I was treading on the frozen pavement above us, I gingerly interjected what I hoped were appropriately amusing remarks into the conversation and was rewarded when Greg's bass laughter boomed enthusiastically in response. I was unsure if it was with sincere amusement or through benevolence of recognising my gaucheness, but I persisted either way. When he rested an arm across my shoulders, I immediately understood that it bore no sexual implication but rather, that it was there in a casually reassuring, relaxed manner. I guessed that he ticked all of the boxes for many gay men as he was classically handsome and owned a noticeable attribute behind the tight, faded jeans. But he wasn't my type. Nevertheless, the placement of his arm suggested acceptance, and I was delighted that it would be winding Vernon up no end.

I pulled out my wallet. "My round. What's everyone drinking?" As there were no takers, I bought myself a pint, but when I turned to rejoin our small throng, Vernon had already slipped in next to Greg and was cosied up so close to him that he could only have been nearer if he'd been inside his Levi's, and those were so tight that there was barely enough room in them for Greg himself. Vernon gazed at him with nauseating, overdone affection and the epitome of saccharine sweetness, yet still managed to throw visual daggers at me.

"That's the second pint she's had in five minutes. She's probably a gin queen as well. Just you look at her eyes. You're the professional, Greg; you must be able to see it. There's lush written all over that innocent face of hers."

I relied on Bill for enlightenment at the unfamiliar word.

"It means alcoholic, dear."

With this new information, I observed his earlier words of advice and turned my back on Vernon.

Bill nodded to someone on the fixed seating. "Back in a minute. I need to talk to Ray."

Within the low-ceilinged, tackily decadent, and adorably alternative world, my eyes continually absorbed everything, and my memory recorded every look I received, wondering if I dared to smile back, and if I did, if would it signify commitment. I had absolutely no idea of the rules.

I continued to steal glances at a man at the end of the bar whose bullish bulk blocked my view of the posters on the wall behind him. His sombre black jacket seemed fit to burst at the seams, and the matching black tie contrasted against the white shirt smeared with blurred colours from the illuminated ceiling. With one forearm resting on the bar, he traced the indents of a dimpled pint tankard with the tip of a thick forefinger, and a few inches away, a fat cigar rested in a plastic Double Diamond ashtray. He periodically huffed at the rising smoke, making it twitch and temporarily dissipate until it resumed its course in a steady grey line towards the foil-covered ceiling. His attire, along with his glum expression, made me wonder if he'd just attended a funeral.

His companion was an equally appealing character, and I stared without caution at the thick-necked, shaven-headed scowling bruiser who leaned his tattooed, gorilla forearms on the bar. His brutish features were enhanced by a black goatee beard scratched with grey. Tiny rings pierced each ear, their colour matching a golden front tooth that was exposed with each of his rumbling guffaws. I imagined he'd be more at home on board a pitching and rolling seafaring galleon during an on-deck melee, gripping a cut-throat dagger between his teeth and brandishing curved scimitars in each hand as he took on all-comers in a one-man mutiny.

The two men were deep in conversation and occasionally, one of them would throw a dark, furtive glance at me, which was as simultaneously unsettling as it was thrilling. As if on a predetermined signal, both looked over at me and chuckled. They were laughing at me, but I couldn't tear my eyes away from the nefarious-looking duo. A jab to my ribs claimed my attention.

"I see you've already got a fan club." Vernon's sneer jolted me from my unsubtle surveillance.

"Eh?"

"You want to watch those two. I know what they're capable of."

"And what's that?"

"You don't want to know."

"I do."

"Believe me, you don't."

"But I do."

Vernon narrowed his eyes and leaned in closer. "A few words of advice, Dorothy. Don't get carried away with the first bloke who looks at you. You're just a novelty that'll soon wear off, and there are people in here who can be real bitches."

Before I could allude to Gran's saying about pots and kettles, his eyes widened as something over my shoulder diverted his attention, and my head seemed cleaved in two halves when he shrieked, "Sister!"

I turned around just as a short, almond-eyed man bearing an alarmingly blond pudding basin haircut pushed me aside. My drink spilled for the second time that evening. Even though they were only inches apart, he greeted Vernon with the same ear-splitting shriek.

I held my pint glass and dripping fingers up. "Oi, do you mind?"

The new arrival looked me up and down, pursed his lips and made kissing noises. "I don't mind at all if you've got the cash to pay for it."

Vernon's return greeting was of more impressive volume down my right ear. "Tanya! Sister!"

"You! Girl!"

The vocal antics of these gay screech owls provoked my temper. "Do you fucking *have* to do that?" As my words shot out, I was aware that I sounded like our Tim when Baz in the local yelled, "We won!" as the triumphant darts team returned from an away match at the Lord Alcester.

Tanya stepped backwards with mouth agape and hands clasping his face in exaggerated dismay, resembling the titular character in Edvard Munch's painting, *The Scream*. He raised his eyebrows and turned to Vernon. "Who's she, then?"

"This is Dorothy, and you can call her Dot." He grasped Tanya's arm. "And she calls herself *a local lad*."

Tanya smiled at me. 'You look the kind of girl who brushes her hair one hundred times before bed. Have you got a nanny? I bet you have; your sort always do." He sounded like he was on drugs.

"You *what*?"

"Are these clip-ons?' His hands flashed up and tugged at the silver rings in my earlobes.

"Ouch! Gerroff!" I jerked my head backwards.

"Oh, obviously not. Well, they look cheap enough for clip-ons." He then took a small step back and squinted at me, the coloured blossoms of light converting his immaculate coiffure into a floral-covered crash helmet. "Wasn't you chucked out of Cha-Cha's the other weekend?"

I shook my head. "Not me. I don't even know where Cha-Cha's is."

Tanya squealed with laughter. "Cha-Cha is a queen, girl, not a place. Where do you live—Mars?"

"No, St. Ann's."

Tanya rolled his eyes. "Same thing."

I needed Bill to rescue me from this frightful pair. Thankfully, he was watching from the fixed seating where he sat next to a man in a burgundy jumper covered with a design of snowflakes and white skiers. He mouthed, "Two minutes."

Greg forcefully pushed Tanya aside and laid a heavy hand on my shoulder. "Simon, we're off down the club at closing time. If you want to come, I'll sign you in as my guest."

"Are you sure? I mean, yes, please. That's fabulous. It's like, well, another dream come true, but only if you're sure it's okay. I don't want to put you to any trouble."

Vernon snorted loudly, glared at Greg, and grasped Tanya's shoulders. "Have you heard that Gerald's back?"

Tanya fanned his face with his fingers. "Gerald? *Really?* Get away."

Vernon held his head high. "Yes, really. I have it on good authority he'll be reclaiming his place on the meat rack tonight."

Tanya gazed at the psychedelic ceiling. "Hm...fancy that then. Back so soon. I thought we'd seen the last of her. Obviously, Earls Court wasn't the success she made it out to be on her postcards. Well, it didn't take her long to come running home, did it? And no doubt she'll be swanning about again like Vivien Leigh, thinking she still owns the place. Well, I've got news for her; things have changed. Let's go down the club and find out what went wrong. But, girl, you must first promise not to be a bitch."

I'd never encountered anyone like these two over-exaggerated caricatures. It was as if they were acting in a really crap play and laying it on thick just for my benefit, what with me being the new meat. Their performance recalled a scene from *The Naked Civil Servant* that was shown on telly a week before Christmas 1975. Although it was school the next day, Dad let me stay up to watch it. On that Tuesday night, I'd sat on the settee in my pyjamas, hugging a saggy turquoise satin cushion and clenching my toes until they hurt. With my imprisoned breath making my chest and head ache, I stared, goggle-eyed at the screen as the inexperienced Quentin Crisp was offered a lipstick to try for the first time by one of the gaggle of painted-faced male prostitutes sitting around a table in the Black Cat Café. A couple of feet away from me, Tim slouched in his chair, staring at the television, his mouth open, and his half-eaten supper of pigs' trotters, pickled onions, and a sloppy mountain of piccalilli on the plate that he balanced on his chest.

He burped, then wiped his fingers on the side of the chair. "Ayup, Dad. You want to come in and see this queer on the telly."

I squirmed as if my nightclothes were filled with dozens of slippery live eels. The reflection in the large picture window showed Dad enter from the kitchen in his royal blue pyjamas and, as was his routine, he sat at the table with his supper and the *Evening Post*. He always liked to do the crossword before going to bed.

"That's not a very nice word, Son, and I wish you wouldn't use it. You must remember how your mother and I were great friends with Reg and Chum back in the sixties."

"I know, Dad. There's nowt up with Reg and Chum. I saw them the other day in the best side of the Corner Pin, and they asked to be remembered to you. It's just this bloke's not bleddy right." He crunched a pickled onion. "Though I suppose you've got to take your hat off to him for having the balls to do that back then in the war." As if he were King Henry at a medieval banquet, he tore at the rubbery flesh of a greasy pig trotter with his teeth, gulped, wiped his mouth with the back of his hand, and gave me a sly look. "It's a bit like you with your Marc Bolan wigs and women's boots and all that, int it?"

If only the settee would turn into a huge mouth and swallow me. "Shush. I'm missing it what with you yakking on. I'm trying to watch."

"Why, are you taking notes?"

Household video recorders were uncommon in those days but seven years later, I retained my admiration for Quentin Crisp, fascinated by the dichotomy of his benign nature and the assertive, confrontational parade of his effeminacy. On telly, I adored the cosy, cup-of-tea-by-the-fireside camp of Larry Grayson, but I was threatened and deeply unsettled by Vernon and Tanya. His bitchy behaviour towards me illustrated how hard as nails Vernon was, and so I must heed Bill's advice to avoid him and his equally unsavoury cohort.

With perfect timing, Bill rejoined our group and squeezed in next to me. "Sorry I had to leave you with that one and his odious friend. This evening hasn't been the best welcome to the gay scene for you."

"Are they always like that?"

Greg had obviously overheard our exchange. "Yes, and frequently worse." He whirled the remaining couple of inches of beer around the bottom of his glass. "But be heartened that they are the exception rather than the rule."

Footfall thundered down the stairs and en masse, heads swivelled towards the doors where the bloody glow of the glass panels bore shadowed figures, immediately reminding me of when Nazi soldiers stormed resistance safehouses in the World War Two drama, *Secret Army*, that Dad and I had avidly watched. Both doors burst open to reveal a trio of men wearing black Harrington jackets. The stubble of their savagely cropped heads glowed as red dust halos from the ruby bulb above them. It was already bad enough having to negotiate the unexpected contretemps with Vernon, but I hadn't considered the possibility of the bar being attacked by queerbashers. My new companions continued chatting, seemingly unbothered by this incursion as the considerably taller of the three pushed towards us, a tightly rolled prison fag of the type smoked by our Steve clamped between his lips. The other two guarded the doors, their sentry-like stance ensuring that no one would escape.

But what was up with the barmen? One polished a glass as he talked to the two bruisers that were the focal point of my lust, whilst his colleague wiped a yellow sponge over the bar top. I shook my head when, in another bizarre example of almost supernatural musical co-ordination, the old ska song, "Skinhead Moonstomp" began to play on the jukebox. The low-key pace continued without any display of alarm at this intrusion and, checking the unconcerned faces mottled from the kaleidoscopic lights, I might as well have been in a surreal scene from the sixties television series *The Avengers*. So disconcerting was the atmosphere, I wouldn't have been surprised to see the leather-clad Emma Peel jump through the door and karate chop these neo-Nazi invaders into submission.

The gangly intruder sucked his roll-up down to the tips of his finger and thumb, both visibly tainted nicotine umber when he squished the soggy fag end into an ashtray on the bar. He threaded towards the bruisers and draped his long arms around their shoulders. He kissed each one, then called across to where we stood, now rejoined by Vernon and his alarming friend.

"Oi, Tanya. You going down the club?"

Tanya coyly fluttered his eyelids. "Only if you promise to have the last dance of the night with me."

"Yer on."

"Did you know Gerald's back?"

"No. What's she come home for?"

Tanya wiggled his fingers at Vernon. "That's just what her and me was going down the club to find out." He blew kisses to the two sentries guarding the doorway. "What's up with them two? Are we suddenly not good enough now they live on Bread and Lard Island?"

Despite the surreal, hallucinatory situation, I chuckled at the colloquialism for the upmarket suburb south of the River Trent, of which local legend proclaimed that the expensive mortgages of those citizens who aspired to better themselves forced them to dine on meagre portions of bread and lard.

"Nah, they got bad colds and don't want to spread their germs."

Some of my magazines mentioned the subculture of gay skinheads, and I'd naïvely assumed that they were a London-based phenomenon. But here they were in my city, referring to other gay men by feminine pronouns and considerately not wanting to pass on their colds. There was so much to absorb in this twinkling seat of my new learning, but when the two bruisers and the tall skinhead laughed and looked over at me, the years rewound to my school days and the conspiratorial glances and whispers of those who had already determined my four o'clock fate. But as the new boy here, I wouldn't let my historic psychological damage taint my first night.

The stark overhead lights rapidly flashed several times, banishing the shadows in temporary, urgent stabs of white, and instead of a sturdy brass bell that I was used to hearing rung in pubs at closing time, one of the barmen tinkled a tiny brass flower. "Last orders, gentlemen."

Carl appeared at my side. "We're off to the club now. Are you coming? Greg's going to sign you in." He rubbed his hands as if anticipating the low temperature outside. "I hope we don't have to queue too long in the cold."

At the end of the bar, the two bruisers drained their pint glasses, stood up from their stools, and lumbered past me. The one in the black suit who looked as though he'd been at a funeral scowled as if he were ready to kill me. Although not up to my height, they were certainly impressive and brought to mind the phrase built like brick shithouses. The gold tooth glinted when the piratey one bumped into me with a deliberation that in no way was accidental. "Catch you later."

Was his growl a threat? Or something else? I was too inexperienced in the etiquette, roles, and rituals. I had no idea how to approach a bloke, what to say, how to respond, or how to behave.

Bill smiled. "Come on. We're off to the club."

So here were the final stages of my introduction to gay life. The culmination of the evening's events was now within walking distance. At last, I was going to enter the inner sanctum, the pinnacle of my ambition, the fruition of taking control of my life. I stepped to the jukebox and slipped in a silver ten pence piece, scanned the name tags, and jabbed down the requisite pair of white plastic buttons. As I passed the barman gathering the empties, "If My Friends Could See Me Now" blasted for the second time that night. Laughing to myself as I climbed the stairs to street level and passed the *Private Party. No Admission* notice, I remembered my misdirected exploration of the upstairs bar. Now I was going to the club as part of a group of out gay men. Its scarlet doors had attained magical, mystical properties, and when I stepped through them, in the words of the song still audible below me, I'd rejoice with all my friends.

28

THE ART OF FALLING APART

THE GLACIAL WIND STOLE my breath like an invisible assailant. I took a couple of seconds to steady myself on the sparkling pavement. I couldn't afford to slip over on the final stage of this evening's journey. The frost-burnished tarmac of the dual carriageway reflected the headlights of the few cars that passed us as we descended to where the ugly road was swallowed by the monstrous concrete mouth of a multi-storey car park. There was only a short distance left until I got to the club, and I imagined my excitement hovering above me in the crystallised night air like an aurora borealis. However, no matter how carefully I trod, the thick rubber ferrule on my walking stick was no match for the polished pavement, and I slipped, lurching against Greg, who quickly grabbed me before I fell.

Vernon was jubilant. "If you can't walk in heels, dear, you shouldn't try. Watch and learn from the expert." With his left hand holding his cigarette aloft and the other hand resting upon his right hip, he began a Mae West sashay. Within seconds, those ridiculous New York cowboy boots became airborne, and he hit the ground next to my feet with a terrible thud. "Help me, Dorothy. I've broken my back."

"Shame it wasn't your fucking neck." But my response horrified me. Oh god, I'd only been out on the gay scene for five minutes and had already become a bitch, just like him. Nevertheless, I bit the side of my bunched fingers, struggling to stifle a joyous laugh as I watched him attempt to stand with the ungainliness of a new-born foal.

He clambered to his feet and glared at me. "Just you remember that you're the new girl in town, Dorothy, so you watch your step."

"I think that you should be watching yours." As if it was my first time on skates, I continued navigating the treacherous black ice towards the level ground. At last I stood outside Part Two, the gay nightclub which I'd yearned to visit since it opened during the furnace of the previous summer when my need to be inside had burned with equal ferocity. Now I shivered, not only from the biting January wind, but also from the memory of a morning six months earlier. I'd signed on the dole at the labour exchange, then walked the several hundred yards along Canal Street until I stopped on the pavement opposite the club. I'd gazed with pathetic longing, desperately needing to be a member of the nocturnal gay fraternity behind those glossy red doors. But the pappy flesh blighting my chest and a headful of hang-ups made that an impossibility until surgery freed me from the physical restrictions. *Then* I'd take charge of my own destiny.

And now I was going in! This was going to be just *so* fabulous.

Bill jabbed his gloved forefinger onto a brass button and kept it pressed down, maintaining the angry buzzing of a million wasps. He placed his face closer to the red doors. "Come on, Tony. We're freezing."

The door opened, and we left the subdued yellow streetlights behind and pushed into the midnight interior, clustering at the red reception counter to pay our entrance fee. Greg signed me in as his guest, and as I proudly printed my name, address, and phone number in capital letters, I was astonished to see that other guests included Liza Minnelli, Margaret Thatcher, and Zsa Zsa Gabor, and that they all shared the same residence.

"Fairy Towers?"

Greg chortled. "It's what we call the Victoria Centre flats; a very high percentage of residents are gay men."

Bill shoved his head between us and winked at me. "And some call it Vaseline Villas."

I slid the change from my fiver into my frayed jeans pocket, already determined to become a member on my next visit. I drew in my breath— maybe tonight I wouldn't leave alone. *No. Don't be daft.* Best not to try and run before I could walk, and my bad leg was already sending a worrying alert that I'd already overdone it.

But how it was worth the wait. I was determined to remember every moment because I was certain that I'd never relive these dizzying first sensations with such knee-trembling intensity again. This was my final rite of passage, a quasi-religious experience, which made me wonder if the throat-choking rush of emotional sensations that overwhelmed me was what the devout experienced when entering a church.

LP-sized windows in the two black doors displayed a crazed artist's palette of distorted colours which pulsed with the attacking bass bump

Chucking Putty at the Queen

from behind them. Compared to the Arctic wasteland outside, the temperature in the reception was that of a hothouse and within seconds, had provoked a popping of sweat on my brow. Most of our entourage were already checking their coats into the cloakroom, their garments snatched by a sallow-faced youth with a greasy fringe. He stared at me sullenly from a pair of black-rimmed eyes as he rammed wire coat hangers into the shoulders of jackets and anoraks.

"Oi, girl, are you checking that stick in or what?"

"No, thanks. I need it to walk with." A rush of pride puffed my chest out from the power of quashing my complexes about relying on it. Following the years of embarrassment and hatred of my disability, I'd really come a long way since I'd phoned Gay Switchboard twenty-four hours earlier.

An uncertain smile crumpled the youth's flat face. "Sorry. I thought it was just for show. You know what posers we get in here. I'll look after it for nowt if you want to dance."

"Cripples dancing. Whatever next?"

I turned and glared at Vernon.

"When will we see your debut on the dance floor, Dorothy?" He nudged a pasty, rat-faced man next to him. "That'll be a cabaret worth getting front row seats for."

Before I could answer, a man pushed past me as he wrestled out of a green padded bomber jacket and thrust it towards the coat check youth.

"That's an original Schott, so you take care of it. There's nothing in the pockets neither, so don't waste your time looking through them."

The youth scowled as he defiantly stuffed a hanger inside the arm holes then handed the man his receipt. "As if I'd do owt like that."

The man snatched the blue ticket. "You usually do."

I nudged Bill and nodded at the youth. "He could cheer up a bit."

"Oh, don't mind her, dear. That's Betty Blue Lips. She has a congenital heart condition and knows that she's not long for this world."

Bill shivered in the blast of frosty air that ushered in a line of men from the street. A pair of cherub-faced blond men in light blue leather "bumfreezer" jackets rushed past and tugged open the doors to the disco, allowing me a tantalizing glimpse of laser colours slashing through the dry ice, along with a deafening blast of a woman singing of a hit and run lover. This was a completely different planet from my Saturday nights in the local pub with its one rope-light draped flaccidly over the dartboard.

279

I eagerly stepped forwards, but Bill grabbed my arm.

"Your eyes are like saucers, dear. Anyone would think you're speeding. You have to do this the right way and build up to it. You will only get this chance once. Little bites first before you dive into the main course. Come on, you can buy me a drink upstairs in the quiet bar."

This delay added to my frustration, but as Bill had been kind enough to take me under his wing, I trusted that he knew what he was doing. We joined the rest of our troupe and climbed metal stairs through the blackness towards a small landing. The door at the end opened, and two men in checked work shirts burst out, their huge black moustaches adding a walrus-like effect to their unshaven chubby faces. In the narrow area, a physical crush was unavoidable, and laughing, they dished out kisses in friendly greeting, including one for me at the back of the queue, before they clumped down the stairs in their sand-coloured work boots. Talk about if my friends could see me now; I'd had my bum pinched in the pub and been kissed by a pair of strangers.

Bill held the door open for me. "Come along, dear."

I stepped into an industrial-inspired elegance that I'd only seen in the American interior design library books that I'd pored over when I was jazzing up my bedroom. The walls and ceiling of this enormous L-shaped room were painted dove grey, with the floor carpeted in a complementary charcoal tone. Dozens of men stood in groups or lounged alone, and as they moved, I glimpsed others relaxing on spacious black leather sofas placed in facing pairs and separated by low, glass-topped tables edged with shining chrome. Wide, white tubs housed sumptuous, towering palms, under-lit to splay spiked shadows onto the ceiling. It was exactly the effect I'd attempted to create in my bedroom, and I adored this chic, harmonic opulence as instantly as I had loved the shabby, ad-hoc glam of the cellar bar earlier.

I thought back to the estate pub that had been my sole nightlife experience when I was younger. Now that I was surrounded by gay men, I inwardly cringed remembering my crush on John, the married man who looked like the models in the gay magazines. How desperate and naïve I'd been. I could have got into a load of trouble, and with that thought at the front of my mind, I jumped out of my skin when a man squeezed past me, making my heart lurch with the recognition of the short back and sides haircut, thick Groucho Marx moustache, steel-rimmed glasses, and checked shirt. But it wasn't John. This man joined two others standing beneath the graceful palm leaves, all uncannily similar in appearance apart from the colour of their hair, moustaches, and plaid work shirts.

And sashaying towards this knot of ersatz masculinity was Vernon. Immediately their heads were together, and eyes darted over at me before peals of laughter erupted. I turned my back on them as Bill sipped from the gin and tonic I'd bought him.

"It's quiet for a Thursday, but it'll be lively tomorrow and wild on Saturday. It always is." His attention focused over my left shoulder, and as I turned, he grabbed my forearm. "Don't look. It's Shane. I got off with him last week and quite fancy my chances again."

"Oh, okay. Sorry."

Bill winked. "It's your first night here. Wouldn't you like to explore?"

I took a draught from my pint. "In a bit. This is ace. I can't believe I'm here."

"Well, you *are*, dear."

"*I know*."

Bill shot another glance over my shoulder and patted my upper arm. "Don't worry about me. I'll be all right here on my own."

"No, this is fine. It's more than I imagined."

"There's plenty more to discover if you want to go off." He motioned towards a long, dark corridor. A dim light source glowed at its end. "Along there is the restaurant and the stairs down to the disco where the real action is. You'll love it."

I sipped my lager. "Mm, it sounds great."

"Yes, you'll love it *when you go downstairs*."

The penny dropped. "Oh, god. Sorry. See you later." The muted tribal thudding from below seemed to grab my feet and propel me forwards, helping me leave my embarrassment behind, but I couldn't resist a backwards glance. Bill was already snogging his friend. Blimey, he didn't hang about. I tried not to stare, even though it was the first time I'd witnessed such an open demonstration of two men kissing. Fighting an unexpected sense of rejection by Bill's abrupt dismissal, I proceeded with the unhurried pace of a processional ceremony that befitted such an occasion. Similar to the New York gay bar described in one of my John Rechy novels, the black walls bore white paintings of a cowboy, a construction worker, a biker, and a muscle man. I paused, contemplating

them as if I were a sophisticated art connoisseur holding a glass of champagne in an upmarket gallery and not a gauche nineteen-year-old clasping a pint of rapidly warming lager on his debut visit to a gay club.
"Hello!"
The voice startled me from my appraisal. I turned and saw a slim, tanned man walking past wearing shorts, striped legwarmers, and a cropped blue sweatshirt bearing the pink appliqued slogan, "Lights, camera, action." I raised my glass and smiled, fit to burst with the joyfulness of gay brotherhood, thrilled that from hidden speakers Grace Jones sang her version of the old Marvelettes song, "The Hunter Gets Captured by the Game." The line about the world seeming like a new place certainly was apt as I watched the man slink with panther-like grace towards the end of the passage and through the doors to the disco.
A few more paces brought me to a cigarette vending machine, the soft blush from its transparent plastic front illuminating a diminutive, skinny figure. I stifled a giggle because, with his spindly legs emerging from skin-tight leather shorts and vanishing into black jackboots, he reminded me of the actor Charles Hawtrey playing Charlie Muggins in the comedy film, *Carry On Camping*. I already thought that Vernon could have been an extra from one of the much-loved film series; how many more lookalikes would I see before the night was out? A hardware store's worth of silver chains looped from each shoulder of his too-big leather waistcoat that partially obscured a bare torso. A pair of mirrored US cop sunglasses obscured his eyes and, like many men I'd already seen so far, a huge moustache adorned his top lip. As I passed, I just knew that he watched my progress from behind the reflective lenses, so I nodded. "All right?"
He stood mannequin still and showed no response as I continued towards the low light at the end of the black tunnel. Ignorant sod, he could have at least acknowledged me. Anyway, I didn't care, this was *my* time, and I was about to descend into the action.
"Excuse me, excuse me."
The sound of faintly tinkling chains made me glance back. He scurried towards me with the tops of his jackboots slapping his thin legs like unenthusiastic applause, whilst the links of his swinging metal ornamentation sparkled as if they were strings of diamonds. "Hang on a minute."
I stopped, expecting him to cadge money for the cigarette machine

Chucking Putty at the Queen

or, even worse, come onto me. But I couldn't have been more wrong.

"Is your name Smalley?"

"You what?" My astonished face reflected in his convex mirrored lenses.

"You're Steve and Tim Smalley's brother, aren't you?"

"Er...well, yeah."

"I thought so. I used to live near you years ago. Like..." He sucked at his teeth as if to stimulate his memory. "1967. You was only a nipper then."

"Yeah, I would have been five."

"And you used to walk up and down Lamartine Street in your mam's shoes, wearing her earrings and carrying her handbag."

"I know."

"People talked about you."

"They still do."

He thrust out a skeletal hand. "I'm Clint."

Despite the heat of the club, his fingers were like ice. "I'm Simon."

"Nice to meet you after all this time. Do you remember Margaret Watkins?"

Oh, did I remember Margaret Watkins? She was roughly the same age as my sisters, one of about ten troublesome kids in her bad news family. Their feckless, light-fingered father frequented the Sir Colin Campbell pub and was a gambling associate of our Steve. Gran warned us that Mrs Watkins was a "foul-mouthed washerwoman," and Dad urged me to avoid their numerous offspring, of which, no doubt this chap was one.

I furrowed my brow as if I were trying hard to recall. "Um, Margaret Watkins. The name seems a bit familiar. Are you her brother?"

"No, I'm her husband."

I floated in a brief vacuum of speechless astonishment until he lowered the sunglasses and looked over the top of them.

"Can I ask, are you secretly gay?"

"I'm not secretly anything, mate."

"Sorry, I didn't mean it rude. It's just that my wife and family don't know I'm gay."

I gawped at his regalia, especially at the kitchen sink plug dangling on the end of a chain from his studded belt. "They *don't?*"

"No, so I have to be careful."

"Your secret's safe with me."

"Ta." He coughed awkwardly, and I pulled back from the smell of a dozen overflowing ashtrays. "Nice meeting you, but don't tell no one you seen me here, 'cos like I said, nobody knows I'm gay."

From the comprehensive explanations within my library of gay magazines, I'd become fully conversant with the inventive hanky code by which some gay men signalled their sexual proclivities. Certain colours correlated with specific sexual tastes. Tucking the relevant handkerchiefs in the back pockets of jeans or leather trousers eliminated unnecessary, time-wasting conversations by blatantly symbolising what was on offer or similarly, what was hoped for. This unique method of advertising ranged from a single handkerchief folded and discreetly visible, to the extremes of the sexually adventurous, whose back pockets resembled the vivid tail plumage of exotic birds. I'd also read of the S&M scene where handcuffs and cock rings adorned the epaulettes of leather jackets and belt loops, but one accoutrement of Clint's regalia confounded my knowledge.

As he turned around to leave, I just had to ask. "Hang on, Clint. I'm new to all this. I know about hankies and what they mean and all that, but what does the sink plug signify?"

He fingered the grey rubber and gave me a wan smile. "Oh, that, I just couldn't get it off the chain with me pliers." With a nod, he strode away and resumed his position at the side of the cigarette machine.

As I neared the restaurant, I cheered inwardly when I saw that some of the gay stereotypes I'd seen in the magazines were out tonight. Inside the subtly illuminated interior, two burly older men in American army uniforms sat at a table beneath yet another enormous palm. They ate with forks as they held hands over the pale grey tablecloth, their peaked caps placed beside the steady flame of a tiny candle in a chromed holder. A slash of white light from the large presentation chiller was the only true brightness in the room, and that was directed onto the prawns and avocado that a thin-face blond man in a chef's uniform was placing onto the aluminium surface.

He smiled and beckoned me to the doorway. "If you're hungry, love, these prawns are delish, and the moussaka is out of this world, even if I do say so myself." He nodded to the men at the table. "Ask them two."

I smiled happily at his friendliness. "No, ta, you're okay. I had something before I came out."

He winked and wiggled a prawn at me. "Well, if you get peckish later, you can always come in for a nibble."

I smiled again at his reassuring demeanour and still consumed by a floating and dreamy sense of ultimate belonging, I turned my attention to the two closed black doors. I leaned towards one of the panes of wire-strengthened glass and peered through into the blackness beyond. The top of a wide metal staircase with red handrails dropped into an ominously dark abyss. I grasped the door handle, then paused, revelling in the momentous occasion. The thudding repetitive bass from beneath my feet and behind the doors transmitted an exhilarating promise that something extraordinary awaited me down there. This was it: my big moment.

Loud, overtly ribald laughter snatched my attention. I turned and looked along the dark corridor back towards the lounge. Vernon and his cronies were watching me. Knife-edge horror stabbed me when one of them walked towards the toilets dragging his right leg in a grotesque limp. I quickly checked myself. *No, don't be stupid.* It's just paranoia taking control and ruining my life again. I don't know the bloke, I've never seen him until tonight, and he could have a leg injury too. After all, I didn't own the rights to being a gay man with a bad leg. But when he returned from the toilet walking with a perfectly balanced gait, my initial suspicions were proved correct.

Despite my titanic achievements this evening, everything counted for absolutely nothing. I'd never escape this sort of shit, and I'd never escape my own hang-ups. Even though it was a different dark passageway, it may as well have been the hate-filled corridors of school. This club was where I'd expected to find acceptance and camaraderie, but it was just the same as the world outside its red glossy doors. Even my own kind hated me. I had to get out. I had to go home but first, I'd have to navigate past that lot. With the cowed shame of a dog that had been thrown out onto the street for defecating indoors, I slunk towards the door, on the alert for a foot to trip me up.

"Are you going back to Kansas, Dorothy?"

A flash ignited Bill's titbit of gossip about Vernon's leisurely lifestyle into a final flame of resistance. I'd never be coming back here again, so what the hell? "Yes. Some of us have to go to work in the morning. We can't all ponce about living off our grandmother's wealth."

The air rippled with a collective intake of breath from his entourage, and a whispered, "Touché" brushed my ears.

I turned to the one who'd limped. "And if I were you, I'd get that leg looked at, or you'll end up like me." I dragged my eyes up and down him and shook my head. "Nah, forget it, mate. You could *never* be like me."

Back out on the small landing, I clutched the banister to steady myself against an unexpected twist of vertigo, anticipating a shove that would send me tumbling headfirst just like at school, but the door behind me remained closed. Finally, with both feet firmly in the reception, Tony the brick-wall bouncer opened the door to the street and looked left and right as if I were an old-aged pensioner who needed escorting across a busy road.

"You're okay; it's clear."

I realised that he was checking that it was safe for me to leave. The last thing I needed was to be attacked by queerbashers.

He clapped my back. "Goodnight then. Take care. See you soon."

"I doubt it."

Just before the door closed, Betty Blue Lips called, "Ta-ra, girl!"

It was a farewell from the gay scene that I'd so desperately yearned to be a part of but from which I was now fleeing. The freezing fingers of the harsh frost drew me out onto Canal Street. The pavements that once shone with promise and excitement were now slippery death traps as I slid further into pathetically woeful self-pity. Knowing my luck, I'd slip and injure my bad leg and end up back in hospital, incarcerated in plaster. Each timorous step was marked by unforgiving self-recriminations as I mentally replaced the ticks of my successes with angry red crosses of failure. After my prolonged and formidable odyssey to reach gay liberation, the glorious yellow brick road had turned out to be made of dirty old cobbles.

29

THURSDAY NIGHT AND SATURDAY MORNING

HOME HAD NEVER BEEN more welcoming than when I arrived back from the club. I hadn't needed my key to get in. Dad's worrying foible was to leave the house unsecured, refusing to relinquish the opinion still held by many of his generation when referring to their shared halcyon history: "We never had to lock our doors back in the old days."

I stood in the dark hall, holding my breath to see if my entrance had disturbed his and Tim's slumber. All was silent, which was perfect for me. The last thing I needed was the third degree about my evening or remarks on the late hour. The luminous hands on my watch showed a quarter past one. As I'd never been out so late before, I should've been rejoicing at sneaking in long after the local pubs had shut, but I just wanted to get into bed and forget the whole debacle.

I crept upstairs and lay defeated and demoralized under my duvet, wishing that the old electric blanket would hurry up and get warm. More than once, Tim had warned me against using it, pointing out the silver wires visible through the perished rubber of the flex, but I didn't care if I was electrocuted or if the whole bed went up in flames. That would be a fitting end to my disastrous night and serve me right for being so wet by surrendering to my mental weakness. Instead of soaring to the zenith of my liberation, my insecurities and over-sensitivity had plummeted me back into the black chasm of paranoia that continued to dominate my psychological being.

Three years ago, my emotionally unsteady life had suffered another upheaval when Jacqui and her family moved away from St. Ann's. Despite the new distance that separated us, we continued to meet in town every Saturday morning. I admired her cosmopolitan weekend existence of being out on the razz, drinking brandy and lemonade and dancing to disco music in the city's nightclubs. More often than not, the mission on our meet-ups was for her to buy something new to wear that evening, which meant a committed trawling of the frock shops. We traditionally accomplished this exhausting feat in two shifts separated by a sustenance break in the cavernous cafeteria above big Woolies, the larger of the two Woolworths stores in town.

    I couldn't wait to unburden myself to her. She'd understand; hers was the voice of reason and rationality throughout the persecution I'd suffered at school and after we left, when I still genuinely believed that my schoolyard enemies hid in the shadows, determined to kill me. And only six months earlier, when I'd told the doctor how the excess flesh on my chest was making me miserable, Jacqui was the only other person in whom I could confide. There would be no ridicule or condemnation from her, and my trust in the strength of our friendship was proved correct. "You should have told me sooner instead of suffering on your own, you big gonk." Her immediate worry about my psychological well-being overrode any sign of her shock at my unusual disclosure, and she took the afternoon off work to accompany me to my appointment with the surgeon.

    During the morning portion of this shopping trip, we'd visited just about every ladies' fashion emporium and boutique in town, including Miss Selfridge, Dorothy Perkins, Etam, and Chelsea Girl. In all of them, she'd dismissively flicked through the assortment hanging from circular chromed racks and tried on garments with mounting frustration. At our first port of call, my attention was grabbed by an elegant black dress with discreet gold thread enhancements. But despite her determined protestations of "No, that's not it" or "it's just not me," when the shops were about to close, we'd end up returning to this one, seconds before the doors were pulled shut and the sign turned to closed. Then, to the visible exasperation of the manageress preparing to cash up the tills, Jacqui would buy the dress several hours after I'd remarked, "What's the point in having a puff as a mate if you don't trust his fashion advice?"

    But before that inevitable conclusion to today's retail therapy, she was impatient to hear a report of my progress two nights earlier. The Woolies cafeteria was busy.

    "Phew, what a pong." Jacqui wrinkled her nose at the odours of frying chips and boiled cabbage, then tutted at the litter of dirty plates from the previous occupants of the only free table for two. "Just look at this lot. Some people are worse than pigs."

    "I think that you're doing a disservice to pigs."

Chucking Putty at the Queen

She gathered the scattered knives and forks, bound them neatly within the constraints of a paper napkin, and laid them upon a tray made of moulded, laminated wood. The sight of this commonplace utilitarian object always roused virulent memories of my foes smashing similar trays on my head in the school dining hall as they called me "fucking queer" and "puffy bastard" and assured me that my life would soon be over.

Jacqui shoved the tidy bouquet of cutlery towards me. "Take that to the dirty plates bit."

"Who do you think I am? Avis Tennyson?"

She threw her head back and guffawed at my reference to the menial character in the soap opera *Crossroads* from years ago. "You plonker! Trust *you* to remember her. Nobody else would."

Fortunately, I was saved from undertaking waitress duties by the appearance of an apron-fronted woman. "Let me take them for you, ducky. You can't manage that with a walking stick."

"Thank you, I'm glad that someone around here cares."

Jacqui raised her eyebrows. "Just shut your gob and sit down. I want to hear all about it. Did you cop off?"

"Hang on. Let's eat first; I'm starving."

After our meal, and with our empty plates shoved to one side, she used the pointed end of a teaspoon to unite two small pools of spilled coffee upon the tabletop. "So, come on, Pie, what's up?"

I smiled at her affectionate nickname for me, based on the old nursery rhyme, "Simple Simon Met a Pie Man." She hadn't used it for ages. When I'd regaled the events of Thursday night and described my new archenemy, Jacqui half-closed her eyes.

"I don't like the sound of him."

I slowly tore a red paper napkin apart and reassembled the ragged-edged pieces into a carnation, then pushed it towards her. "I'm not his number one fan either."

She rapped my knuckles with the teaspoon and leaned forwards. "Listen. I'm not being horrible, but you've never been out with anyone, have you? It's as plain as owt that he's jealous of you because his boyfriend paid you some attention. Ignore him. He's a prat. You get out there tonight and start again. You can't go back in the cupboard now."

"Closet."

"Eh?"

"It's closet, not cupboard."

"Don't split hairs. It's the same difference."

She dropped the teaspoon and grabbed my hand. "Do they let women in?"

"I dunno. I didn't see any, but I wasn't there that long. It's supposed to be blokes only. Why?"

"I'll wear a false moustache and a flat cap and go in with you. Then you point him out to me, and I'll warn him off."

"What, will you give him one of your *Hong Kong Phooey* kung fu chops?" I sniggered because she actually *was* an accomplished practitioner of martial arts. "I shouldn't need you to be fighting my battles for me like you and Ju did at school."

"Listen, Pie, you're acting like a divvy. Stop being so sucky and do summat about it. Ignore him and find yourself a boyfriend." Sitting back, she brushed her hands briskly together to remove wayward grains of sugar. "And preferably not his." She tidied the crockery and stood up. "Do you really want another cuppa? I'm not that fussed. We'll go back up to Dorothy Perkins for that black and gold dress you like."

After its successful purchase, we stood at her bus stop. She opened her purse and scratched about inside for her fare. "You *are* going back down there tonight, aren't you?"

"Yeah."

"You'd better. You can't let a tosser like him put you off, not after all you've been through. It's time to move on."

"I hear you."

She snapped her purse shut. "Have you got a five pence piece?"

I dug into my pocket. "Here you are."

"Ta. So what you going to wear then?"

"That orangey checked shirt that you hate."

"Oh god, they won't miss you in that. I hope they've got their sunglasses ready."

"Ha ha."

"I'll tell you what: wear some of that Aramis that I got you from duty free when I went to Tunisia. It smells dead nice; you're bound to pull."

I smiled and shook my head. "I think it'll take more than aftershave to do that."

She boarded the bus, and as her coins clattered into the fare slot, she turned around and winked. "Gimme a ring tomorrow, first thing. I want a full report."

"First thing on a Sunday? Give over, you'll still be in bed."

"Not if me mam tells me it's you on the phone, I won't." The back seat was empty, and with her shopping beside her, she sprung up and tugged open the strip of hinged window. "And don't worry about that puffy prat. He's only jealous of you. And if he says owt tonight, you know what to do, dontcha?"

The air brakes expelled snaky hisses, and the wheels began to slowly turn. "No, what?"

She blew me a kiss as the bus pulled away from the pavement. "Hit him with your handbag."

30

FIRST NIGHT IN SODOM

THE PEP TALK FROM Jacqui did the job, and a reinvigorated, brilliant confidence powered me that early evening when I got ready to go out. I needed something to represent the heat of my determination, so yes, I *would* wear the shirt that she thought was too loud. When I reached into my rickety wardrobe, the warning creak of its unstable joints denoted how its strength was forever weakened since I'd hidden inside from my phantom foes four years earlier. I'd cowered amongst my clothing in the darkness, convinced that they'd got into the house and were creeping up the stairs to kill me. Although that experience was behind me now, the psychological bonfire of the persecution I'd suffered at school still smouldered. But I could not–*would not*–permit it to be reignited into full flame by another enemy, especially one as ridiculous as Vernon.

The cotton work shirt of lava-hued checks slid easily from the wire hanger, its hook a metal question mark as to how I'd fare this evening. Success or another failure completely depended upon me. One thing was certain: I must claim this night as my own.

Only six months ago, I could never have dreamed that what I was doing now would be possible. How momentous it had been to undergo surgery to remove the pappy flesh on my chest that had been the pivotal source of my misery. My self-energisation had been no flash in the pan, and my resolve remained unshakable. I'd been to Gay Switchboard and taken my first steps into the nightlife so previously alien to me. So what that I'd already made a new enemy? Vernon could take a running jump off Trent Bridge. I chuckled at Jacqui's advice about hitting him with my handbag.

I ironed a white T-shirt that would show off my taut chest and prodded the silver spear-shaped point around where the arms joined the body in a seam of neat stitches, determined to remove every minuscule crease as if I were smoothing away my mistakes from Thursday night. The soundtrack to my sartorial preparations was Pete Shelley's *Homosapien* album, and from the speakers of my Sanyo music centre, he assured me "Yesterday's Not Here." No, it wasn't, and with the warm cotton now adorning my torso, its dried-outside-on-the-washing-line freshness reassuringly hugged my newly flat chest. I finished my third glass of Dad's homemade wine that he'd brewed several years earlier. At family get-togethers, the cumulation of its delicious but sneakily powerful kick left most of us reeling with an unexpected upsurge of rhapsodic elation and a shared love for the world and humanity, and when he'd presented bottles to a few select friends in the local, his friend Ken reported its effect on his usually meek wife. "I don't know what you put in that wine, Sid, but Evelyn got up on our dining table in the middle of Antiques Roadshow and started singing 'We'll Meet Again.'"

I hoped that I'd never meet Vernon again. But who cared about him? This was *my* Saturday night. I poured a fourth glass and slipped into the brightly coloured shirt, and with my brain and veins fizzing, I was soon in full choral agreement with the former Buzzcocks lead singer that yesterday was indeed gone for good. I tucked the tails into the waistband of my jeans, then buckled my black leather belt before admiring my trim torso in the mirror. The puppy fat that had hung around like a hungry dog waiting to be fed was gone. I was ready, and it was time for my glittering gay future to really begin. Jacqui was right. I couldn't allow my past misery to define my future happiness. I had to lock my Thursday night failure into a mental safe box, throw away the key, and start again. I needed to do this solo, to prove to myself that I could, and as testimony to the successful surgery that had empowered me to ring Gay Switchboard in the first place. Tonight would be my *real* debut.

Tony the doorman greeted me with a warmth befitting old friends reuniting and this time, the upstairs lounge was absolutely rammed. Apart from my childhood sufferance of attending football matches with Nick, I hadn't been in the company of so many men en masse. I scanned the sea of faces but was unable to locate one from Thursday night to whom I could anchor myself. At least that dreadful creature Vernon wasn't here— or was he? I chided myself. No, I wouldn't enter that endless dark alleyway of paranoia again because it was a one-way route. Let him make bitchy remarks; I didn't give a shit. A few weeks earlier, I'd read *The Picture of Dorian Gray* for the fourth or fifth time. On this feverish peak of the weekend, Oscar Wilde's words provided literary encouragement: "There is only one thing in the world worse than being talked about, and that is not being talked about." Taking on board that sentiment tonight, I embraced the courage to enter the arena, and I *would* emerge triumphant.

When I squeezed through the melee and reached the bar, two bronzed, muscular men in matching white vests emblazoned with the Bundeswehr emblem parted to allow me through. "You're new meat, dear." I silently repeated Bill's words as if I were a monk chanting a devotion. I reassured myself that I looked good, and my bad leg didn't matter. I was tall and broad-shouldered, my shirt was dazzling, and the tight triangle of T-shirt at my neck was whiter than white above my flat chest. I gulped my lager and half-emptied the glass. I'd have to watch the alarming habit that I'd picked up from Nick: walloping off a pint in record time before quickly buying another. I'd already bolstered my resolve to enjoy tonight by recklessly consuming Dad's wine and, as well as the sensation that the carpet beneath my feet was made from jelly, the mildly hallucinatory effects of the inebriant concoction transformed the pervasive thumping from the disco below into the heartbeat of an unseen beast trapped underground. A surge of alcohol-induced confidence stiffened my backbone into a steel rod. I was the lone adventurer who must free it.

For the second time in forty-eight hours, I embarked on my odyssey along the dark corridor, passing the masculine murals until once more, I stood before the black doors. I relished my magnificent moment, the incessant thudding insisting that I make my inaugural descent into the lascivious underworld that the articles and photos in my gay magazines promised awaited me. I shook my head and blinked. I was far from drunk, but I was cresting on the silver peaks of an adrenaline wave that was about to break. I glanced back. It was difficult to see the lounge area through so many men, but at least there was nobody laughing at me, and no Vernon and his checked-shirt cohorts lampooning my limp.

The chef from Thursday night looked up and gave me a wave. Other than him, nobody disturbed my most precious, intimate moment of ceremony here in front of the doors. I had achieved this reward on my own. I deserved it and this time, I would not turn tail and take flight. The emotional ache of needing fulfilment would finally be soothed. I placed my empty glass on a low table in a shadowed alcove where a pair of denim-clad men sat with their arms around each other, their legs visible through violent rips in their jeans. I hoped that this wouldn't be the only flesh on display tonight.

I pulled the door open and recoiled from the upthrust of heat as if the door belonged to a blast furnace. A fuggy, not unattractive, chemical odour engulfed me. I bet myself that it was amyl nitrite, the poppers so frequently referenced in my gay porn magazines and of whose heart-racing euphoric rush I'd vicariously experienced from those licentious tales. In this darkened area, the ultra-masculine brand names beckoned from adverts in those pages: Bolt, Bullet, Hardware, Locker Room. Each overtly macho moniker assured sexual power would be initiated by the inhaled instant kick.

The force of the frenetic synthesised music whooshing up the metal stairs overwhelmed me, and I nearly fell down them in my eagerness to be absorbed into the core of its source. Beefy bass bumped with increasing rib-shaking intensity with each of my descending steps, and the treble peaks drilled my ears as percussion hooks pierced me, pulling me down until my feet could go no further.

Blades of fragmented coloured light stabbed through the darkness, allowing me to distinguish an ocean of men, ebbing and flowing as if tugged by an unseen current. The velvet blackness was unlimited, and I slowly became aware of more figures pinpointed by glints of silver illumination on the rims of drinks glasses and the cigarette tip fireflies that flitted to and from mouths hidden in darkened depths. The pounding bass and amyl odour amalgamated in a dulled throb trapped by my skull. When two men in front of me moved, I stared at the back of a sturdy six-footer standing apart from the others—a difficult accomplishment in this overpopulated area. A trio of coloured handkerchiefs stuffed into his back left pocket signalled his sexual preferences, but they were difficult to determine in this environment. With the reverence of a zoo visitor standing before a wild creature in its cage, I cautiously manoeuvred to get a better view. Clad in lustrous black leather, he stood with a military assertiveness as if his beefy weight forced his heavy steel toe-capped boots onto the floor. Enhancing this regimental impression, a shining metal crescent edged the peak of the Muir cap that shadowed his eyes and below that, his broad face bore a dense black beard. His unzipped leather biker jacket revealed chest hair erupting above a vest that changed colours, chameleon-like under the lights. The shine on the handcuffs hanging from the belt loop of his leather trousers forced the blood through my veins as if they were lengths of hot wire. This was a real-life leatherman who had stomped straight from a Tom of Finland illustration. When he turned and slowly moved deeper into the darkness where the disco lights failed to penetrate, I didn't dare to follow him.

The relentless fury of a synthesizer raced above a mammoth drumbeat as the song's clattering, hysterical percussion sounded as if someone was maniacally hammering on a metal sheet. The bass surged from the floor and climbed up my body as a male voice urged me to come on.

A corner of black wall hid the source of the interstellar illumination and hypnotic music where I was about to attain utter spiritual and sexual freedom. Apprehension iced my skin in this overheated foreign landscape as I shuffled forward between the wall and jammed bodies, and the effort of my awkward movement manifested in jerky spasms in my bad leg. With my back pressed against the wall, I gripped the curved wooden handle of my walking stick, not only to aid my stability but also for reassurance.

I closed my eyes and groped my way to the corner. But my potent moment was ruined when my bad leg crumpled beneath me, forcing me against the wall as if I'd been pushed.

Hands grabbed my shoulders. "Are you all right?"

Inches from my ear, the voice was just audible. Its owner was a smooth-faced man of around my age and height, frowning beneath a blond-streaked fringe. The fusion of anticipation, alcohol, and elation increased my urge to confide. I shoved my head forward as if in a confessional. "It's my first time here, and I want it to be perfect."

"*Really?*" His astonishment seemed a condemnation.

"I know it sounds stupid."

"If you want it to be perfect, you need this." He held up a stubby brown bottle. "You'll feel like you can dance barefoot on broken glass."

My baptism had taken a new turn, and multifaceted fear provoked my awkward reticence. "I don't know... I've never done drugs before. I don't even smoke."

He giggled. "It's not drugs, silly. It's only poppers. They sell them behind the bar."

"But it's illegal, isn't it?" I could already see the local gossips shaking their heads, tutting as they read the headline of the *Nottingham Evening*

Post: "Local Man In Gay Club Drug Death."

His eyes shone below the golden fringe. "How old are you?"

"Nineteen."

"Same here. So we're both underage and illegal. If we got caught with a bloke, we'd go to prison, and he would an' all. Fuck that rubbish. Come on, it's time to let yourself go."

He was right. This was the spark to ignite the new epoch of my life. My chance to break out of my constrictions, to celebrate, to stick two fingers up to the bastards who had bullied me, to those who beat me not only with their physical attacks but also with their verbal vilification. Could I never be free from the horrors of my schooldays? Denunciation from my sports teacher and my deputy headmaster flashed across my memory: *Lazy. Does not apply himself. Fails at all physical activity. Simon is easily led.*

Well, fuck them all. Instead of the stupid sports they'd forced me to participate in, there were other physical activities into which I was more than willing to be easily led. "Show us then."

He unscrewed the lid and raised the bottle to his nose. Pressing one nostril closed with his thumb, he deeply inhaled, then repeated the procedure with his other nostril. Even in the velvety shadows, his face seemed to darken with a deep rose blush. He offered the bottle to me as the recorded voice continued to encourage my progress.

His hands cupped mine as I copied the action. Within seconds, the muscular beat magnified and pummelled my whole being, reverberating against my cranium as magenta pulsed behind my eyelids. My heart banged against my ribcage and down my legs as the synthesizer galloped around my veins and spiked along my arms to trace the whorls of my fingerprints.

"Keep your eyes closed; I'll tell you when to open them."

He gently turned me around and with one hand on my shoulder and the other pressed flat against my back, he manoeuvred me forwards. "Now!"

31

MENERGY

THE STORIES AND ARTICLES in my magazines were inadequate preparation for the Dionysian display of ecstatically dancing men, several shirtless in the steamy heat. Atop one of the cabinets housing a mammoth speaker, a slim skinhead wearing a yellow jockstrap stomped his cherry red Doc Marten boots as he rapturously thrust his arms upwards and twitched his fingers as if trying to reach the inky midnight beyond the swirling, flashing lights. Pulsing colours morphed from apricot to lime to turquoise, then tangerine into flamingo pink and blood red, smearing his sweat-drenched body with stained-glass colours in this carnal cathedral. His taut body awakened a childhood memory of a disturbingly erotic illustration in a library book, where confident black ink strokes depicted a deranged religious disciple clad only in a loin cloth, stretching towards thunderous clouds as he desperately beseeched his unseen god for salvation. From beneath the altar where the DJ controlled the musical excitation, clouds of manufactured fog billowed, spreading and churning the colours, elevating them into prismatic swirls split by bolts of white lightning and neon lacerations of crimson. Misted from the jungle temperature and dripping with teardrops of condensation, a mirrored wall doubled the crowd, boosting the flashing, whirling, disorientating lights. Incredulity stretched my eyelids wide, and I looked around to thank my new friend, but he was gone, absorbed in the undulating crowd.

We never met again.

Diffused reflections of the carnival colours bounced from the mirrors onto what I later learned was the "meat rack," the prime location where you stood to be noticed. This blatant advertisement of availability was evidenced by the long line of men. Although most wore conventional garb, some were in vests and others were bare chested beneath leather waistcoats. Others posed shirtless in army gear, police uniform, or cropped sweatshirts with gym shorts, and as anomalies to the bold freedom of expression surrounding them, a couple of heavily moustached men stood in full formal dinner dress, each holding a champagne flute as if they'd popped in after an evening at the opera. The motorized beat paused, and the lights died, offering a second of black respite until all was resurrected in an atomic flash of liberating white illumination coinciding with the affirmation that this native love was restless, and that the singer was just not satisfied. I'd never heard anything so primitive, so urgently sensual before, and instinctively understood that it was undoubtedly, unequivocally gay music.

At the vanishing point of this vista, a horizontal strip of low light glowed as a sunset above the heads of the surging ocean of men. This was obviously the bar, and although my sandpaper throat needed soothing with a pint of cold lager, I doubted that I'd make it through the crowded channel. Having come this far, I wasn't going to give up, so I squeezed through the bodies, first acknowledging, then succumbing to my innate urge to dance, to join the fiesta of freedom erupting in this neon-flashed mayhem. Because of my bad leg, I'd never danced before, but the irresistible pull of the urgent, exciting music overrode the first chip of concern that I might show myself up. There was so much lost time to make up. At the end of the meat rack, I headed to the cloakroom, recalling Betty Blue Lips's offer to look after my walking stick without charge. He smiled and nodded over the heads clamouring to check in outdoor garments. I raised my stick and winked as if we were established friends and was rewarded when he grinned and stretched an arm above the waiting men.

"Giz it here then, girl."

He grabbed my walking stick, causing the line of men to turn and glare disapproval at my queue-jumping. Betty Blue Lips's small example of preferential treatment washed over me in a wave of belonging and acceptance that was almost as heady as the poppers I'd inhaled. My head swelled as if I were suddenly granted status as gay nightclub royalty, and I joined the line of men shuffling and shoving to get through the doors. By careful negotiation, I ascended past the crowd on the several wide steps to the bar, where the lighting behind me ricocheted from the mirrors at the rear of the optics. This fabulous gay galaxy was a million light years away from that stifling New Year's Eve at the local pub when I promised myself that something had better change with my life, and it bloody well had.

I clutched my cash in preparation for my first purchase of amyl nitrite.

Chucking Putty at the Queen

Behind the bar in the pubs I usually frequented, I was used to seeing plates bearing cheese or ham cobs sweating within their transparent cling film shroud, boxes overstuffed with packets of crisps, and dangling pennants adorned with gleaming blue sachets of peanuts. But here, the supplementary recreational wares on offer consisted of cardboard trays filled with bottles of poppers. Their familiar names jumped from my softcore porn bibles that described the promised land in which I now stood, my hands trembling with the anticipation of buying a bottle.

Just as in pubs and clubs all over the city on the other side of the shiny red doors, the bar staff here were constantly run off their feet, competently serving multiple customers. For me to gauchely request a recommendation of which brand to buy would be madness and proclaim my virgin status in this wonderland. I squinted at the shallow cardboard trays beneath the parade of shining spirits optics and decided on the more direct, aggressively named Rush, because Liquid Gold reminded me of the antique furniture restorative wax that Tim used. Already the spectre of sibling disapproval hovered on my shoulders. I remained forever moored to my status as "the baby of the family," rendering me unable to completely unhitch the mental tether and float away from the harbour of my younger years. I was caught unawares by a memory of my sister Marge flicking through my LPs during her return visit home from Australia when I was fifteen. Upon reading *Now I Wanna Sniff Some Glue* on the debut release by The Ramones, she'd nodded toward Dad and whispered, "Does he know you've got this in the house?"

Toxic culpability consumed me. The lastborn of Sid & Betty Smalley's children just didn't buy illicit chemicals to inhale in homosexual nightclubs.

Until now.

I parted with a crumpled, well-used fiver. A couple of years earlier, the same sum had bought me juicy, jungly plants for my bedroom, and now here I was buying drugs. How easy it was to step from innocence to decadence.

I'd promised to jettison the past. Revelling in my scandalous behaviour, I slit the tight plastic wrapping around the lid with my left canine tooth, and with the slyness of a junkie scoring smack in a litter-strewn alley, I slid the small bottle into my jeans pocket, where it pressed against my upper thigh like a thumb reminding me of its presence.

From this vantage point, I indulged my obsession with records as I attempted to scrutinize the DJ's technique. With his headphones askew and covering only one ear, he reversed and halted the twelve-inch discs, cueing with fingers on the rims of the black platters as if he was a sorcerer casting spells over two dark cauldrons. Although I'd read about the pioneering gay technique of mixing records, I'd never witnessed the practice, and from my raised perspective, I observed his method with thrilled fascination as the beats never deviated, despite his ushering in of a new song. At his side, an unshaven, cropped-haired man whose top half was tautly bound by a black rubber T-shirt enthusiastically flicked switches, jabbed buttons, and twisted knobs on a console. His manic actions reminded me of Dr Frankenstein raising his assemblage of body parts to the colossal storm that raged above his castle, waiting for lightning to energise his creation with life. Walking from pub to pub in town with my straight mates I'd become accustomed to drunken beer-boys shouting "Herman Munster" and "Frankenstein" at me. I gingerly descended the steps. An awkward journey without the support of my stick, but I was determined to join the jubilant, gyrating congregation because it was time for this monster to come to life beneath the dynamic electrical flashes.

When I reached the perimeter, I remembered Vernon's remark about cripples dancing and hoped that my bad leg wouldn't let me down. For me to collapse during my debut amongst this excitable melee would be catastrophically embarrassing, and knowing my luck, he'd appear to laugh at my downfall, just as I had when he'd slipped over on the icy pavement. Hang on, what was I doing? Here I was bothering about him again when I was surrounded with everything I'd ever dreamed of—and more.

I effortlessly fitted in amongst the dancing men like a cog in a well-greased machine. The pervasive odour of poppers increased and before I could reach into the pocket of my jeans, a man with a huge ginger moustache appeared in front of me, his ripped T-shirt revealing pierced nipples. He grinned and held his own bottle to my nose. For the second time that night, I inhaled and instantly became a part of the perfect pandemonium. When my dancing partner thrust his arms aloft to the kaleidoscopic lights, I followed suit and was submerged in a visceral, chemical-driven commotion, an overwhelming, beautiful bedlam where the thrusting beats per minute determined the increased tempo of my heart as I pounded away my years of frustration and anger. Sweat stung

Chucking Putty at the Queen

my eyes, and as I wiped my forehead with the back of my hand, I spotted the neighbour from our old way, perched on top of a speaker box at the far end of the meat rack where I'd begun tonight's adventure. Clad in leather shorts, he shimmied like a 1920s flapper girl, the multiple thin chains attached to his belt thrashing in silver blurs as he waved a shining gold fan in each hand.

The crowd moved as an organic mass of infectious excitement, whooping encouragement when, wearing just work boots and a black leather jockstrap, an athletically muscular Black man clambered onto a speaker box at the opposite end of the meat rack to my ex-neighbour and began to gyrate, his sleek ebony skin turning aubergine beneath a spotlight. The man with the enormous ginger moustache mouthed along with the song about there being a fire in his heart tonight, which I didn't take to be a proclamation of his desire for me. Finally, my bad leg pulsed an SOS telling me it was time to quit and replenish the fluid I'd lost. I'd have to retrieve my walking aid before I could climb the steps to the bar and get a pint.

In the cloakroom, Betty Blue Lips grinned as he presented me with my stick. "Well, somebody's having fun."

"Not half. It's the best Saturday night I've ever had!"

Back at the bar, I surveyed the men all around me, many of whom had their arms around each other. Yet disenchantment defeated me amidst the wonder of this clamorous, celebratory confederation of gay men, because there was nobody that I fancied, no one man that adhered to the unbending criteria of what I considered attractive. True, I admired many handsome faces here and more so, adored the freedom of those bold men dancing shirtless with sweat-sheened torsos, ecstatically throwing their arms aloft as if twenty-pound notes were falling from the darkness beyond the lights. But the fussy boxes on my list of what I found desirable remained unticked. So what? I was here, living my dream, and I didn't care if the grand Saturday event never happened tonight because I'd made it this far. My triumph sparkled with the radiance of the strobe lights as I surveyed the spectacle like Caligula, rejoicing in the uninhibited exhibition beneath me.

The door to the reception area opened and into the arena came a middle-aged, bearded man, just like the ones who had dominated the sensual dreams of my slumber for as long as I could recall. Above a strong nose that verged on being bulbous, this new gladiator's short hair semi-circled his bald pate as if it was the plaited leaves of a laurel wreath. His broad shoulders and wide chest were sheathed in a light blue V-neck jumper. I initially thought that he wore a dark T-shirt beneath it until I realised that the black triangle was chest hair. Could everyone around me hear my heart frantically thudding above the music? The new entrant bulldozed through the men populating the bottom of the wide stairs and determinedly climbed as if he was a triumphant warrior preparing to receive decoration for his valour. When he reached the top step, we connected as he brushed past me. Unlike the pubs that I usually frequented, here I had no need for caution, of being frightened that my yearning, covert looks would be noticed and that trouble would ensue. Now that I'd passed through the red doors and become a participant in this homosexual haven, I was instantly bestowed with free rein to stare if I so wanted. And therefore, when he was on the same level with me seconds later, separated by several men, stare I did. He glanced, then looked away as if disinterested. New to the game, I was uncertain of how to proceed and so pretended to observe the frenzy. But unable to resist, I cast a quick look over, admiring his bearded, brutish profile before I returned to my sham scrutiny of the psychedelic Mardi Gras below me.

Two of the muscular men between us removed their vests, tucked them into the back of their jeans and descended to the dance floor, allowing a slim chap in a battered denim jacket to immediately occupy the vacant space as if he'd been waiting for his chance. The man whom I'd now named the Roman Centurion entered my peripheral vision just as the chap in the battered denim jacket moved away. As if a human game of chess was being played, the position was rapidly occupied by a moustached man whose yellow tank top fitted his well-developed torso as smoothly as a second skin. His adroitness in slipping beside me made me wonder if this was the most desired spot in the club as the locomotive music chugged and urged me to take a trip to another dimension and leave my troubles far behind.

When the bloke in the yellow tank top threaded down through the compact cram and became surrounded by dry ice, the vacuum created by his call to join the gyrating mass seemed to have sucked the Roman Centurion into it. His burliness was too substantial for the space vacated by the slim man, and when his upper arm pressed against mine,

Chucking Putty at the Queen

nervousness twitched my bad leg like a taut wire being plucked. The lights below pulsed in dark bruises of indigo and burgundy on the white fog as a robotic voice initiated a countdown from ten. At its climactic lift off, synths squirted in electronic ecstasy as the strobes slashed the chemical clouds, with dozens of pumping fists puncturing the mists in celebration of the euphoric, flickering madness.

I moved to allow yet another man through to the bar and then resumed my position, hoping to inconspicuously shift towards the Roman Centurion. But before I could dare to try and make contact with him, two men slick with sweat climbed the steps, and I let them pass between us. I was getting seriously pissed off with moving from side to side every few seconds like a supermarket's malfunctioning automatic doors and decided to plant myself firmly. This tactic successfully forced the next man expecting me to shift out of his way to divert around my left side, and by pretending that I was giving him space, it allowed me to move to the right. Immediately, the Roman Centurion's upper arm was against mine. The pressure remained steady. A cold adrenaline rush of fight or flight that I recognised from school crawled up my back. I was no scrapper, and fleeing was my default reaction. In those days, it had preceded yet another bout of violence against me, but this freezing fizzing sensation was different because I wasn't scared for my life.

But I didn't know what to do and pulled away. I'd never been in this situation, and I grasped the enormity of what was happening to me: the real conclusion of my bedsheet-tangling, sweat-drenched teenage dreams. This man was signalling his interest in me. Or was he? The place was packed, crammed with men. Inevitably, there'd be contact but nevertheless, I wished I could stop my shivers despite the high heat of the nightclub. I moved my upper arm and tentatively made contact. The pressure that was returned bore no ambiguity. His knuckles brushed against the back of my hand and unleashed my courage, and I pressed back against them. His big, hot hand wrapped around mine, and I revelled in the rediscovered comforting connection with male adult skin far rougher than that of my own. He nudged me with his shoulder, and I looked at his broad, hirsute face, the subdued lights filtering from behind the bar smearing the skullcap of his baldness. Mournful dark eyes regarded me as I stared unashamedly at this amalgamation of every hefty road-digger, gas fitter, rugby player, and builder that I'd ever fancied. And here I was in a gay club holding hands with him.

He nodded towards the doors and began to descend the steps, still firmly gripping my hand as he bowled through the men as if they were ninepins. "Simon is easily led." *Yes, I am.* I complied with the willingness of a pup following its new master, keeping as awkwardly close as possible to maintain our bond without stumbling to the bottom of the steps. I trusted that the swirling illumination would decorate my progress because in my unbelievable triumph, I needed every pair of eyes to witness that I was leaving with someone.

Oh, how wonderful! There at the end of the meat rack was Vernon, staring at our progress. Cockiness consumed me, and I hoped that my smirk boasted, *Yeah, look at me. I've copped off with this bruiser.* The dance floor exploded when a familiar shimmering synth intro charged across the fade from the existing record. "You Make Me Feel (Mighty Real)" by Sylvester; the first time I'd heard it was on the radio in 1978, when I was a sixteen-year-old printing apprentice and had audaciously informed the workforce of my homosexuality. The song had electrified me then, but although my announcement had been empowering, it had taken over three years for me to act on it. And now look at me. *I've done it.* I was on the gay scene, and I'd got off with a bloke, and not just any bloke, but one who exceeded any expectations that I'd dared to dream were possible.

In contrast to the frenetic hubbub of the disco, the silence of the empty reception was an ear-numbing airlock, and in the brighter light, the dormant volcano of my historical insecurities erupted, spewing toxic negativity that incinerated my arrogant self-congratulation of seconds earlier. This burly thug would now see that I used a walking stick and wore a raised shoe, and he'd change his mind and make an excuse to return to the melee of the disco, where he'd find someone better.

Tony the doorman's even white teeth gleamed against his swarthy face. "Taxi, gents?"

The beefy man didn't desert me but nodded once and gripped my hand harder with his substantial paw. Tony tugged open the door and raised his arm before he let us step out onto the frosty pavement. Once more, I was beneath the portal that I'd stared at from over the road months ago, wishing that somehow I could become a part of what unimaginably fabulous activities went on inside. Not only had I succeeded, but I was leaving with *a man*. And he'd chosen me when there were so many others for him to pick from.

A fleet of the city's trademark black and white cabs lined the kerb like neatly arranged dominoes. My new friend lumbered around to the far side of the front one and squeezed into the back. The restrictions that my bad leg caused meant that I struggled to get in until Tony strode over, took my walking stick, and helped me into the back, then thrust his hand forward.

"Your cane, sir." He nodded before slamming the door shut.

The man beside me took no notice as I got myself as comfortable as I could in the cab that stank of stale cigarette smoke and the Feu Orange air freshener dangling from the rear-view mirror. The cabbie turned the knob on his radio cassette player, reducing the volume of the banging tabla drums and wildly plucked sitars that matched the frenzy of the music I'd just left behind inside the club. He twisted around and looped his left arm around the headrest of the front passenger seat. I was surprised that he could lift his hand considering the amount of thick gold rings that adorned his fingers. He nodded to my companion. Maybe as he was the older of us, the driver automatically identified him as the authoritative half.

"Good evening, sir. To where are you going?"

"Broxtowe."

I realised that his gruff baritone was the first time I'd heard him speak, and what's more, I didn't know his name, nor did he know mine. And when the taxi pulled away, gaining speed beneath the sodium streetlights of Castle Boulevard, I realised something else: I had no idea what would happen to me once we arrived at our destination and no matter what, I couldn't wait to find out.

32

THE WORLD IS FULL OF MARRIED MEN

"LISTEN. I'M NOT BEING horrible, but you've never been out with anyone, have you?"

Jacqui's words echoed across the four years since our lunch in the Woolworths cafeteria when I'd confessed my disastrous debut at the club. And her rhetorical question still remained true. However, I was no innocent; I'd relished innumerable recreational liaisons, but none had developed into a relationship. When I copped off with a bloke that I *really* liked, the hopeful seeds of potential boyfriend I scattered never blossomed into anything other than non-committal sowing and reaping. Not having a gentleman friend wasn't the be-all and end-all of my life, and I continued to have a whale of a time, but every man that I especially liked invariably had an affair, as we called partners in those days. Either that or he was married with kids and living what the puritanical Sunday tabloids called "a secret life." I yearned for someone whose love and companionship would banish the loneliness of Sunday afternoons, those morose, dragging hours that rubbed my nose in my single man status. With a dedicated lover at my side, the journey onwards would be transformed into a golden road of unlimited devotion.

Yet that perfect man remained elusive. Some queens on the scene branded me aloof and stuck up because I was pretty choosy about the men that I got off with. The ones I engaged with had to fit a certain profile: older, masculine, and balding or with short hair. A moustache or beard was almost essential. Bonus points for a beer belly. However, my picky requirements were not particularly omnipresent on the scene. Therefore, when a man of this type who was, in personal ads parlance, "straight acting," appeared and showed interest in me, it was as if the row of ripe red cherries on a fruit machine reels aligned, and I was rewarded with a joyous jackpot payout of masculine riches.

Since my mid-teens, I'd habitually indulged in amateur self-analysis. Many years earlier, I concluded that the traumatic situations in my formative years shaped my preferences, the strong father figure of a particular visual profile, but it certainly hadn't determined my sexuality. I'd read what I regarded as misguided propositions on what "caused" homosexuality in men; most theses concluded that the "blame" was the presence of an overbearing mother and a distant, spineless father. Others proclaimed the reverse theory, that an emotionally remote mother thrust the male child towards his father for love and affection. What rubbish! I *knew* that I was born homosexual, and I became aware of my attraction to men with strong, masculine attributes a long time before Mam died. I'd received equal amounts of love and attention from both of my parents, and I'd instinctively known that society's names of sissy, pansy, fairy, and queer defined me as bad and unnatural, so I'd kept my trap shut.

It turned out that Mam and Dad knew all along. In my late twenties, I learned that, when the cancer which eventually killed my mother was wreaking its terminal havoc, she called my sister Marge to her bedside and tearfully admitted her worries that I would grow up not only motherless but facing abuse and violence for "being different." She never lived to witness the torment that I suffered, but nor did she see me grow into a proud gay man who took control of his destiny and actively converted his dreams into reality.

And in that reality, if I didn't cop off with someone then I'd return home to spend the night as a single man in a double bed. I adored the *actual* sleeping with another man and concluded that this was a throwback to after Mam died, when I'd begun to sleepwalk. Due to his fear of me falling down the stairs whilst engaging in my somnambulistic wanderings, Dad had insisted that I spend my nights with him, where he could keep an eye on me. "I've just lost your mother. I couldn't bear it if I were to lose you as well because of my negligence."

When demolition of our area forced our move to a new three-bedroomed council house, Tim and Nick both had their own rooms. Dad and I shared the front bedroom as we had at the old house, and as there was no spare money for an extra bed, I continued to sleep with him until I was fifteen. Nothing was ever mentioned by my brothers about this situation. I never considered it unusual that Dad and I slept in the same bed, but I did understand that I had needed to be wrapped in the psychological comfort blanket that Dad provided for far longer than the immediate months after Mam's death.

Chucking Putty at the Queen

At fifteen, when my hip injury was finally correctly diagnosed and I was admitted to hospital for urgent surgery, my prime source of anxiety was not the impending operation but how on earth I'd be able to sleep without Dad next to me. A few weeks after enduring eight hours of punishing surgery, I was allowed home on crutches for a fortnight respite. With my body encased in plaster from chest to toes, this presented difficulties at night as I needed to lie diagonally across the double bed. Nick had recently moved out, so Dad relocated to the back bedroom. He saw my alarm, and in wartime terms he reassured me, "It's only for the duration, Son." But when I was freed from my plaster constraint and discharged from hospital, I was dismayed that the arrangement of separate rooms continued, which killed the joy of being in the peace of home after my prolonged incarceration on the sterile but noisy ward.

Therefore, years later when I went back to a man's house, the turning out of the light and snuggling up with him would have me rejoicing in the blissful physical warmth of that masculine presence next to me, and of knowing that I wouldn't wake up alone. Tellingly, the difference as I lay beneath the strange duvets and unfamiliar sheets of these men was that I never obsessively listened to their breathing as I had every night with Dad. That is, until one evening when I took a train to the Leicester scene.

I'd be an unfamiliar face, and you never knew your luck. My optimism was proved right when I left the club at two a.m. accompanying a stout, balding man with a handlebar moustache and whose comforting smell of cigars and Old Spice aftershave awakened my not-too-dormant insecurities. His bedroom curtains were not pulled together fully and in his tight embrace, I stared at a pearly crescent moon that reclined upon a pillow of deep lilac cloud in the inky sky. Once sleep claimed him, my childhood terror held me tighter than his arms ever could as, enveloped by those two familiar fragrances, I vigilantly monitored his breathing pattern.

Old habits and memories die hard.

If it was a weeknight pick-up, I became used to standing self-consciously in a stranger's kitchen the following morning, shuddering at the bitter tang of black coffee but not wanting to ask for milk and sugar when I should be on my way. Our shared night was nothing more than that and had already become the embodiment of the Jean Carne song, "Was That All It Was," a momentary thing that wasn't worth remembering in the morning. I'd dodge him as he darted back and forth getting ready for work, with both of us awkwardly aware that my presence had caused his morning routine to descend into anarchy. I had no such timetable to dominate my existence, having the louche luxury of being on the dole, and I'd hover as he knotted his tie and slid into his suit jacket if he was an office worker or executive, or wrestled himself into overalls if he was a lathe operator on the factory floor. Once, to my immense surprise on a dark Wednesday morning in Leeds with rain thrashing the windows, the taciturn man sporting Victorian lamb-chop whiskers who the previous night had told me, "I sort of work for the government," turned out to be a police sergeant.

I was too familiar with the rude interruption of another man's alarm clock which brought the dry mouth of early mornings, when I'd work my jaw and lips like a toothless hag sucking a boiled sweet, wondering if there'd be a spare toothbrush, or if I'd have to once more resort to smudging my forefinger with Ultrabrite to rub around my teeth. Always, a list of *woulds* flew around my mind as I tried to remember what part of town I was in: would I be offered a shower? Or would we share one? Would I be driven home? Would I need to get a bus or walk (depending on how far away from home I'd found myself)?

But regardless of these immeasurable encounters, Jacqui was right; I'd never had a boyfriend. The dates I had weren't the *proper* dates that I'd seen portrayed in the 1970s sitcoms. I'd had no assignations in garlic and herb-fragranced basement bistros where Mantovani provided an easy listening soundtrack, and flickering candles stuck into wine bottle necks added life and movement to frescoes portraying the terracotta tiled roofs of whitewashed villas on the Sardinian coastline. I'd yet to encounter a fawning waiter proffering an oversized phallic peppermill, or my companion buying me a rose from the flower seller who hawked her wares around the pubs and restaurants. None of that had occurred because my pseudo-dates were merely an arrangement to get it on with each other again. I wasn't *really* complaining as I frequently experienced enough ephemeral excitement and relished the consequences of simultaneously being the hunter and the hunted in those chance connections that provided transitory thrills for both parties. And so I remained a lone wolf constantly prowling.

Until Hugh.

Hugh was married with kids about my age, both of whom were at university up north. After several impromptu, passionate meetings over the years, I began to see him on a regular basis. I fancied him very much, he fitted the requisite physicality, and he was emotionally stable, kind, considerate, and loving. Despite the age gap of some twenty-five years, we were never stuck for conversation, interacting with an easy familiarity rather than being relative strangers bound only by lust. But it wasn't the heart-stopping, breath-taking, all-consuming rapturous love that I desperately craved. Perhaps the inspiration from having submerged myself with the covers of *English Romantic Poetry* too many times, I hungered for a relationship where, when we parted if only for a few hours, my heart would sink like the Titanic slipping beneath the icy black waves of the Atlantic. I was desperate for a man whose appearance would make my spirits soar like doves sparkling white against an endless cerulean sky of the hottest English summer ever. He would be a man to celebrate life with, a beau to take home to my dad and show off how proud I was to be with him. However, there was a polarity in that. Although I ached for someone special to share even the most banal aspects of life, I was not prepared to rescind my recreational activities, believing that monogamy was a fate worse than death. I'd waited such a long time to get onto the gay scene, and the mindset of a huge majority of gay men was the freedom of not being shackled by the restrictions that the heterosexual world had. Most of us didn't have offspring and consequently, we were without the ties that bind with the role of a parent. We were free agents, rejoicing in our sexual liberation and of "getting it everywhere," as one straight pal described my behaviour.

I was very fortunate to have not one but two best gay friends—sisters—in Patrick and Andy. I'd met Patrick on my second visit to the social gatherings at Gay Switchboard. Andy was introduced to me by a mutual acquaintance shortly before my twenty-first birthday the following year. It was evident upon their first meeting that he and Patrick were poles apart, and I learned to juggle my time between them to prevent any unnecessary friction. Liking me didn't mean that they liked each other.

By this time, I was seeing Hugh. Following an acrimonious split with his boyfriend, Patrick had given up his Fairy Towers flat and moved to Brighton. We corresponded frequently, with our gossipy letters often crossing in the post. In his most recent, he'd told me that he was returning to Nottingham for a few days to see his mam. He called me when he arrived, and we arranged to get together when I wasn't seeing Hugh.

"It'll be just like old times," Patrick almost sang once we decided where and when to meet up. "Tish and Simone on the town."

As well as having what he called "a girls' night out," I was looking forward to seeing who was around. But Hugh put a spoke in my anticipatory wheel when he announced that he wanted to meet my much-talked-about friend and insisted on breaking his home obligations to join us in the pub. When Hugh went to the bar, I had the peculiar sense of someone looking at me and turned to see the grinning, unshaven face of a bloke I'd met a couple of weeks earlier. On that night, the man mountain with cropped hair and brutishly handsome features was dressed in a black leather bomber jacket and had been standing to attention by the door. I'd sighed, thinking that the AIDS-phobic aggression towards the men visiting the gay pub must have increased to such a level that they'd had to employ security. Yet before my lips had touched the froth topping my pint, he was at my side, chatting me up. It transpired that he was no bouncer but a punter from Manchester called Ian who'd recently split with his boyfriend, Scott. In order to get over him, he'd relocated to Nottingham with his work because he had an aunt, or cousin, or something here; I was so turned on by him that I wasn't really paying attention. The next morning I realised just how hung up he was.

"Do you want coffee?" he shouted through from the kitchen.

Before I could answer, he called louder, "Scott! Do you want coffee or what?"

"I'm Simon, not Scott!"

The naked bruiser stood in the doorway with staring eyes and red cheeks. "Oh, god, I'm sorry. I'm so sorry. That's really rude of me."

I chuckled. "It doesn't matter. He's obviously still on your mind."

"It's just that you remind me of him."

To add weight to this statement, he took a photo in a tortoiseshell-effect frame from the bookcase and handed it to me. We could have been twins. "So you only got off with me 'cos I remind you of your ex?" I was only joking, but he dropped to the edge of the sofa and put his head in his big hands. Between sobs, he told me how much he missed Scott. I sat next to him and laid my arm over his broad shoulders, and for the next forty-five minutes, my role changed from one-night stand to relationship break-up counsellor.

Nevertheless, he was a real bit of all right and on this evening in the pub with Patrick and Hugh, when he winked across the room and smiled at me, of course I went over to have a word to see how he was doing and to establish if he was up for round two at some point. Hugh's presence scuppered any direct action, and as Ian was so not his type, suggesting a threesome was out of the question.

The next afternoon, I met up with Patrick in Farmhouse Kitchen beneath the WHSmith store. The underground restaurant had become the go-to place for me and my pals, both straight and gay, and I adored the cosiness of the booths separated by pale pine dividers, their tops containing troughs of compost from where small spider plants hung and ivies tumbled amongst a variety of shade-tolerant foliage. Soft illumination glowed behind dark cream shades atop lamps fashioned from sawn minor branches of trees.

Patrick spooned coleslaw onto his buttery jacket potato and got more on the tabletop than on the steaming spud. "I enjoyed it last night, but girl, that Hugh's got it *really* bad for you."

"Did he tell you that?"

"He doesn't have to. When you went to the loo, he gave me a real intelligation."

Despite my unease, I smiled at another of his dyslexic mispronunciations. "What about?"

"About you, of course. Questions, questions."

"Such as?"

"Such as who's that man last night? You know. That bouncer you got off with. Trust you to get picked up by a bouncer."

"He isn't a bouncer; he just looks like one."

"Well—this coleslaw is delicious, by the way—he wanted to know who else you're meeting, where you go when he's not seeing you, where do you go in the daytime, who do you *meet* in the daytime, and do I know how many other blokes you get off with." He pointed with his fork. "I'm telling you, girl, he's got you really bad."

I used my teeth to rip open a sachet of vinaigrette, then dribbled it over my green salad as Patrick continued to wave his fork around.

"So how do you feel about him?"

I peered into the wooden bowl. "They're getting a bit stingy with the cucumber. There are only about three slices in here."

"Simone..."

My sigh trembled the fronds of ivy at the side of my face. "I like him, I really do. He's a lovely bloke, and I enjoy being with him, and it's great fun...but there's just summat that's not there. One bit that doesn't click. I really wish it was there because on paper, he ticks all of the boxes."

Patrick looked over the top of his spectacles. "All of the boxes but the most important one."

A few evenings later when I was getting ready to go out, Dad offered me a glass of his homebrew. "Who are you seeing tonight, Son?"

"Hugh."

"I've not met him, have I?"

"No, not yet."

"Invite him in for a beer sometime."

Two nights later, Hugh came to the house. Dad was at the kitchen worktop carefully unscrewing the stone stopper in a big brown bottle. "Steady as she goes, Sidney, we don't want beer all over the place."

"Dad, this is Hugh."

When he turned around, I was sure there was the slightest flicker of surprise at the well-groomed, immaculately attired burly man who held out his beefy paw in greeting. In his smart salt and pepper dogtooth check jacket, brilliantly white shirt, and dark blue tie, he looked every bit the successful executive that he was.

"How do you do, Mr Smalley? Simon's told me a lot about you."

"How do you do? It's nice to meet another of Simon's many friends."

Diamonds danced in Hugh's dark eyes as he shot me a glance. "He's a very popular lad."

The next morning as I sat at the table eating my cornflakes, Dad came in from the kitchen.

"Another cuppa, Son?"

"Ooh, yes, please." I watched the steaming brown flow and waited for whatever else was forthcoming.

"Hugh seems a pleasant chap."

"Yes, he's great."

"What your mother used to call a 'man's man.'"

How was I supposed to answer that? Say, "Yeah, he's dead butch. Just how I like my men."

Dad cleared his throat.
Here we go.
"He's quite a bit older than your other pals, isn't he?"
"Yeah, he's just a few months shy of fifty."
"And you were twenty-four in March."
"Yep."
Dad rotated my cup until its handle aligned with the gap between the stylised flowers on the saucer, turned the spoon until it was parallel with the handle, and then did the same with the other three cups on the tray. Perhaps that was where my moderate OCD originated.
"So about twice your age."
"Something like that."
"I was quite surprised when I saw him."
"Oh, really?" I stoppered my mouth with cornflakes, but Dad's words demanded further response. "Why?"
"Because I wasn't expecting him to be so old."
I didn't think that this was the time to tell Dad that I was attracted to older men, so enthusiastically spooned more cereal into my mouth.
"I noticed he wears a wedding ring."
"Yeah. He's married and has twins about my age. They're at uni in Newcastle."
I gulped the crunchy cereal down too quickly and coughed.
Dad thumped me between the shoulder blades several times. "And no wife around?"
"Yes. Monica's lovely. You'd like her, she's very tall and elegant. You'd probably call her an English Rose."
"You've *met* her?"
"Oh, god, yeah." I scooped up the few remaining cornflakes and slid them into my mouth. "Actually, she introduced us."
Despite my ostentatious nonchalance, I thought it best not to say that when I first met Hugh in the club, he told me, "My wife said, 'If you don't go and ask that handsome young man for a date, then I'll do it for you.'"
Dad replaced the tea cosy onto the pot and looked out into the garden. "I do worry about you, Son. I sincerely hope that there will be no...*unpleasantness* with his wife."
I stood up and laid an arm over his shoulder. "Don't worry, Dad. I know what I'm doing."

He didn't look around. "I really hope that you do, Son."

And so Hugh and I ticked along easily until he declared his love for me and enthused about getting a flat for us. I was no marriage-wrecker and would not allow any unpleasantness to arise. It was unfair on Hugh to continue our relationship knowing that I was unable to reciprocate the blistering fervour of his adoration. It was an uncomfortable and unfamiliar situation I found myself in; it was usually me being rebuffed by someone that I wanted to be more involved with, someone onto whom I tried to project my own white-hot love only for it to be blackened by their determined rejection. Until I had to tell Dad of Patrick's death to AIDS three years later, letting Hugh know my decision was the most heartbreaking thing I'd ever done.

My routine changed without the three nights of the week when I'd usually see Hugh.

From the kitchen came the familiar hiss of a bottle being opened and seconds later, Dad walked to the sideboard and picked up two half-pint glasses. "You've not seen so much of Hugh lately, Son. Have you had a falling out?"

"No, not at all."

"I hope that your friendship hasn't caused any problems between him and his wife."

"Honestly, Dad, it's nothing like that. It's just something that I had to do."

"So you won't be making an appearance in the divorce court?"

I couldn't believe that I was having this conversation and laughed at how outrageous a situation it was. "Not a chance. Like I said, it was just something that I had to do."

He placed the glasses on the table and stepped over to me. "I hope you're not too unhappy, Son. Perhaps it's for the best." He squeezed my shoulder. "Now, how about a glass of this lager that's ready?"

Once more, the Smalley panacea was called into action.

"Cheers, Dad, that'd be lovely. You really mustn't worry about me."

"But I do, Son. I'm your father. I've worried about you since your mother died. All I want is for you to be happy." He stepped towards the kitchen, then turned around and smiled. "If I didn't worry about you then something would be terribly wrong with me."

We were as bad as each other because all I wanted was *his* happiness. We'd been through so much together. But although he'd asked to meet Hugh, he deserved better than to be worrying about me having a relationship with a married man.

33

FRIENDS OF MINE

How CERTAIN PEOPLE ENTERED my life was a question that I often pondered. I accepted that, frequently, you were forced cheek-by-jowl with others due to unavoidable circumstances such as in the classroom, workplace, or by being neighbours. Sometimes those interactions proved to be a case of right time, right place; on other occasions, the opposite was evident: wrong time, wrong place. Thankfully for me, the former is truer, and I consider myself incredibly fortunate having had good friends as I navigated my path through the years. Some travelled with me in a manner similar to the moment during a train journey when a locomotive pulls alongside on an adjacent track and runs parallel with your carriage. You progress side by side until that train accelerates and moves ahead, and the distance between you increases with the divergence of your routes. Occasionally, those tracks would come to run side by side again, despite the passing of miles and years.

When I bump into people from my early days of going to the social group at Gay Switchboard, I'm reminded of how those men had been so warm-hearted in welcoming the nineteen-year-old me. That is, all of them apart from the ghastly Vernon. Thankfully, as he lived an hour's drive from Nottingham, our paths barely crossed, which suited me fine. I heard that he'd succumbed to AIDS in 1989, and it took me straight back to my first evening in that small room filled with the comforting aroma of hot coffee and the less welcoming fug of cigarette smoke. His snarky "Well, keep it to yourself. We don't want to catch it" had become tragically foretelling, and despite his antagonism towards me, I was saddened that this drama-loving character had such a devastating finale to his one-man show. Never again would he wear those stupid boots emblazoned with *New York* in cut-out leather letters.

Amongst my gay sisters were Jon and Paul who lived in Oxford, whom I saved up to visit in springtime and the run-up to Christmas. Whilst they were at work, I spent my days in tourist mode, wandering with my head in the clouds above Matthew Arnold's dreaming spires, trying to imagine life as a scholar there and, not for the first time, rueing my inadequate education. Inevitably, my meandering terminated on Paradise Street in the city's gay pub, the Jolly Farmers, where I'd enjoy a lunchtime pint and an appropriately named Ploughman's Lunch.

It was Jon and Paul who took me to the ultra-club Heaven in London, and when I returned to Nottingham, Patrick was beside himself with envy. "I always thought that I'd be the first of us to get to Heaven." Since meeting at the switchboard socials, we'd become "best sisters" and often took the train together to experience gay nightlife in other cities. We even had Saturday nights in smaller towns, whose sole club seemed to be in someone's front room. We journeyed to London for Gay Pride marches, and when he relocated to Brighton, our friendship never diminished.

Throughout these years, Jacqui was my stalwart confidante, and I remained unshakeably firm friends with Tony, the first of my straight male mates to whom I'd come out in autumn 1981. At the start of the following year, he'd jacked in his job and as we were both on the dole, we met up five afternoons each week and scoured the second-hand record stores, charity shops, and vintage clothing emporiums in town.

As well as us having the same birthday (although I was a year older), we liked similar groups and travelled down to London, where we saw Soft Cell; up to Sheffield for a gig by The March Violets; and crossed over the border to Leicester for a concert by Siouxsie & The Banshees, whom I was hooked on since I bought their debut single, "Hong Kong Garden," when I was sixteen. Otherwise, we stayed in Nottingham, where we feasted upon the banquet of groups who appeared at Rock City: Play Dead, New Model Army, Danse Society, Zodiac Mindwarp, Sisters of Mercy, and in an astonishing coup for Nottingham, a favourite from my teenage punk years, The Ramones.

The absolute pinnacle of bands we saw together came on November 5 1985, when we went to the Royal Centre and took our seats in the middle of the front row for Siouxsie & The Banshees. Immediately afterwards, hastened by booming artillery explosions and zooming skyrockets which split the Bonfire Night sky into a big neon glitter, we undertook a hundred-yard dash to Rock City to see The Cult perform. For days afterwards, we fizzed as if we were the very fireworks that Siouxsie had sung of during her first encore.

My weekend nights remained dedicated to the gay scene, although I once succumbed to Tony's suggestion that I change my routine.

"Come on, give Part Two a break for once and come to Rock City on Saturday night. You'll have a great time. They always play a couple of T. Rex songs and a load of glam rock."

The following Saturday I found myself in the middle of a slow-moving snake of punters shuffling closer towards the brightly lit entrance when I was gripped by the panic of what—or who—I was missing by not going to the gay club. I didn't want to be here, amongst the lacquered and knackered backcombed Goths, the psychobillies, and the rockabilly rebels, nor the spiky old punks and Mohican-topped new punks. I wanted to be with my own tribe, where wearing black leather adhered to a completely different code. I grabbed Tony's arm. "No, sorry, I can't."

"Can't what?"

"I can't go in. I need to go to Part Two."

"Aw, don't be a sap. Come on, listen to what's on."

The doomy bass of "Bela Lugosi's Dead" by Bauhaus took me back to when I'd bought the white vinyl twelve-inch single in the summer of 1979 from the now-demolished Selectadisc only a hundred yards away. Within two years, its rarity had assured a good price when I sold it to pay Dad's overdue gas bill. But what was now considered a Goth classic wasn't going to uplift me. I needed a fix of dancing to pumping, loud Hi-NRG.

"No, sorry, I'm off. I'll see you tomorrow night." Within fifteen minutes, I'd raced as best as I could down streets and through dark alleys until I arrived at a different black chasm, this one filled with men and the pulsing synthesised songs that were such a huge part of the soundtrack to my gay liberation.

Despite my friendships, a fulfilling, reciprocal romance remained elusive. Phrases and voices from my teens resurfaced. Johnny Rotten's vitriolic assurance of "No future for you" and the school careers teacher's judgement that I wouldn't come to much seemed to point my way forward.

After another of our afternoons in town, Tony unexpectedly commented, "You know, I've been thinking. We can't go on like this forever. One of us is going to have to get a job."

He was right, of course, and when he met Paula, who lived twenty-five miles away in Leicester and began spending more and more time there, I realised that the gap between the parallel tracks of our friendship was already widening. Yet, a bond had been forged, and several years later when Tony and Paula announced they were to be married, he exemplified the uniqueness of our friendship as we shook hands.

"When we first met, I never thought that I'd end up having a big queen as best man at my wedding."

On their special day, the photographer decided to take a couple of what he called "fun snaps" and directed us into our positions.

"Right, I want the best man to be like he's making a move on the bride, whilst the groom is grabbing his arm and trying to pull him away."

Tony shook his head. "Pull him away? I'd have to push him *towards* a woman, mate."

Such a close friendship between a gay man and a straight man must have not been a rarity, but I believe that it was certainly uncommon when the heightened fear of AIDS was being fanned into a homophobic firestorm by irresponsible press reportage. Tony defended me if anyone made derogatory remarks or when idiots voiced their opinion that he should be scared of catching AIDS from me. And how I'd guffawed when he relayed an incident in Rock City after a woman asked him if he was worried that I'd make a pass at him.

"Of course he won't."

"How can you be so sure?"

"Because I'm not a twenty-five stone, hairy-faced slob."

I hosted small get-togethers for my birthday, and as the date grew closer, I'd return from an afternoon in town to be enveloped by the delicious aromas from the kitchen, indicating that Dad was baking in preparation for the celebratory gathering. When the day arrived, he'd organise a selection of his beers and wines, and in the evening, he'd don his suit and stay to have a glass of his wine and "a natter with your chums." Tim always popped up from the local to have half an hour with us, laughing and joking without embarrassment or nervousness, and he was particularly fond of Jon and Paul. That was quite a turnaround from my twenty-first, when they called me but Tim had answered before I could get to the phone. I stood impatiently holding my hand out until, after several seconds of him frowning with the receiver at his ear, he finally thrust it at me.

"Some of your fuckin' puffy mates for yer."

Thinking it was me on the phone, Jon and Paul had sung "Happy birthday, dear Cissy" and followed that with a barrage of ribald remarks about what they expected me to get up to that night at Part Two.

When I returned to the living room he was examining my cards, holding the one from Chris which bore his unambiguous, succinct message, "You're legal now."

Tim harrumphed and replaced it on the shelf, then picked up another. This one was from Jim, the burly man with the CHE badge whom I'd met on my inaugural visit to Gay Switchboard. His assertive, masculine hand scribed the more political missive, "No longer illegal, just partially decriminalised. Keep fighting for our rights." At my theatrical cough, Tim spun around, his face so red that I feared he'd drop dead on the spot.

He replaced the card on the shelf. "Who was that on the phone?"

"Jon and Paul from Oxford."

"Didn't they send a card?"

"Yeah, it's this one." I reached past him and tapped the overly floral front amongst which shiny gold letters proclaimed, "Happy 21st Birthday, Dear Daughter."

"Daughter? And you've got some here that say Happy Birthday, Sister. Are all your puffy mates fucking barmy or what?"

Dad entered from the kitchen balancing three plates of food with the practised ease of a waiter. "Birthday tea coming up. And please leave off, Tim, they're only having a bit of fun."

"Well it don't seem right to me."

Nevertheless, each time that Jon and Paul drove up to see Jon's parents in Derbyshire, they always came to see me and Dad, who thought that my heavily moustached Oxford pals were wonderful. Tim was of the same opinion and visibly cheered up when I told him of an impending visit. He'd make the effort to come and see them, making me wonder if he'd finally realised that my "puffy mates" were just regular blokes after all.

Of these soirées, my *Simone's Birthday Bash 1986* remains the most poignantly memorable. I played "Heat You Up, Melt You Down" by Shirley Lites, one of my favourites from around the time of my twenty-first, and when she hit and held an eardrum-bursting high note, Dad exaggeratedly grimaced.

"Whoever she is, she's got a strong voice...that is, if she *is* a she."

The laughter of my guests prompted him to play to the gallery.

"Well, you never know these days, do you? When Simon's mother and

I were younger, we used to mosey into town for a drink."

What was he up to now?

He puffed his Hamlet cigar until all eyes were on him. I'd seen this before; he was in the limelight and knew it.

"Simon's Aunt Lu would babysit. This is when we only had Penelope and Margery, so my wife and I could go into town for a drink. She used to love the Peach Tree opposite the Theatre Royal because a lot of what we used to call 'theatricals' drank in there." He rested his cigar in the glass Home Ales ashtray that Tim had pinched from the pub and gripped his lapels as if he was the prosecutor in a court case. "The County Hotel next door to the theatre used to hold a Gentlemen's Hour every evening. We couldn't go in, of course, as the notice on the door proclaimed it to be just that. But one evening I told Betty—that's Simon's mother, as I'm sure you all know—that I was going to go in. 'Oh, no, Sid, you mustn't.' But I grabbed the handle and popped my head inside. Do you know what I saw?"

"What, Mr Smalley? *What* did you see?" Patrick asked, his usually strident Irish brogue softened by his curiosity.

"Well, let's just say that I've never seen so many handsome, immaculately groomed, Brylcreemed men gathered in one place, even when I was in the RAF during the war. I pulled the door open a bit more so that we could listen to them."

Then to my astonishment, he placed his right hand on his hip and with the other hand, he lightly patted the side of his head as if he were delicately tidying a coiffure.

"'Ooh, Queenie, would you like a pink gin? Ooh, yes, please, dear, and don't go too heavy on the angostura bitters. Ooh, Queenie, have you seen Mildred lately? Oh, yes, ducky, have I ever! I told her she should never have shaved off her moustache; she was the spit of Errol Flynn, but now she just looks like Hedy Lamarr when she's been on the sauce.'"

My mates gawped with obvious confusion at this unseen side to Dad, then burst into laughter. Patrick spluttered and began to choke until Stuart bashed him on the back. Dad maintained a poker face as he adjusted the carnation in his buttonhole, twisted the ends of his handlebar moustache, and cleared his throat. What was coming next? Surely he couldn't top that little performance.

"Okay, lads, I'm going to buzz off and leave you to it. But before I do,

I'd just like to say that if Simon's mother was alive, she'd be as proud as I am of what a fine man he's grown into and of what a wonderful group of friends he has."

He lifted his cigar from the ashtray, turned smartly, and stepped into the hall. I looked around to my guests and saw eight pairs of glistening eyes staring as Dad closed the door behind him. My father certainly knew how to make an exit worthy of the theatricals that he and Mam used to see in the Peach Tree, that's for sure.

34

I'M THE ONE YOU WANT

How did everything become so bloody boring? My Saturday nights used to be completely different, when Miquel Brown's Hi-NRG anthem, "So Many Men, So Little Time" was the perfect soundtrack. But as I handed over £2.50 to enter L'Amour, Nottingham's newest gay club (which was somewhat uncharitably, but not without good reason, nicknamed La Morgue), was the effort was still worth it? There'd been a couple of venues since the closure of Part Two the previous year: Penelope's in the Lace Market, the Catacombs on Byard Lane, and Casablanca on Greyhound Street. But despite these valiant attempts to provide fabulous gay nightlife in our fair city that was known, not ironically, as Queen of the Midlands, nothing could touch the days of Part Two.

The old Sherwood Rooms was now the Astoria, which held a massively popular Monday gay night once a month. Punters flocked to it from across the Midlands, and despite many of my friends raving about the capacity crowds, I doggedly refused to go, my argument being that when the straight management held a gay event on a Saturday night, then I would. But until then, I could not participate in such blatant exploitation, using gay people to fill a cavernous 1920s ballroom that would otherwise be closed on a Monday. And so I stayed away, feeling righteously principled as I sat at home drinking Dad's homemade beer and playing the Hi-NRG records that my friends would be dancing to. Furthermore, having heard from pals of the shameless comments made by the bouncers about AIDS and queers to the queuing revellers, and that the staff requested latex gloves to wear on the Monday nights in case they "caught anything," I was amazed at the fickle treachery of those gay people who went, willing to suffer overpriced drinks served by hostile bar staff.

So when I wasn't hopping on a train to Leicester, Manchester, or Birmingham on a Saturday night, I frequented L'Amour. If I was going to be ripped off with high-priced, watered-down drinks, then I'd rather it be done by my own kind. Once more, my glum outlook weighed me down as I climbed the stairs to the upper bar and surveyed the same old jaded gene pool. Andy was there with a couple he knew from Derby, so I chatted with them. But I was totally bored. Perhaps I should just give up and go home. There was nothing here for me, and my despair deepened when "American Love" by Rose Laurens came on. In my opinion, the dismal dirge epitomised the malaise that had stricken the gay scene, and it depressed the hell out of me. Others obviously thought differently. They writhed and whirled beneath the flashing lights with such enthusiasm that you'd think it was a qualifying round for the UK Disco Dance Championship.

Andy gyrated on the spot. "Are you coming to bop?"

"No, I can't stand this." I adopted a husky, exaggerated vibrato. "*Ah-merr-ikkun luh-huv*. I hate it."

Andy smirked and poked my chest. "You're only saying that 'cos you had your heart broken by American Tim."

"Fuck off, Andy. I hate it because it's crap. It's nothing at all to do with Tim. I'm over him now. *Totally* over him."

"But you're not though, are you?"

He dashed towards the dance floor, and before my still shredded emotions could slide into the memory hole that led to the deliciously handsome man I'd met in Oxford whilst he was stationed there with the US Air Force, two men came through the arched entrance. I'd seen them once or twice before in the Admiral Duncan but hadn't taken much notice of them. They weren't regulars like most of the faces here tonight, and actually, thinking about it, they weren't too bad. One was tall, balding, and unshaven, and the other was shorter, with cropped grey hair and matching beard. Our eyes met, and he spoke to the taller man. Within seconds, they were at my side and introduced themselves as Tom and Peter.

"You here with somebody?"

"No, on me tod."

Tom laid his arm over Peter's shoulders. "We've been together eighteen months."

"Congratulations."

Peter nodded. "We're committed to each other."

"That's nice."

"Yeah, we're monogamous. But we've been talking, and we think that at this stage of our relationship, we're ready to introduce someone else into it. But we'll only do safe sex."

"It goes without saying." I didn't know if I had the fatal virus circulating in my body, gathering its destructive strength and wreaking unstoppable havoc on my immune system. A close friend was succumbing to the ravages of the disease, and several familiar faces had become gaunt before disappearing from the scene completely. The new script of my life was underlined by constant fear, obsession, and worry that a dry cough was indicative of infection, or that an underarm gland was more swollen than usual. And did my sweating at night mean nothing more than it was time to remove the heavy ex-army blanket covering my quilt? And what about the consuming lethargy? Was it a result of my disability or something far more sinister? Was that a bruise where I must've banged my arm? Or was it a Kaposi's sarcoma blemish? I despised succumbing to this whole new strain of paranoia. Regardless, the inside pocket of my leather biker jacket always contained rubber johnnies, lube, and a bottle of poppers. I was a cruising boy scout, always prepared, because we'd all learned that safe sex didn't mean no sex since the arrival of AIDS.

"So how about it? We're very inventive and experimental, and we've got loads of equipment and videos."

Half past twelve on a Saturday night. It wasn't going to get any better than this, so I might as well go back with them. Like the song said, nothing's worse than being alone. "Yeah, okay. Where do you live?"

Big smug smile from Tom as if he'd been waiting for the chance to go into estate agent mode. "In an *enormous* house in Edwalton with two reception rooms, four bedrooms—en suite, of course—a utility room, dressing room, walk-in pantry off the Scandinavian kitchen, a gravel drive, and a double garage."

The pulse of the music speeded up into Earlene Bentley's enduring romper, "The Boys Come To Town."

"We *love* this! Wanna dance?"

As much as I adored the song, I wasn't in the mood. "No, ta. I'll miss this one out."

"But you won't leave, will you? You *are* coming back with us?"

Was I that much of a catch? Or were they just determined that they'd liven up their Saturday night in their big house in Edwalton and thought I

was their best option? "Yeah, I'm coming back."
"You promise?"
"Of course."

They leaped up onto the dance floor, but unlike those around them who were lost in music, Tom and Peter were a pair of hovering hawks with their eyes focused on me, the prey beneath them. A rapid exodus to join the dancers gave me an uninterrupted view towards the passage leading to the stairs. As in moments of revelation in corny horror films when the music becomes muted and the surroundings blur, I watched the arrival of a giant of a man so tall that he had to duck his head to pass under the doorway. Cropped red hair gave him the appearance of a farmer from the Scottish Highlands, albeit one who wore a leather biker jacket over what looked like one of those olive-green German soldiers' shirts that the Army & Navy stores sold for a couple of quid. A pair of faded jeans with rips in the knees encased sturdy legs that I thought any rugby prop would be proud of. As the bodies moved and my greedy view travelled further south, I had to know what size his enormous black Doc Martens were... At least size thirteen or fourteen? He ducked back under the arch into the small dark area between the bar and the top of the stairs. Within seconds, several gawping queens were gathered around him.

Andy appeared and grabbed me. "Look at *him*! Who is he?"
"Dunno, but I'm going to find out."
"Not before me, you don't."

I sighed as he rushed away. This was the trouble having a best friend who fancied the same type of man as me. Sometimes, nights out became a competition. I wasn't about to be an also-ran in the race, but just when I'd moved towards the goliath, my progress was thwarted by Tom and Peter, fresh from the dance floor, their scarlet faces glistening with sweat, and their eyes wide.

"Hey, you're not leaving, are you?"
"No, I–"
"Thank God for that. We thought we were losing you. Are you ready to go?"

Damn. I watched Andy flirting with the big man while Tom and Peter's hands moved under my leather jacket as if they were store detectives frisking me.

Tom licked my ear. "Dancing makes me randy."

Chucking Putty at the Queen

From behind, Peter groaned. "You won't regret you met us."

The trouble was that since the arrival of the big man, I already did. Ordinarily, their handsy attention would be welcome, but my eyes were on the one person that I needed to meet, and this couple pawing me was really irritating.

Tom squeezed my shoulder. "Just you wait here, tiger. We'll go down and ring for a taxi."

Jesus, did he really just call me 'tiger?' "Okay. Whilst you're doing that, I'll go over and say ta-ra to my mate." This was the only chance to get myself noticed by the big bloke before I embarked on a threesome that I now wished I hadn't agreed to. The closer I got, the more that I realised his size. I was six feet five and still looked up at him. A skinny queen known as Gwendoline simpered from beneath the fringe of his peroxide-streaked wedge haircut. He'd once taken the piss out of my limp when he was with his gaggle of hairdresser friends in the pub and had loudly asked me, "Are you mentally disabled as well as physically disabled?" so there was no way I was going to let that little scrag-end get a look-in. I elbowed him aside and thrust my hand towards the stranger. "Ayup, I'm Simon."

Andy was obviously eager to show off that he'd already made a connection. "He's called John, and he's from London." As if to establish some kind of possession, he linked his arm through John's.

I smiled up at the big man. "I know this is naff, and I bet you get asked this all the time, but how tall are you?"

John's eyes danced with sapphire sparkles in the shadows. "Six foot ten."

I fought the urge to push Andy backwards down the stairs, and for the umpteenth time in five minutes, I cursed myself for promising to go back to Edwalton with Tom and Peter. I couldn't back out of it because I'd never be so cheap as to renege.

As if my thoughts had transmitted to them through the ether, they rushed up the stairs and flanked me, glaring at John and Andy as they tugged at the sleeves of my jacket.

"*Here* you are! Let's go, the taxi's outside." Tom smirked at the crescent of men. "Too late; he's coming home with *us*!"

They trotted down the darkened steps to the foyer as John stared at me.

Andy gave me a shove. "Go on then. Don't hang around." His delight at my departure was evident.

John grinned. "Have fun. See you later."

"I hope so." I rolled my eyes to convey my remorse at leaving. "I mean, I hope I see you later."

Andy followed me to the top of the dark stairs. "I beat you to him. I've got off with him, and you haven't."

I feigned an elaborate yawn. "Don't you worry yourself about me, girl. I'll have fun."

"Phil knows them; he reckons they're a right pair of gin queens."

Tom came back up the stairs. "Hurry up, the taxi's waiting. *We're* waiting."

Andy poked me in the ribs. "Aren't you jealous I beat you to him?"

Refusing to admit how right he was, I smiled around my clenched teeth. "I told you, don't worry about me. Everything comes to he who waits."

The unignorable urges that were the prime motivation for me to venture out tonight had completely vanished as I followed Tom and Peter into the summer night heat.

"Why do you use a walking stick?"

Peter nudged his partner. "Don't be rude."

Tom placed a forefinger to his bottom lip and pulled a comedy sad face. "Sorry, I didn't mean to offend you."

"You haven't. It'd take a lot more than that to offend me, and I'd rather you ask than guess. I've heard all sorts of rumours: that I had polio as a kid, or that I was a Hells Angel stabbed in the leg during a knife fight."

"So what's the truth?"

"I was a victim of PSD."

"What?"

"Platform Shoes Disaster. When I was fourteen, I tripped in a pair of five-inch heels and dislocated my hip. But it went undiagnosed for ages and just ended being fucked up."

They exchanged glances again. "It doesn't stop you having fun though, does it?" Tom asked.

"If it did I wouldn't be here, would I?"

At the bottom of the narrow street stood a mobile fast-food van. A bag of chips and a battered sausage seemed a much more preferable option than my eager new playmates. I awkwardly crumpled next to

Tom into the back of the waiting cab. Peter slammed the front passenger door and instructed the driver to our destination, which was populated by big posh houses with gardens that stretched forever. Rapping on the side window made me jump. It was Andy, blowing me kisses. As the car gathered speed, I twisted around and watched through the back window as he and John walked off down the street. Damn!

I didn't do jealousy, believing it to be a negative, futile emotion, but on this occasion, it overwhelmed me. Struggling to suppress my unexpected, irrational anger of Andy copping off with John, my night went from bad to worse. Phil had been right. Tom and Peter mixed drinks that were substantially more gin than tonic. It was only when Tom repeatedly dropped the lime he was slicing onto the marble tiled floor that I realised the level of their inebriation. After they necked their drinks, they poured more before taking me on a guided tour of the house, pointing out the expensive items with levels of superiority and increasing obnoxiousness.

The circuitous route returned us to the kitchen, where, as they mixed even more drinks, they began bickering about which one of them I preferred. It was like a really crappy television comedy featuring exaggeratedly camp queens, and if it wasn't so tragically real, it would have been amusing. "Look, I'm not being rude, but I think it best if we do this another time."

Tom took a glass-draining slug of his drink. "Be like that then." He wrinkled his nose. "You're nothing special even if you think you are."

So within less than an hour of arriving at the opulent house, I left them at each other's throats. I doubted that they'd even noticed my departure. Thank goodness I'd not touched the tenner I kept for emergencies. At the first call box, I phoned for a cab to take me home.

35

BRAND NEW LOVER

THE NEXT DAY, I met Andy for our traditional Sunday afternoon postmortem of the previous night, but on this occasion, he was untypically unforthcoming about what happened. He was more interested in how my night had played out.

Summer and autumn passed with a sense of me treading water. One week before Christmas, Andy and his boyfriend, Alan, invited me to join them on a visit to Lincoln to see the festive lights and market. On a bitingly crisp day under a pale blue sky, we mooched around the stalls laden with homemade jams, mustards, conserves, and one bearing only bottles of parsnip wine. Others displayed nativity tat made from badly painted offcuts of wood, and the only bookstall proved a dud as it sold only religious publications. Nevertheless, I bought Dad an embossed bookmark bearing one of the cathedral's stained-glass windows, knowing that he'd love the colours.

Urgent repair work precluded admittance to the hallowed premises, meaning that our intention to sit within its majestic interior was thwarted. Being a believer, Andy was particularly disappointed, and although Alan and I were atheists, it was hard not to be impressed by the architectural grandeur.

Finally, the aroma of hot food was no longer possible to ignore, and the ever-generous Alan insisted that he'd treat us to lunch. His and Andy's relationship had entered its second year, and this offer was typical of him. Andy, captivated by all things historical, just had to visit the Henry VIII Steakhouse, which was nothing more elaborate than a converted caravan painted with wobbly lined approximations of a Tudor hall. Beneath the coloured lights of the fast-food wagon's extendable awning, Andy and I dined on what the *Ye Olde Menue* board proclaimed to be "genuine" venison burgers. God knows what they actually contained. I was famished and didn't care to examine the meat too closely, reassuring myself that they couldn't be any worse than the ten-for-a-quid ones that Dad bought from a bloke in the pub. A few feet away, the staunchly vegetarian Alan stood next to the throbbing diesel generator of the Nut Cutlet Diner, tucking into a wholemeal cob stuffed with a chickpea and mung bean rissole. By the time I'd wiped my greasy lips on the festively coloured red and green paper serviette, the sharpness of a knife-edge east coast wind had ushered in slate-grey clouds that eradicated the delicate blue, and from them, fine snow fell, dusting the dirty paving slabs with the exquisite white traceries of Nottingham lace. I scrunched the serviette into a ball and successfully lobbed it into a nearby litter basket. "Cor, that was lovely. Thanks, Alan."

"You're welcome. I just hope that it's not the only meaty mouthful you have today."

"*Alan!*" I guffawed in delighted surprise at his untypically ribald remark. I examined the crowd. Cutting through mercury clouds of expelled breath as if I had laser-guided vision, my focus zoomed in on a hefty bloke in a donkey jacket, who looked as if he'd just stepped out of the expansive flatlands of the Lincolnshire potato fields. One of his big paws rested on the handle of a pushchair in which sat an infant, well-wrapped in heavy woollens. His other hand clasped that of a petite woman. As he stared to the heights of the cathedral, she gazed adoringly up at him. A sombre cloak of maudlin envy swathed me. Well, I was going out when we got back home, so maybe tonight would be *the* night.

The clouds fractured and separated, permitting insipid sunshine to illuminate our afternoon. Shadows gradually lengthened on the cathedral's patchwork of masonry, altering its appearance as would the slow, unstoppable advance of a tide soaking a beach, transforming the sand from honey gold to chocolate brown. A distant bell chimed the three-quarter hour, commanding our hasty return to the car park.

When Alan pulled into the parking area behind my home, the snow was coming down but not too severely to worry about, so we agreed to meet at nine in Gatsby's. It was evident that the effect of our exposure to the perishing wind cutting over from the North Sea had taken its toll. Alan looked as if he'd just driven from the east to west shorelines of the USA rather than to Lincoln and back.

Andy yawned, then frowned at me. "What's up with you?"

"Are you coming out tonight or what?"

"Yeah, of course. Don't get your knickers in a twist. I'll have a kip when we get back to Alan's and see you later."

"Okay, see you in a bit."

Alan's car tyres squished thick black lines through the sloppy new snow, and they disappeared into the dark evening. Would they keep their promise? Of course they would. I could count on Andy, at least; he'd never miss a night out, whereas the more academic Alan wasn't a fan of noisy pubs and clubs and preferred literature over loudness.

I went indoors to tell Dad about my day and to present him with his bookmark. Lethargy quickly overtook me in the dry warmth. We watched the telly until I decided that if I didn't shower immediately, then I'd fall asleep. As I dressed to go out, I played a tape that I'd made a few weeks earlier. The second track was "Hold On To What You Believe" by electro-pop duo, the Technos. I thought back to the sturdy farmer type man earlier and in my irritable inertia, I jabbed the pause button after a couple of minutes. "Yeah, it's all right for you to tell me it won't be long. It's a bit late now, and I'm fed up with holding on. *It* won't be long because *it* won't ever happen."

I needed to stop talking to inanimate objects. My bed looked far too inviting. No, I couldn't give in. I held my forefinger down on the fast forward button, making the tape speed through the remaining minutes of the song, converting it into the high-pitched, garbled effect of a complaining person on a telephone in a comedy programme. After a brief second of silence and the squiggly noise of the next track, I removed my finger. In her unique Liverpudlian tones, Cilla Black assured me "Something Tells Me Something's Gonna Happen Tonight."

I resumed my dialogue with the tape recorder. "It better had happen tonight, if I ever get there." I was overtired, and a few minutes later when I was downstairs, a prolonged yawn almost dislocated my jaw.

Dad turned around from the kitchen worktop where he'd been labelling jars of onions that he'd pickled that afternoon. "You sound all-in, Son."

I clamped a hand over my mouth to muffle another yawn. "I could do with an early night, but I told Andy and Alan I'd meet them at nine."

"You don't sound too enthusiastic, Son. Are you sure that's all? Because if you're short, I can let you have a couple of quid until your next giro. You're young; you should be out enjoying yourself with your pals, especially in the run-up to Christmas."

"No, ta. You're all right, Dad, I don't want a sub."

He dug into his trousers pocket, then held out his upturned palm. A pair of golden one-pound coins shone like the foil-wrapped decorative chocolate currency dangling from the tinselled branches in the living room.

"Go on, Son. Have a pre-Christmas pint on me. You never know who might be out tonight."

"Honestly, Dad, it's okay. I'll just go up and clean my teeth."

Back in the living room, I put my black leather biker jacket on, hauled my heavy overcoat on top of it, and headed out. Small, dryish snowflakes fell prettily like spring blossom from the apple trees up at the allotments, but there was no promise of summer now as we headed into the bleak midwinter. The raw air scraped my cheeks as I looked back at my footsteps and the alternating punctuation from the rubber ferrule on my walking stick along our otherwise undisturbed wintery path. The curtains remained open, and the Christmas tree lights were comforting blobs fuzzed by the condensation shrouding the big picture window. It would be so easy to turn around and return to the warmth of the house, but I'd never stand anyone up and just hoped that I'd make it to the pub without slipping over. When I reached the main road, I slid my chilled right hand into the overcoat pocket and felt what I immediately knew were two one-pound coins nestling at the bottom. *Oh, Dad.*

I reached Gatsby's without accident despite the increase in the dimensions and velocity of the snowflakes, which were settling worryingly. The red wine velour curtains of the lounge were drawn as I passed towards the side doorway, and I smiled, remembering Patrick asking me why I always entered this way instead of diving through the corner doors straight into the livelier side.

"Because when you go into the disco, it's dark and crowded, and nobody can see you."

"They always see *you* because you're head and shoulders above most people in there."

"That's not the point. In the quieter bar, it's always well lit. So you can see who's in but more importantly, they can see you. It's called 'making an entrance.' I go in that way to be seen."

I lightly smoothed the snow from my head, careful not to disturb my quiff despite there being enough hair gel there to keep it rigid for weeks.

Chucking Putty at the Queen

How my life had bloomed from the tight bud of paranoia during my school days when I'd hidden from the bullies who were out for my blood. Now my petals were fully, gloriously opened and turned skywards. I threw the door open and strode into the greenhouse heat of the lounge and, not for the first time, congratulated myself on selling my unused racing bike and some of my record collection to finance contact lenses. No more of that embarrassing routine of waiting for spectacles to de-mist. That was completely unconducive to entrance-making. When I was sure that nobody had missed my arrival, and with the door to the disco area in my sights, I stopped to chat to several older men that I knew until the clock showed dead on nine.

"Mind your backs. Coming through, coming through."

A grey-bearded man holding a tray of drinks reversed in a clumsy three-point-turn from the counter, forcing me to make a quick sidestep to avoid a collision. The backs of my legs connected with a stool and when I turned around, there was John, the big man from the summer. Before I left the house Dad told me, "You never know who might be out tonight."

The disco door opened, and a man wearing a Santa hat covered with small flashing red lights stepped aside to let me pass through. I hesitated, not wanting to miss a chance to reacquaint myself with John but equally reluctant to let my friends down. Although I didn't want to be disloyal to them, I really hoped that they weren't waiting, because knowing my sodding luck, Andy would cop off with John again.

They were nowhere to be seen, and I slipped back into the quiet bar. What a mammoth visual feast awaited my eager eyes. *Blimey, he is a big bloke.* My nerves jangled like wind chimes in a stiff breeze, and I hoped he couldn't see my hands shaking as I ordered a drink.

Peggy flipped the switch on the beer pump and leaned forwards. "Simon, do you know that big bloke who's sitting behind you? I've seen him at the Turkish baths a couple of times."

"No, I don't. Well, I sort of do, if you count meeting him for about two seconds at the club in summer. Why d'you ask?"

He placed a pint of lager in front of me. "Well, don't look now, girl, but he ain't half staring at you."

Oh, please don't let my mates arrive right now and ruin this moment. I hadn't been so wired since that night four years ago, when I met the Roman Centurion and had left the club with him without us exchanging a word. The song from my tape echoed through my mind: "Hold on to what you believe." In my heart of hearts, I was sure that I would meet my equivalent of the mythical Great Dark Man, and I remembered Irish Mary in the pub telling Dad, "Every old sock finds an old shoe." Right now, I sensed that something was *happening*, something different. Or was that merely tiredness clashing with the heightened emotions surrounding Christmas?

I turned back to the bar and took a sip of my drink.

Peggy widened his eyes. "Bloody hell, Simon, you're not usually backwards at being forward. What you waiting for? Go on!"

When I looked again, John's grin was the green light I needed; it was all systems go. I took a deep breath, stepped over to the table and lowered myself onto a stool opposite the big man.

Although I'd been in a similar situation countless times, the next morning was different. This wasn't just lust. We chatted with the ease of two people who had known each other for decades, yet the memory of past knock-backs made me unable to ask to see him again. I was sure that we'd forged a spiritual and emotional connection and couldn't bear it if this gentle goliath made it clear that our time together was only a one-off.

I stood in the kitchen, reluctant to drain my coffee from the mug as it would signify another step closer to the end of this liaison. Each tick of the wall clock tormented me with the countdown to when I'd have to take the bus back into town. He'd offered to drive me, but I'd declined, knowing that if I was just a one-nighter then it would be too hard for me to leave the intimate confines of his car. And if I was going to cry, then I'd rather do it privately on public transport.

"I think there's a bus soon, but I can't remember if it's ten to and twenty past the hour, or twenty to and ten past." He placed his mug on the countertop. "Or it could be five to and twenty-five past. I'll walk you down to the request stop on the main road."

The snow was a slushy memory, only sparkling white in the darkest shade as we crunched down the gravel-covered driveway. I could usually rely on myself to come up with all sorts of chit-chat to fill these awkward moments after such an encounter, but bashfulness rendered me tongue-tied, and I couldn't ask him the one question that I really wanted to.

He stopped and raised a hand to shade his eyes from the sharp winter sunlight and looked to the horizon. "I can't see a thing, let alone a bus."

Chucking Putty at the Queen

Good. I hoped that it had broken down, or was hijacked, or had blown up—anything to delay me leaving him. In the near distance over the road, a two-carriage train was swallowed by the blackness under a humpbacked bridge. Crossing it, a narrow lane twisted as a thread of pewter ribbon through the acres of untilled earth delineated into fields by bare, blackened hawthorn hedgerows. The train was heading to the city, a destination to which I didn't want to return. I was convinced that, in more ways than the obvious visual one, John stood head and shoulders above any man that I'd met before and believed that something emotionally unique had occurred during the past few hours. Through the blinding glare of sunshine came a streak of red as a single decker whooshed past. It seemed that neither of us had heard its approach.

"Oh. There goes your bus."

I didn't care because I didn't want to be on it.

"There'll be another, but I don't know when because I drive everywhere. You'd better get yourself a timetable for the future."

I dared not look at him. Instead, I focused on the brown field where the sun glinted silvery-yellow on the blades of a plough being pulled behind a tractor, its progress followed by a grey and white trail of shrieking seagulls divebombing the freshly turned soil. *The future?* I grasped my courage and looked up into his eyes that had changed from sapphire into the soft hyacinth blue of the December sky. "Are we going to have a future?"

He gripped my hand and smiled. "That's what I'm hoping."

EPILOGUE

WHAT HAVE I DONE TO DESERVE THIS?

FROM THERE ON, MY life changed stratospherically for the better in ways that were unimaginable to me. I'd never met anyone so fascinating as this sculptor who adored opera and classical music, was an aficionado of the Victorian music hall, and whose bookcase included unusual titles that aroused my curiosity: *A Short Walk In The Hindu Kush*; *Modern Poultry Husbandry*; and *The Complete Book of Self-Sufficiency*, whilst the inherent bibliophile in me thrilled at the orange-and-white Penguin editions of the entire collections of Evelyn Waugh and P.G. Wodehouse.

His property stood on eight acres which enabled him to keep goats, ducks, ornamental chickens, guinea pigs, rabbits, and several species of parrots including an impressive blue and gold macaw.

I'd laughed. "Everything but a partridge in a pear tree!"

Until he moved to Nottingham, he'd been a keeper at London Zoo, and my amazement multiplied when he told me that he was a championship dog judge and travelled the country exhibiting his pedigree Bearded Collie and Belgian Shepherd. However, before I met his canine companions, I quickly feigned nonchalance, not letting on how terrified I was of dogs. I'd spent years avoiding the large packs that freely roamed our part of St Ann's after they were kicked out of their respective homes each morning.

Early in the new year of 1987, he announced returning to Hampstead for a week to visit his mother, and I eagerly agreed to his suggestion that I join him and meet her. I scribbled a card announcing this thrilling development and mailed it to Patrick, whose reply arrived by return post. "Wow, Simone. He must be serious if you're meeting the mother-in-law already."

I didn't have much to share with John, only the limited treasures of my life thus far: walks around those precious woods, visiting the countryside hamlets untroubled by reconstruction, and of course, Dad, the jewel in my crown.

In return, John shared his bounty of being born in the affluent, village-like environs of Hampstead, with its treelined pavements flanked by attractive Georgian, Victorian, and Edwardian houses; some elegantly tall and stately and others stolid and imposing, with the occasional charming cottage tucked away. I adored the architectural antithesis of the uniform, pebble-dashed modern boxes of my own locality, and especially loved the atmospheric descent of night's inky canopy when milky light from the original gas streetlamps pooled on the paving slabs, although the illumination was now created by electricity instead of flame.

To a lover of literature like me, the fact that previous Hampstead habitues included Keats, Daphne du Maurier, DH Lawrence, Evelyn Waugh, and Stella Gibbons immediately increased its allure. Twice each day, when we took the dogs for long, leisurely walks over the famous rolling heath that lay at the end of John's road, I imagined those esteemed wordsmiths seeking inspiration as they had wandered along the twisty-turny paths through the abundant, ancient woodland.

On subsequent visits to London, I soon saw how beloved and popular John was when he introduced me to his expansive network of friends, a cosmopolitan and Bohemian circle of creative individuals, all of whom welcomed and accepted me without question. I met writers, painters, poets, and ceramicists; physicists, university lecturers, and surgeons; zoologists, horticulturists, opera singers, and theatre designers. Then there were his neighbours! Film stars, composers, members of parliament, and there were even a couple of real lords and ladies too. And John's cachet with Dad increased tenfold when I casually let it slip that he was friends with Maria Callas's pianist. My head spun at being surrounded by such knowledge and celebrity, and I knew that Patrick would be wildly jealous when I told him that I'd spoken to Dusty Springfield and Boy George, both of whom lived nearby.

Initially, I was overawed by his friends. Embarrassed by my inadequate education, I remained mindful of making faux pas which would reveal me as gauche and foolish. However, all of them treated me without judgement or condemnation for my origins, and I soon became less wonderstruck and more relaxed in their company. This exposure to the wider world exemplified the opportunities therein, and back in Nottingham, I barely ventured onto the gay scene, tired with how mundane it was in comparison with my new experiences in the metropolis.

Chucking Putty at the Queen

Supported by the positivity of John's encouragement and love, I began to value myself and started a career in music retail. John moved to the city and bought a tall Victorian house which we renovated to free it from the ugly 1960s modernisation imposed on it, and best of all, it was a ten-minute walk from the woods where I'd spent so many glorious hours as a child.

On his suggestion, I applied for a passport. Me, having a passport! For my debut journey outside the UK, we visited Paris for a long weekend. In the heat of a summer Sunday morning, we waited beneath the royal blue and gold striped canopy of a side street café, squinting in the sunlight that reflected on the steaming pavements following an unexpected rain shower. Eventually a haughty, pencil-moustached waiter showed us to a circular table covered with an immaculate white cloth. We lounged in creaky but comfortable wicker chairs, quickly sitting upright with the arrival of our earth-dark coffee and plates of golden croissants. From a passing vendor, I bought a postcard depicting the Eiffel Tower that I'd just been to the very top of, and in the most minuscule handwriting that I could manage, I penned a report to Dad, enthusing how we'd dined at a seafood restaurant opposite the legendary Moulin Rouge theatre, where, wrapped in a heavy fog from dozens of Gauloises, we feasted on garlicky escargots and moules mariniere, mopping up the creamy, herby sauce with chunks of warm crusty baguette and shared a bottle of red wine with an unpronounceable name ("No *vin ordinarie* for us," John said). With immense pride, I signed the card, "Lots of love from Simon and John," wishing that everyone around us could look over my shoulder and witness this first time of writing the salutation. After a sip of coffee, I drew an asterisk that looked like a tiny, squashed spider and added the postscript, "French bread isn't a patch on yours!"

Thereafter, we travelled to Holland, Germany, Belgium, Switzerland, Canada, and extensively across America, explorations that further widened my cultural and social horizons, and my delight was compounded when we flew business class to San Francisco for the first of numerous visits to the city I'd been obsessed with since my childhood. I basked in similar wonderment as I stood beneath the voluptuous foliage outside Ernest Hemingway's house in Key West. In my early teens, I'd read Dad's copy of *The Sun Also Rises* with no possible idea that such an incredible experience would happen to me in my mid-twenties.

John was a member of the Royal Horticultural Society, and my newfound happiness bloomed when he took me to the Chelsea Flower Show. In the stifling heat of a crowded white marquee, the extraordinary blue exquisiteness of a wave of delphiniums washed over me. I burst into tears.

John put his arm around me. "What's the matter? Is your leg hurting you?"

"No, it's not that." I sobbed. "It's just all too beautiful. I can't believe this is happening." His strong hug told me that he knew it was not only the floral flamboyance to which I was referring.

And when I reported to my dad of evenings attending the opera in London, he beamed and squeezed my shoulder.

"I do wish your mother could see this. Our son going to the opera. It's incredible, and it's all happened because of you meeting John." He winked. "I can't make my mind up if you're Pygmalion or Cinderella. Perhaps a bit of both!"

"Cheers, Dad. I'll be whoever has the prettiest frocks."

Five years later, I stood with him at the bar in the Sycamore Inn. Even though I lived with John, I visited Dad three or four nights a week. I was relating an incident at my work in a record store in the city; it was nothing important, just an anecdote about an awkward customer who demanded a refund because she didn't like the songs on the album she'd bought even though the previous day she'd assured me that she was Phil Collins's number one fan.

He took a draught of his beer and then, as I'd seen him do hundreds of times, darted his tongue around his handlebar moustache to remove the froth. Looking straight ahead, he cleared his throat in the way that always preceded him offering an opinion, making a judgement, or contributing a wry aside.

"If you ask me, Son, fate dealt you a really bad hand."

"*Pardon?*"

"Fate dealt you a really bad hand. You were such a happy child, and your mother and I knew that you were different to your brothers and sisters. She was over the moon when you were born."

Where the hell had this come from?

"No boy should lose his mother when he's eight years old. If that wasn't enough for you to contend with, you had all the problems with

Chucking Putty at the Queen

the injury to your leg and being hospitalized, then the unfortunate thing with your chest that made you so miserable. And on top of that, being bullied at school for who you are. You had so much weight to bear on your young shoulders." He sighed and laid a hand on top of mine. "But do you know what I believe?"

I didn't know if I *wanted* to know what he believed.

"That despite all of those...tragedies, Son, the best thing that ever happened to you was the day that you met John."

When a tear rolled down his cheek, panic raced through me. We were back on the night that Mam died, just the two of us sitting in his car beside the burned-out garage at the end of our street, surrounded by darkness. "Dad..."

Still staring ahead, just as he had on that terrible night, he squeezed my hand. "Remember what I used to tell you when you were growing up: I'm your father, and I know you better than you know yourself." He beckoned to the barmaid. "Same again, please, Tina." He wiped his cheek with a forefinger. "But I still had to let you find your own way to be yourself without too much of my interference. That's how your mother and I agreed we'd raise you long before she became ill. I'm so proud of you, Son, and I'm delighted that you've found happiness with John after all that you've been through. And if she was here, your mother would be too, and she'd love John as much as I do." He placed a note on the bar. "Get them in, Son. I'll be back in the shake of a lamb's tail."

Dazed by this frank outpouring, I watched him go to the door leading into the corridor, and for the first time since Mam's death, the suffocating fear that he wasn't returning was absent. At ten thirty, when the landlord covered the beer pumps with bar towels, I accompanied Dad home. I usually popped in for a nightcap of his homemade brew but this time, I didn't join him in the memory-filled house. Instead, I began walking to where John and I had already begun creating our own memories as a couple. Only the day before, I'd rooted around in the attic and tugged out one of the many boxes crammed with the ephemera and minutiae of my earlier life that had accompanied my moving in with John. I soon found what I was looking for: my pocket diary for 1986. I'd flicked through until I reached New Year's Eve. I knew full well what I'd written back then but still needed to see it. The blue-inked entry seemed to glow on the cheap, thin paper. "I think that at long last, this is it."

My thought had been proven correct and, further embracing my romantic nostalgia, I went downstairs and played "Hold On To What You Believe," the record that I hadn't heard since that night five years earlier when I'd almost not gone to the pub, recalling Dad's prescient proclamation, "You never know who might be out tonight."

I didn't give credence to mystical forces, but how prophetic his words and the song title had proved to be. Despite my numerous misguided hopes of reciprocal feelings from so many other men, I'd held on to my belief that I would one day meet the love of my life, and I had.

I passed along the maze of walkways, taking familiar shortcuts down steep, shadowy steps leading to the narrow, pitch-black canyons between blocks of flats. No longer was I squeezed by the childhood terror of being jumped and beaten up here by youths who hated me. Those years were behind me now, and each of my echoing footsteps took me further from my past and closer to my present. I quickened my pace and emerged from the darkness to head toward the bright lights of the road. The fresh memory of Dad's words powered my strides homewards to the man who loved me.

"The best thing that ever happened to you was the day that you met John."

Glossary

A bit black over Bill's mam's – dark storm clouds gathering
Adrian Street – flamboyant TV wrestler in the 1970s
Ain't – is not
Anyroad – anyway
Ayup/eh up – hello
Barmy – mad
Beer rinse – beer-enhanced shampoo
Biro – ballpoint pen
Bleddy – bloody (but not describing blood covered objects)
Bleeder – someone regarded with contempt or pity
Blimey – exclamation of surprise (from gor blimey, from god blind me)
Bog – toilet
Bogeys – hardened nose snot (US boogers)
Bogger – rascal
Boggering about – messing around
Bogger it/bugger it – exclamation of annoyance
Bonfire night/ Guy Fawke's night – November 5th fireworks commemoration of 1605 attempt to blow up the Houses of Parliament
Bumboy, bum boy – male homosexual
Bumfreezer jacket – British adaptation of continental styles, particularly Italian, of the late 50s and early 60s, favoured by Mods, with a shorter back panel leaving the bum more exposed to cold weather.
Bummer – male homosexual
Chippy – chip shop
Chips – sliced lengths of deep-fried potato, thicker than French fries
Cilla Black – English pop singer & TV celebrity
Clothes' horse – foldable wooden frame for drying clothes on usually in front of a coal fire
Co-Op – grocery store (Co-Operative supermarket)
Cob – a circular, domed bread similar to a burger bun, but not a bap, which is larger and more flattened.
Daft – foolish
Deffo – definitely
Doccos – Dr. Marten boots

Dolly tub – usually galvanized metal barrel used for laundry
Duck /ducky – informal of friend
Dusty Springfield – English pop singer 1960s-80s
Faffing about – messing about
Fag – cigarette
Fry-up – fried breakfast
Gob – mouth
Gobstopper – solid confectionary ball
Gonk – idiot, fool
Gorblimey – exclamation, from God blind me
Gormless – vacuous, foolish
How do you do – the correct response when someone greets you with 'How do you do."
Int – is not (variation of ain't)
Jubbly – triangular frozen drink
Larry Grayson – camp celebrity comedian known for catchphrase, "Shut that door" and The Generation Game
Leathering – punishment administered by means of whipping a person's backside with a leather strap or belt
Lippy – cheeky, insolent
Loo – toilet
Lulu - Scottish pop singer
Marc Bolan – English musician and pioneer of the Glam rock movement of the early 1970s
Mithered – worrying about something
Nanar – grandmother
Navvy – road diggers/workmen
Nits – eggs of head lice
Nowt – nothing
Oi – exclamation to attract someone's attention (Oi, watch out!)
O-levels – school examinations
Owt – anything
Pig bins – containers for waste food from schools/hospitals that were taken to feed pigs
Pissed – drunk
Ponch – conical copper device attached to long pole to assist laundry washing

Poncing/poncing about — aimless behaviour
Pots and kettles (pot calling the kettle) — English proverbial idiom in which somebody accuses someone else of a fault which the accuser shares, and therefore is an example of hypocrisy.
Potty — eccentric, crazy
Prat — idiot, fool
Puff — effeminate man, slang for homosexual
Quentin Crisp — inspirational homosexual English raconteur and boundary-pusher
Rezillos, the — Scottish pop group with camp/kitsch appeal
Rock — novelty stick of sugary confectionary usually a souvenir of a holiday, with location going through it in red or pink letters (e.g., Mablethorpe rock)
Sandie Shaw — English pop singer prevalent in 1960s
Shippo's — Shipstone's brewery beer
Sucky — see gormless
Summat — something
Summat and nowt — dismissive term, something to be unbothered by
T. Rex — Marc Bolan's musical group
Tabs — ears
Taking the mickey — to make fun of someone
Tom Robinson — English musician & gay rights advocate
Tomorrer — tomorrow
Top of the Pops — weekly television music programme
Touched (a bit) — mentally weak
Trap — mouth
Uns — ones (green ones — green uns)
Wazzy — weak (usually in relation to tea or coffee)
Yakking — gossiping/talking
Yard, the — area at work usually builder's yard, joiner's yard
Yobs — aggressive person, usually male
Zebra crossing — painted black and white striped pedestrian crossing on a road

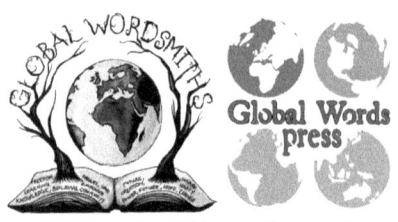

What's Your Story?

Global Wordsmiths, CIC, provides an all-encompassing service for all writers, ranging from basic proofreading and cover design to development editing, typesetting, and eBook services. A major part of our work is charity and community focused, delivering writing projects to under-served and under-represented groups across Nottinghamshire, giving voice to the voiceless and visibility to the unseen.

To learn more about what we offer, visit: www.globalwords.co.uk

A selection of books by Global Words Press:
Desire, Love, Identity: with the National Justice Museum
Times Past: with The Workhouse, National Trust
World At War: Farmilo Primary School
Times Past: Young at Heart with AGE UK
In Different Shoes: Stories of Trans Lives

Other Great Butterworth Books

That Boy of Yours Wants Looking At by Simon Smalley
A riotously colourful and heart-rending journey of what it takes to live authentically.
Available from Amazon (ASIN B09V3CSQQW)

Unwritten by Helena Harte
No strings is fun 'til it unravels.
Available from Amazon (ASIN B0DGQFFHYB)

The Promise by Addison M Conley
When the world keeps pulling you under, who do you reach for?
Available on Amazon (ASIN B0DDY9FH6Z)

Back to Back by Jo Fletcher
When Fred and Ruby's worlds collide, can love rise from the rubble?
Available on Amazon (ASIN B0D6M499K2)

Heart of the Storm by Ally McGuire
Sometimes a storm is just what you need to clear the skies ahead.
Available on Amazon (ASIN B0CYTSQXWW)

Sanctuary by Helena Harte
Passions ignite and possibilities unfold. Welcome to the Windy City Romance series.
Available from Amazon (ASIN B0D4B42RRW)

Brave Enough to Love by Valden Bush
In a dance between truth and sacrifice, can they rewrite the rules of love?
Available on Amazon (ASIN B0CQP8PMVB)

Dead Ringer by Robyn Nyx
Three bodies. One killer. No motive?
Available on Amazon (ASIN B0CPQ8HFK7)

Medea by JJ Taylor
Who will Medea become in her battle for freedom?
Available from Amazon (ASIN B0CK2FB7GW)

Virgin Flight by E.V. Bancroft
In the battle between duty and desire, can love win?
Available from Amazon (ASIN B0CKJWQZ45)

Fragments of the Heart by Ally McGuire
Love can be the greatest expedition of all.
Available on Amazon (ASIN B0CHBPHR6M)

Here You Are by Jo Fletcher
Can they unlock their hearts to find the true happiness they both deserve?
Available on Amazon (ASIN B0CBN935ZB)

Stunted Heart by Helena Harte
A stunt rider who lives in the fast lane. An ER doctor who can't take chances. A passion that could turn their worlds upside down.
Available on Amazon (ASIN B0C78GSWBV)

Dark Haven by Brey Willows
Even vampires get tired of playing with their food...
Available on Amazon (ASIN B0C5P1HJXC)

Green for Love by E.V. Bancroft
All's fair in love and eco-war.
Available from Amazon (ASIN B0C28F7PX5)

Call of Love by Lee Haven
Separated by fear. Reunited by fate. Will they get a second chance at life and love?
Available from Amazon (ASIN B0BYC83HZD)

Where the Heart Leads by Ally McGuire
A writer. A celebrity. And a secret that could break their hearts.
Available on Amazon (ASIN B0BWFX5W9L)

Stolen Ambition by Robyn Nyx
Daughters of two worlds collide in a dangerous game of ambition and love.
Available on Amazon (ASIN B0BS1PRSCN)

Cabin Fever by Addison M Conley
She goes for the money, but will she stay for something deeper?
Available on Amazon (ASIN B0BQWY45GH)

Breakout for Love by Valden Bush
They're both running from their pasts. Together, they might make a new future.
Available from Amazon (ASIN B0CWHZ4SXL)

The Helion Band by AJ Mason
Rose's only crime was to show kindness to her royal mistress...
Available from Amazon (ASIN B09YM6TYFQ)

Sapphic Eclectic Volume Five edited by Nyx & Willows
A little something for everyone...
Available free via the Butterworth Books website

Of Light and Love by E.V. Bancroft
The deepest shadows paint the brightest love.
Available from Amazon (ASIN B0B64KJ3NP)

An Art to Love by Helena Harte
Second chances are an art form.
Available on Amazon (ASIN B0B1CD8Y42)

Music City Dreamers by Robyn Nyx
Music brings lovers together. In Music City, it can tear them apart. Available on Amazon (ASIN B0994XVDGR)

Let Love Be Enough by Robyn Nyx
When a killer sets her sights on her target, is there any stopping her?
Available on Amazon (ASIN B09YMMZ8XC)

Dead Pretty by Robyn Nyx
An FBI agent, a TV star, and a serial killer. Love hurts.
Available on Amazon (ASIN B09QRSKBVP)

Nero by Valden Bush
Banished and abandoned. Will destiny reunite her with the love of her life?
Available from Amazon (ASIN B0BHJKHK6S)

Warm Pearls and Paper Cranes by E.V. Bancroft
A family torn apart by secrets. The only way forward is love.
Available from Amazon (ASIN B09DTBCQ92)

Judge Me, Judge Me Not by James Merrick
One man's battle against the world and himself to find it's never too late to find, and use, your voice.
Available from Amazon (ASIN B09CLK91N5)

Scripted Love by Helena Harte
What good is a romance writer who doesn't believe in happy ever after?
Available on Amazon (ASIN B0993QFLNN)

Call to Me by Helena Harte
Sometimes the call you least expect is the one you need the most.
Available on Amazon (ASIN B08D9SR15H)

Milton Keynes UK
Ingram Content Group UK Ltd.
UKHW041021171024
449721UK00008BA/80